Third Edition

Appleton & Lange's Review of

INTERNAL MEDICINE

Third Edition

Appleton & Lange's Review of
INTERNAL MEDICINE

Barry J. Goldlist, MD, FRCPC, FACP
Professor of Medicine, Head Division of Geriatric Medicine
University of Toronto
Member, Division of General Internal Medicine, University Health Network
Head Conjoint Geriatric Program
University Health Network and Toronto Rehabilitation Institute
Toronto, Ontario
Canada

Appleton & Lange Reviews/McGraw-Hill
Medical Publishing Division

New York   Chicago   San Franciso   Lisbon   London   Madrid   Mexico City   Milan
New Delhi   San Juan   Singapore   Sydney   Seoul   Toronto

McGraw-Hill

A Division of The McGraw·Hill Companies

Appleton & Lange's Review of Internal Medicine, Third Edition

Copyright © 2003 by Appleton & Lange. All rights reserved. Printed in the United States of America. Except as permitted under the United States Copyright Act of 1976, no part of this publication may be reproduced or distributed in any form or by any means, or stored in a data base or retrieval system, without the prior written permission of the publisher.

Previous editions copyright © 1999, 1996 by Appleton & Lange

2 3 4 5 6 7 8 9   VHVH   9 8 7 6 5 4 3

ISBN: 0-07-138524-X

This book was set in Palatino at Rainbow Graphics.
The editors were Catherine A. Johnson and John M. Morriss.
Project supervision was done by Rainbow Graphics.
The production supervisor was Lisa Mendez.
The cover designer was Elizabeth Pisacreta.

Library of Congress Cataloging-in-Publication Data
Goldlist, Barry J.
 Appleton & Lange's review of internal medicine / Barry J. Goldlist.—3rd ed.
  p. ; cm.
 Includes bibliographical references and index.
 ISBN 0-07-138524-X (alk. paper)
 1. Internal medicine—Examinations, questions, etc.   I. Title: Appleton and Lange's review of internal medicine. II. Title: Review of internal medicine. III. Title.
 [DNLM: 1. Internal Medicine—Examination Questions. WB 18.2 G619a 2003]
RC58. G59 2003
616'.0076—dc21
                                                                     2002016667

Contents

Preface

The practice of internal medicine requires both breadth and depth of knowledge. To acquire mastery of the subject requires extensive reading and clinical experience. The knowledge base is also constantly expanding and changing as medicine enters the era of molecular biology and large, randomized clinical trials. This textbook provides a review of the major issues in internal medicine by presenting a wide variety of typical examination questions and referenced answers.

The text is organized by topic to facilitate in-depth review but contains a large comprehensive test that mimics the typical examination format. The content has been organized to reflect the areas tested on Step 2 of the United States Medical Licensing Examination (USMLE Step 2). The format of the questions is modeled after the format used on the USMLE, making it an ideal study guide for individuals preparing for licensing exams.

The questions and answers reflect the increasing growth of knowledge in the field of internal medicine. As a result, reviewing the answers give the reader a "mini-review" of basic concepts and pathophysiology in internal medicine, allowing the reader to approach clinical problems in an appropriate manner.

Finally, since the last edition was published, the list of references has been expanded and updated to reflect current knowledge in the field of internal medicine.

Barry J. Goldlist, MD, FRCPC, FACP
August 2002

Acknowledgments

I would like to thank my family, particularly my wife Helen, for their support and understanding during those long hours I spent in the library. Thanks also to my secretary, Sue Woodard, whose efficiency and accuracy in transcribing my seemingly random jottings is nothing less than miraculous.

CHAPTER 1

Cardiology
Questions

DIRECTIONS (Questions 1 through 61): Each of the numbered items or incomplete statements in this section is followed by answers or by completions of the statement. Select the ONE lettered answer or completion that is BEST in each case.

1. A 62-year-old man with coronary artery disease presents with heart block. Wenckebach's type atrioventricular (AV) block would cause

   (A) progressive P-R shortening
   (B) progressive lengthening of the P-R interval
   (C) tachycardia
   (D) dropped beat after P-R lengthening
   (E) fixed 2:1 block

2. A pacemaker that functions when the ventricular rate falls below a preset interval is called

   (A) asynchronous
   (B) atrial synchronous
   (C) ventricular synchronous
   (D) ventricular inhibited
   (E) atrial sequential

3. A 42-year-old man develops shortness of breath (SOB) and chest pain 7 days after an open cholecystectomy. The most common electrocardiographic (ECG) finding would be

   (A) a deep S1
   (B) depressed ST in leads I and II
   (C) prominent Q1, and inversion of T3
   (D) sinus tachycardia
   (E) clockwise rotation in the precordial leads

4. A 63-year-old woman develops exertional angina and has had two episodes of syncope. The most likely diagnosis is

   (A) mitral stenosis
   (B) mitral insufficiency
   (C) aortic stenosis
   (D) aortic insufficiency
   (E) tricuspid stenosis

5. A 42-year-old man with known valvular heart disease develops a fever for 1 week. Most of the physical findings are secondary to

   (A) direct bacterial invasion
   (B) immune response
   (C) vascular phenomena
   (D) valvular damage
   (E) pre-existing cardiac dysfunction

6. Which of the following antiarrhythmic drugs mediates its effect by interfering with movement of calcium through the *slow channel?*

   (A) phenytoin
   (B) verapamil
   (C) lidocaine
   (D) amiodarone
   (E) bretylium

7. A 67-year-old man develops chest pain and friction rub 3 days after admission to a coronary care unit. The most likely diagnosis is

    (A) misdiagnosis of infarction
    (B) chest trauma
    (C) viral infection
    (D) transmural infarction
    (E) dissecting aneurysm

8. The effect of calcium ions on the myocardium can best be described as

    (A) positively inotropic
    (B) negatively inotropic
    (C) positively chronotropic
    (D) negatively chronotropic
    (E) excitation contraction uncoupling

9. A 22-year-old woman develops hypertension in the second trimester. This hypertension

    (A) improves in the third trimester
    (B) leads to large-birth-weight babies
    (C) should be rigorously controlled with drugs
    (D) spares the placenta
    (E) spares maternal kidney function

10. A 61-year-old man has an acute myocardial infarction (AMI) and bradycardia. He has no symptoms of bradycardia. Temporary pacing may be indicated for

    (A) persistent bradycardia
    (B) Mobitz type I block
    (C) first-degree AV block
    (D) new fascicular block
    (E) left bundle branch block (LBBB) and first-degree AV block

11. Auscultation of the heart of a 17-year-old boy reveals an increased intensity of the pulmonary component of the second heart sound. The most likely cause is

    (A) pulmonary stenosis
    (B) aortic stenosis
    (C) myocardial infarction
    (D) pulmonary hypertension
    (E) systemic hypertension

12. A 22-year-old woman with a regular heartbeat at a rate of 170/min that abruptly changes to 75/min after applying carotid sinus pressure most likely has

    (A) sinus tachycardia
    (B) paroxysmal atrial fibrillation
    (C) paroxysmal atrial flutter
    (D) paroxysmal atrial tachycardia
    (E) paroxysmal ventricular tachycardia

Questions 13 and 14

13. A 73-year-old man has angina pectoris, but angiogram reveals normal coronary arteries. This occurs most frequently with

    (A) mitral stenosis
    (B) mitral insufficiency
    (C) pulmonary stenosis
    (D) aortic stenosis
    (E) aortic insufficiency

14. The patient in the above question has a harsh systolic ejection murmur at the base, radiating to both carotids. Auscultation of the second aortic sound at the base reveals that it is

    (A) accentuated
    (B) diminished
    (C) normal in character
    (D) widely split due to delayed ventricular ejection
    (E) showing fixed splitting

15. A 69-year-old woman is found on ECG to have fixed P-P and R-R intervals but varying P-R intervals. This is most likely caused by

    (A) surgical removal of an atrium
    (B) independent beating of atria and ventricles
    (C) a re-entry phenomenon
    (D) a drug effect
    (E) a heart rate under 60 beats/min

16. A 57-year-old man has an anterior myocardial infarction. Nitroprusside would be a useful first medication under which circumstances?

(A) severe pulmonary congestion, blood pressure 80 mm Hg systolic

(B) clear lungs, blood pressure 120 mm Hg systolic

(C) clear lungs, blood pressure 80 mm Hg systolic

(D) minimal pulmonary congestion, blood pressure 160 mm Hg systolic

(E) severe pulmonary congestion, blood pressure 130 mm Hg systolic

17. A 28-year-old man develops *Streptococcus viridans* septicemia. The underlying cardiac lesion with the highest risk of endocarditis would be

(A) ventricular septal defect

(B) atrial septal defect, secundum type

(C) mitral valve prolapse with regurgitation

(D) pure mitral stenosis

(E) asymmetric septal hypertrophy

18. Echocardiogram in a 47-year-old woman reveals a cardiac tumor. The most likely cause is

(A) myxoma

(B) sarcoma

(C) rhabdomyoma

(D) fibroma

(E) lipoma

19. Several patients of varying ages in your practice intend to pursue exercise programs. In these patients, exercise electrocardiography

(A) is an invasive procedure

(B) is contraindicated in patients over 65 years of age

(C) detects latent disease

(D) has a morbidity of approximately 5%

(E) is used in pulmonary embolism

20. A 58-year-old man is undergoing cardiac catheterization. As part of obtaining informed consent, you advise that the procedure

(A) is contraindicated in the presence of cyanosis

(B) is considered noninvasive

(C) is generally performed with cardiopulmonary bypass

(D) may cause renal failure

(E) requires carotid artery puncture

21. A 23-year-old man, otherwise well, develops pleuritic chest pain, fever, and a friction rub heard at the lower left sternal border, unaffected by respiration. The most likely cause is

(A) rheumatic fever

(B) tuberculosis (TB)

(C) herpes simplex virus

(D) myocardial infarction

(E) coxsackievirus

22. A 72-year-old woman with angina undergoes cardiac catheterization. The pulmonary capillary "wedge" pressure is an approximation of pressure in the

(A) pulmonary artery

(B) pulmonary vein

(C) left atrium

(D) right atrium

(E) vena cava

23. A 17-year-old girl has fixed splitting of her second heart sound. Investigation would likely show that

(A) pulmonary blood flow is greater than systemic blood flow

(B) pulmonary blood flow is less than systemic blood flow

(C) pulmonary blood flow is equal to systemic blood flow

(D) the left ventricle is enlarged

(E) the systemic blood pressure is elevated

24. A 19-year-old man develops typical angina pectoris. There is no family history. Possible diagnosis includes

   (A) mitral stenosis
   (B) coronary artery aneurysm
   (C) coarctation
   (D) atrial septal defect
   (E) Werner syndrome

25. A 32-year-old asymptomatic woman has a rapidly rising, forceful pulse that collapses quickly. The most likely diagnosis is

   (A) mitral stenosis
   (B) mitral regurgitation
   (C) aortic stenosis
   (D) aortic regurgitation
   (E) coarctation of the aorta

26. A 63-year-old woman on digitalis develops a regular rapid supraventricular tachycardia without visible P waves. The appropriate response is

   (A) an increase in digitalis dose
   (B) complete cessation of digitalis
   (C) withdrawal of digitalis for one dose
   (D) addition of a beta blocker
   (E) addition of a calcium channel blocker

27. A 47-year-old man is found to have edema, ascites, and hepatosplenomegaly. The examination of his neck veins reveals elevated venous pressure with a deep "Y" descent. Heart size on x-ray is normal. The most likely etiology of this syndrome is

   (A) rheumatic fever
   (B) tuberculosis
   (C) unknown cause
   (D) previous acute pericarditis
   (E) neoplastic involvement of the pericardium

28. A 63-year-old woman with atrial flutter is given digoxin. She is likely to develop

   (A) atrial asystole
   (B) atrial bigeminy

   (C) atrial tachycardia
   (D) paroxysmal atrial tachycardia with block
   (E) atrial fibrillation

29. A 62-year-old man has chronic congestive heart failure (CHF). Which one of the following may be implicated in fluid retention?

   (A) decreased renin
   (B) increased aldosterone
   (C) increased estrogen
   (D) increased growth hormone
   (E) decreased vasopressin

30. Three months after an AMI, a 73-year-old man has a follow-up ECG. The sign most characteristic of a ventricular aneurysm is

   (A) ST elevation
   (B) RS-T depression in V5 and V6
   (C) inversion of T waves in one precordial lead
   (D) presence of an RS in a VL
   (E) tall, peaked T waves

31. On physical examination, a 79-year-old man is found to have a slow upstroke in his pulse and a diamond-shaped basal systolic murmur. His chest x-ray (CXR) is most likely to reveal

   (A) right ventricular dilatation
   (B) stenosis of the proximal ascending aorta
   (C) left atrial hypertrophy
   (D) normal overall cardiac size
   (E) displaced apex

32. A 49-year-old man has his serum lipids measured. Which pattern suggests the lowest risk for coronary artery disease?

   (A) total cholesterol 215, high-density lipoprotein (HDL) cholesterol 28
   (B) total cholesterol 215, HDL cholesterol 43
   (C) total cholesterol 180, HDL cholesterol 29
   (D) total cholesterol 202, HDL cholesterol 45
   (E) total cholesterol 225, HDL cholesterol 40

33. A 16-year-old boy has a higher blood pressure in his arms than in his legs. The most likely diagnosis is

    (A) aortic insufficiency
    (B) coarctation of the aorta
    (C) normal variant
    (D) ventricular aneurysm
    (E) severe juvenile diabetes

34. A 79-year-old man with a 40-year history of hypertension and cardiomegaly on CXR is likely to show which of the following on ECG?

    (A) counterclockwise rotation of the electrical axis
    (B) rSR pattern in V1
    (C) right axis deviation
    (D) high-voltage QRS complexes in V5 and V6
    (E) prolonged P-R interval in the limb leads

35. A 59-year-old woman presents for the first time with untreated, uncomplicated CHF. Which of the following is most likely to occur?

    (A) increased urinary sodium content
    (B) low urine specific gravity
    (C) increased urinary chloride content
    (D) anemia of chronic disease
    (E) albuminuria

36. A 60-year-old woman develops goiter, weight loss, and symptoms of anxiety. The most likely cardiac finding is

    (A) prolonged circulation time
    (B) decreased cardiac output
    (C) paroxysmal atrial fibrillation
    (D) pericardial effusion
    (E) aortic insufficiency

37. A 47-year-old woman develops accelerated hypertension. Retinal findings will likely include

    (A) retinitis obliterans
    (B) cotton wool spots

    (C) retinal detachment
    (D) optic atrophy
    (E) foveal blindness

38. A 32-year-old man presents with exertional chest pain. Physical exam reveals lumps on his Achilles tendon, yellow lesions around his eyes, and pigmentation of his iris. This syndrome is likely due to

    (A) type I hyperlipidemia
    (B) an abnormality on chromosome 19
    (C) myxedema
    (D) chronic renal disease
    (E) an inherited defect of glycogen utilization

39. A 22-year-old woman develops idiopathic pericarditis, with a resultant pericardial effusion. The clinical course and prognosis are determined largely by the

    (A) specific gravity of the fluid
    (B) presence or absence of blood in the fluid
    (C) presence or nature of any underlying disease
    (D) cellular count of the fluid
    (E) viscosity of the fluid

40. A patient has postural hypotension with dizziness. This finding indicates a

    (A) better prognosis than hypertension
    (B) correlation with younger age
    (C) previous myocardial infarct
    (D) possibility of diabetes mellitus (DM)
    (E) rare variant of essential hypertension

41. The echocardiogram of a 22-year-old woman reveals mitral valve prolapse. The most common physical finding is

    (A) diastolic rumble
    (B) absent first heart sound
    (C) diastolic click
    (D) aortic regurgitation
    (E) late systolic murmur

Questions 42 through 46

A 36-year-old man is seen because of palpitations. He admits to precordial discomfort, weakness, and anxiety. His pulse is 150, and his blood pressure is 100/70. Heart sounds are normal. Carotid sinus pressure changes the rate to 75, but when released the pulse rate returns to 150.

42. The most likely diagnosis is

    (A) atrial flutter with 2:1 block
    (B) paroxysmal atrial tachycardia with 2:1 block
    (C) sinus arrhythmia
    (D) atrial fibrillation
    (E) nodal tachycardia

43. Prior to the use of drugs, which of the following procedures may be helpful in converting the above to a sinus rhythm?

    (A) carotid sinus pressure
    (B) gagging procedures
    (C) Valsalva maneuver
    (D) eyeball compression
    (E) electrical cardioversion

44. Which of the following drugs is the best choice for treatment?

    (A) digitalis
    (B) mecholyl
    (C) aminophylline
    (D) ephedrine
    (E) atropine

45. This tachycardia is commonly associated with

    (A) hypertensive disease
    (B) a normal heart
    (C) syphilitic heart disease
    (D) coronary disease
    (E) congenital heart disease

46. The chronic form of this arrhythmia is managed by

    (A) combination antiarrhythmic therapy
    (B) surgical ablation
    (C) controlling the inevitable heart failure
    (D) chronic anticoagulant therapy
    (E) beta blockers

Questions 47 through 51

A 25-year-old man complains of left precordial chest pain that radiates to the left shoulder but not down the left arm. The pain is accentuated by inspiration and relieved by sitting up. The pain is accompanied by fever and chills. His blood pressure is 105/75, pulse 110/min and regular, and temperature 102°F. Aside from the tachycardia, there are no abnormal physical findings in the heart or lungs. The ECG shows ST segment elevation in all leads except aVR and VI. On the third hospital day, the patient's blood pressure falls, venous pressure rises, and he goes into congestive heart failure and shock.

47. The most likely diagnosis is

    (A) pulmonary infarction
    (B) myocardial infarction
    (C) pericarditis
    (D) myocardial infarction with secondary pericarditis
    (E) viral pneumonitis

48. The underlying etiologic factor is

    (A) coronary atherosclerosis
    (B) thrombophlebitis
    (C) neoplasm
    (D) unknown but probably viral
    (E) an arteritis

49. The events of the third hospital day were probably caused by

    (A) a second pulmonary embolus
    (B) extension of a myocardial infarct
    (C) cardiac tamponade
    (D) secondary bacterial infection
    (E) rupture of a chordae tendineae

50. The correct treatment on the third hospital day would be

    (A) ligation of the inferior vena cava
    (B) pericardiocentesis

(C) anticoagulation and pressor amines

(D) penicillin and oxygen

(E) coronary endarterectomy

51. The chest roentgenogram on the third hospital day would probably reveal

(A) a wedge-shaped area of consolidation in the left lung field and a left pleural effusion

(B) no abnormal findings

(C) a "water-bottle" heart

(D) patchy areas of consolidation in the left lung field

(E) hypervascular lung fields

52. The laboratory results shown in Table 1–1 are obtained from the investigation of a 37-year-old black woman who has a blood pressure at rest of 140/100 mm Hg. The most likely diagnosis is

(A) Cushing syndrome

(B) primary aldosteronism

(C) essential hypertension

(D) pyelonephritis

(E) bilateral renal artery stenosis

53. Figure 1–1 is the x-ray of an 8-year-old boy who had easy fatigability and a soft, continuous murmur in the upper back. ECG revealed minimal left ventricular hypertrophy. What is your diagnosis?

(A) aortic stenosis

(B) patent ductus arteriosus

(C) coarctation of the aorta

(D) pulmonary valvular stenosis

(E) peripheral pulmonary stenosis

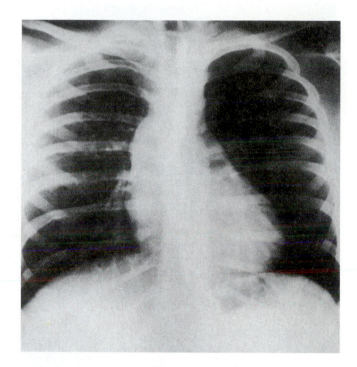

Figure 1–1.

TABLE 1–1. LABORATORY INVESTIGATIONS

Urinalysis	
pH	5.2
Albumin	Negative to trace
Serum Na	140 mEq/L
K	3.5 mEq/L
Cl	100 mEq/L
CO_2	25 mEq/L
Creatinine	1.0 mg/100 mL
Fasting sugar	90 mg/100 mL
Calcium	9.0 mg/100 mL
Uric acid	5.0 mg/100 mL

54. Figure 1–2 is an x-ray of an asymptomatic 48-year-old male executive coming in for his regular annual medical checkup. What is your diagnosis?

    (A) calcific pericarditis
    (B) left ventricular aneurysm
    (C) hydatid cyst
    (D) pleuropericarditis
    (E) normal

55. A 70-year-old man has dyspnea, orthopnea, and paroxysmal nocturnal dyspnea. He has generalized cardiomegaly and pulmonary and systemic venous hypertension. The ECG is shown in Figure 1–3. What is the cardiac rhythm?

    (A) ectopic atrial tachycardia
    (B) atrial flutter with 2:1 AV conduction
    (C) sinus tachycardia
    (D) supraventricular tachycardia
    (E) atrial fibrillation with rapid ventricular response

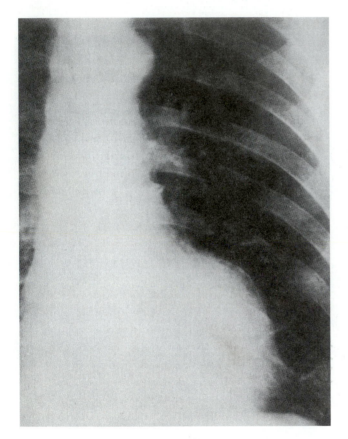

Figure 1–2.

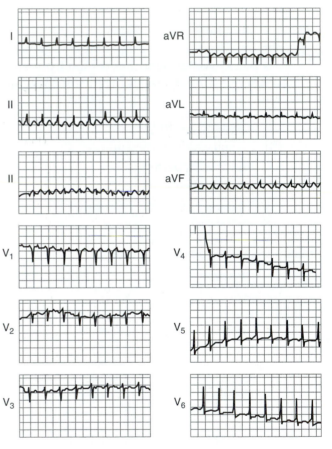

Figure 1–3.

56. What is the rhythm in the lead tracing shown in Figure 1–4?

    (A) first-degree heart block

    (B) second-degree heart block

    (C) third-degree heart block

    (D) premature ventricular beats

    (E) premature atrial beats

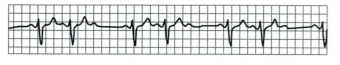

Figure 1–4.

57. The patient is a 42-year-old woman with a history of many years of anterior chest pain of a somewhat atypical nature. The patient's pain has been present and relatively stable for a number of years, and the ECG picture shown in Figure 1–5 is a stable one. What is the diagnosis?

    (A) inferior wall infarction

    (B) anterior wall infarction

    (C) ventricular aneurysm

    (D) nonspecific changes

    (E) pericarditis

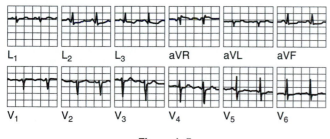

Figure 1–5.

58. The ECG shown in Figure 1–6 was obtained during the initial stages of an AMI. What is the rhythm?

    (A) atrial fibrillation

    (B) atrial flutter

    (C) second-degree heart block

    (D) Wenckebach phenomenon

    (E) ventricular tachycardia

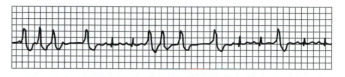

Figure 1–6.

59. A 78-year-old man with advanced renal disease has the ECG shown in Figure 1–7 (lead II). What is the diagnosis?

    (A) hyperkalemia

    (B) hypercalcemia

    (C) hypernatremia

    (D) pericarditis

    (E) ventricular aneurysm

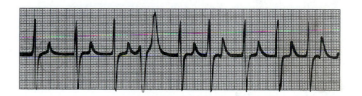

Figure 1–7.

60. A 58-year-old man whom you have followed dies suddenly, spurring you into doing some research on sudden death. Your readings will suggest that sudden death

    (A) is invariably due to cardiac cause
    (B) is rare in infants and children
    (C) has a bimodal distribution in the population
    (D) is defined as death within 24 hours of onset of symptoms
    (E) when caused by cardiac disease is most commonly characterized by coronary thrombi

61. You have a large number of patients in your practice with hypertension. If the diagnosis in an individual is essential hypertension, which of the following statements is correct?

    (A) Over 95% of patients are salt sensitive.
    (B) It comprises about 75% of hypertensives seen in a specialty clinic.
    (C) Renin levels are invariably high.
    (D) Women have a poorer prognosis.
    (E) Alcohol reduces risk.

DIRECTIONS (Questions 62 through 121): Each set of matching questions in this section consists of a list of lettered options followed by several numbered items. For each numbered item, select the appropriate lettered option(s). Each lettered option may be selected once, more than once, or not at all. EACH ITEM WILL STATE THE NUMBER OF OPTIONS TO SELECT. CHOOSE EXACTLY THIS NUMBER.

Questions 62 through 64

    (A) shortened P-R interval
    (B) lengthened P-R interval
    (C) lengthened Q-U interval
    (D) shortening of the Q-T interval
    (E) shortening of the Q-U interval
    (F) broad-based (> 0.20 sec) peaked T wave
    (G) narrow-based (< 0.20 sec) peaked T wave
    (H) widened QRS
    (I) flattened P waves

62. An 80-year-old man with renal impairment taking spironolactone (SELECT FOUR)

63. A 52-year-old woman with severe hyperparathyroidism (SELECT ONE)

64. A 64-year-old man with heart failure taking 80 mg of furosemide per day (SELECT ONE)

Questions 65 through 68

    (A) low right atrial pressure
    (B) normal right atrial pressure
    (C) high right atrial pressure
    (D) normal or elevated gradient between pulmonary artery (PA) diastolic pressure and wedge pressure
    (E) low pulmonary artery wedge pressure
    (F) normal or high pulmonary artery wedge pressure
    (G) low cardiac output
    (H) normal or high cardiac output
    (I) low systemic vascular resistance
    (J) normal or high systemic vascular resistance
    (K) normal or high pulmonary artery diastolic pressure

65. A 52-year-old man with alcoholic cirrhosis develops a variceal bleed with hypotension. Central hemodynamic monitoring would reveal (SELECT FOUR)

66. A 73-year-old man has an inferior infarct with ST elevation documented on right-sided precordial leads. He is hypotensive. Central hemodynamic monitoring would reveal (SELECT SIX)

67. A 20-year-old man is being treated for acute lymphoblastic leukemia. While neutropenic, he becomes severely hypotensive with a temperature of 103.5°F. Central hemodynamic monitoring would reveal (SELECT SIX)

68. A 78-year-old woman has an acute anterior wall myocardial infarction with hypotension and pulmonary congestion. Hemodynamic monitoring would reveal (SELECT FIVE)

Questions 69 and 70

- (A) high-pitched holosystolic murmur
- (B) early and midsystolic murmur
- (C) rapid decompensation with pulmonary edema
- (D) diminished S_1
- (E) may be tolerated without loss of cardiac reserve for years
- (F) diminished forward stroke volume

69. An asymptomatic 19-year-old student with a murmur is found to have mitral regurgitation on echocardiogram. The physical findings might include (SELECT THREE)

70. A 60-year-old man with an acute myocardial infarct develops a new murmur. Echocardiogram reveals acute mitral regurgitation. The findings might include (SELECT THREE)

Questions 71 through 75

- (A) mitral stenosis
- (B) acute rheumatic fever
- (C) hypothyroidism
- (D) hyperparathyroidism
- (E) Wolff–Parkinson–White syndrome
- (F) hypokalemia
- (G) hyperkalemia
- (H) aortic stenosis

71. Broad-notched P wave (SELECT ONE)

72. Prolonged P-R interval (SELECT ONE)

73. Short P-R interval (SELECT ONE)

74. Short Q-T interval (SELECT ONE)

75. Left ventricular hypertrophy (SELECT ONE)

Questions 76 through 79

A 68-year-old is on verapamil for control of hypertension and metoprolol for post-MI therapy.

- (A) true of propranolol but not verapamil
- (B) true of verapamil but not propranolol
- (C) true of both verapamil and propranolol
- (D) true of neither verapamil nor propranolol

76. Useful in heart failure (SELECT ONE)

77. The effects on the heart result in a prominent negative inotropic effect (SELECT ONE)

78. The treatment of choice in chronic atrial flutter (SELECT ONE)

79. Mechanism of action is calcium blockade (SELECT ONE)

Questions 80 through 84

- (A) hydralazine
- (B) enalapril
- (C) aldosterone
- (D) metoprolol
- (E) nifedipine
- (F) digoxin
- (G) furosemide
- (H) metolazone
- (I) amlodipine
- (J) nitrates

A 69-year-old man with CHF is being assessed for possible therapy. Match the medication(s) with the appropriate question.

80. Direct action on vascular smooth muscle (SELECT FOUR)

81. Inhibition of angiotensin I converting enzyme (SELECT ONE)

82. Myocardial stimulant (SELECT ONE)

83. Used for primary pulmonary hypertension (SELECT ONE)

84. May decrease mortality by direct myocardial protective action against catecholamines (SELECT ONE)

Questions 85 through 89

    (A) pulsus tardus

    (B) pulsus paradoxus

    (C) hyperkinetic pulse

    (D) bisferiens pulse

    (E) dicrotic pulse

    (F) pulsus alternans

    (G) delayed femoral pulse

    (H) pulsus bigeminus

This finding would be evident on the examination of the peripheral pulse of a 32-year-old woman with

85. Patent ductus arteriosus (SELECT ONE)

86. Dilated cardiomyopathy (SELECT ONE)

87. Hypertrophic cardiomyopathy (SELECT ONE)

88. Aortic stenosis (SELECT ONE)

89. Superior vena cava obstruction (SELECT ONE)

Questions 90 through 94

    (A) Cannon "A" wave

    (B) prominent "X" descent

    (C) Kussmaul's sign

    (D) slow "Y" descent

    (E) prominent "V" waves

    (F) positive abdominojugular reflux

This finding would be evident on examination of the jugular venous pulse (JVP) of a 57-year-old man with

90. Tricuspid regurgitation (SELECT ONE)

91. Right atrial myxoma (SELECT ONE)

92. Right ventricular infarction (SELECT ONE)

93. Right-sided heart failure (SELECT ONE)

94. Complete heart block (SELECT ONE)

Questions 95 through 99

    (A) aortic stenosis

    (B) hypertrophic cardiomyopathy (HCM)

    (C) mitral regurgitation (chronic)

    (D) tricuspid regurgitation

    (E) mitral valve prolapse

    (F) pulmonary stenosis

Evaluation of a 63-year-old man reveals a systolic ejection murmur. He has no symptoms at the present time. Further physical examination reveals the following findings. What causes of murmurs do these findings suggest?

95. The murmur increases with standing (SELECT TWO)

96. The murmur decreases in length and intensity with the Valsalva maneuver (SELECT FOUR)

97. The murmur decreases with exercise (SELECT ONE)

98. A double apical impulse is felt (SELECT TWO)

99. Transient external compression of both arms with blood pressure cuffs 20 mm Hg over peak systolic pressure increases the murmur (SELECT ONE)

Questions 100 through 105

    (A) cardiac tamponade

    (B) constrictive pericarditis

    (C) restrictive cardiomyopathy

    (D) right ventricle myocardial infarction (RVMI)

A 59-year-old man has SOB and mild peripheral edema. The following constellations of signs would suggest which diseases?

100. Prominent "Y" descent of neck veins, Kussmaul's sign, low voltage on ECG (SELECT ONE)

101. Pulsus paradoxus, low ECG voltage, negative Kussmaul's sign (SELECT ONE)

102. Elevated neck veins, abnormal ECG, third heart sound (S3) present (SELECT ONE)

103. Electrical alternans on ECG (SELECT ONE)

104. Pericardial knock (SELECT ONE)

105. No pulsus paradoxus, prominent "X" descent of neck veins, no Kussmaul's sign (SELECT ONE)

Questions 106 through 110

   (A) diabetes mellitus (DM)
   (B) thiamine deficiency
   (C) hyperthyroidism
   (D) hypothyroidism
   (E) malignant carcinoid
   (F) pheochromocytoma
   (G) rheumatoid arthritis (RA)
   (H) seronegative arthropathies
   (I) systemic lupus erythematosus (SLE)

The following cardiac abnormalities are characteristic of which systemic disease?

106. Endothelial plaques (SELECT ONE)

107. Proximal aortitis (SELECT ONE)

108. Focal myocardial necrosis (SELECT ONE)

109. Systolic scratchy sound (SELECT ONE)

110. Restrictive cardiomyopathy (SELECT ONE)

Questions 111 through 116

   (A) fibric acid derivatives (clofibrate, gemfibrozil)
   (B) nicotinic acid
   (C) bile acid-binding resins (cholestyramine, colestipol)
   (D) hepatic hydroxymethylglutaryl-coenzyme A (HMG-CoA) reductase inhibitors (lovastatin, simvastatin, pravastatin)
   (E) probucol
   (F) estrogens (Premarin, estradiol)

A 63-year-old woman with elevated cholesterol is assessed for therapy. Which drugs are associated with the following statements?

111. Associated with malignancy (SELECT ONE)

112. Can cause gallstones and myopathy (SELECT ONE)

113. Minimal absorption and no systemic toxicity (SELECT ONE)

114. Block the rate-limiting step in cholesterol synthesis (SELECT ONE)

115. Can lower HDL levels (SELECT ONE)

116. Probably can lower mortality associated with coronary artery disease (CAD) (SELECT TWO)

Questions 117 through 121

   (A) thiazides
   (B) spironolactone
   (C) clonidine
   (D) prazosin
   (E) beta blockers
   (F) hydralazine
   (G) angiotensin-converting enzyme (ACE) inhibitors
   (H) calcium channel blockers

A 67-year-old is referred to you for management of hypertension. For which drugs are the following statements correct?

117. Particularly useful in DM (SELECT ONE)

118. Most extensively studied, with proven effect on morbidity and mortality (SELECT ONE)

119. Drug of choice in unilateral renal artery stenosis (SELECT ONE)

120. Older people and blacks respond particularly well (SELECT ONE)

121. Edema without congestive heart failure (SELECT ONE)

Answers and Explanations

1. **(D)** Wenckebach, or type I second-degree AV block, is characterized on ECG by progressive lengthening of the P-R interval until there is a nonconducted P wave. The magnitude of P-R lengthening declines with each beat, so the R-R intervals characteristically shorten prior to the dropped beat. It is almost always caused by abnormal conduction across the AV node, and the QRS complex is usually of normal duration. *(Fuster, p. 857)*

2. **(D)** The ventricular inhibited (VVI) pacemaker functions when the heart rate falls below a preset interval. If a QRS is detected, the pacemaker is inhibited. If a QRS is not sensed, the pacing stimulus is not inhibited and the ventricle is stimulated. *(Fuster, p. 976)*

3. **(D)** The specific ECG signs of pulmonary embolism are rarely seen except in cases of massive pulmonary embolism. In submassive pulmonary emboli, the ECG may show nonspecific ST changes and sinus tachycardia. On occasion, pulmonary embolism can precipitate atrial flutter or fibrillation. One of the most useful roles of the ECG is to rule out myocardial infarction when a massive embolism is present. *(Fuster, pp. 1628–1629)*

4. **(C)** Aortic stenosis is most likely to be associated with angina pectoris, syncope, and exertional dyspnea. Exertional syncope is caused by either systemic vasodilation in the presence of fixed or inadequate cardiac output, an arrhythmia, or both. Syncope at rest is most frequently a result of a transient ventricular tachyarrhythmia. *(Fuster, pp. 1670–1671)*

5. **(C)** Common findings in infective endocarditis include petechiae, Roth's spots, Osler's nodes, Janeway lesions, splinter hemorrhages, stroke, and infarction of viscera or extremities. Many of the complications are thought to be embolic but may include vasculitis. Autopsy studies reveal that many systemic emboli go unrecognized. Brain, lung, coronary arteries, spleen, extremities, gut, and eyes are common locations for emboli. *(Fuster, pp. 2099–2100)*

6. **(B)** The slow channel for calcium assumes considerable importance in the region of the sinus node and AV node. For verapamil, this results in both antiarrhythmic and negative inotropic effects. Different classes of calcium channel blockers have differential effects on these slow channels, explaining the different clinical properties of the various calcium channel blocking drugs. *(Fuster, pp. 911, 1224)*

7. **(D)** Pericarditis secondary to transmural infarction is very common and most cases appear within 4 days. The most common manifestation of pericarditis is a friction rub along the left sternal border. It is evanescent, lasting only a few days. The pain is usually perceived by the patient to be different than that of the infarct. It is worsened by inspiration, swallowing, coughing, or lying down. It frequently is associated with a low-grade fever. *(Fuster, p. 1318)*

8. **(A)** Positively inotropic is the best description of the effect of calcium ions on the myocardium. Calcium plays a role in excitation–contraction coupling and in possible drug effects and heart failure. *(Fuster, p. 108)*

9. **(C)** In the past, there was concern that rigorous drug treatment would harm the fetus. Studies now show benefit in controlling pressure with drugs, but ACE inhibitors are contraindicated because they might cause renal abnormalities in the fetus. Women who develop hypertension during pregnancy have a higher risk of developing hypertension in later life. *(Fuster, p. 1588)*

10. **(E)** There is a possible indication (but not an obligation) to insert a temporary pacemaker if a new LBBB occurs. If LBBB and a Mobitz II AV block occur, there is general agreement on the usefulness of pacing. Temporary pacemaker is not required for first-degree block. For second-degree block of the Wenckebach type (usually with an inferior infarction), pacing is only required if symptoms of bradycardia and hypotension cannot be controlled medically. The necessity for temporary pacing during an AMI does not necessarily indicate that permanent pacing will be required. *(Fuster, p. 965)*

11. **(D)** Pulmonary hypertension is associated with an increased intensity of the second heart sound, which coincides with the end of the T wave on ECG. It is the pulmonic component of the second heart sound that is increased. As well, there may be prominent A waves in the jugular venous pulse, a right ventricular heave, an ejection click, and a right ventricular fourth heart sound. When signs and symptoms are apparent, the pulmonary hypertension is usually moderate to severe. *(Fuster, p. 252)*

12. **(D)** The patient most likely has paroxysmal atrial tachycardia. Sinus tachycardia differs from atrial tachycardia in that it does not start or stop abruptly. In paroxysmal atrial tachycardia, the QRS is usually narrow without clearly discernible P waves. A wide QRS in paroxysmal supraventricular tachycardia can result from a pre-existing bundle branch block, or a functional bundle branch block secondary to the tachycardia. This can make the distinction from a ventricular arrhythmia quite difficult. *(Fuster, pp. 809–812)*

13. **(D)** In the absence of coronary artery disease, angina pectoris occurs most frequently with aortic stenosis. Acute myocardial infarction is usually due to associated atherosclerotic coronary occlusion. *(Fuster, p. 1670)*

14. **(B)** In aortic stenosis, the first sound is usually normal; the second sound is characteristically diminished. There can be a single S_2 either because A_2 and P_2 are superimposed or A_2 is absent or very soft. Severe aortic stenosis may be accompanied by paradoxical splitting of S_2. *(Fuster, p. 1671)*

15. **(B)** Atrioventricular dissociation is the independent beating of atria and ventricles and is recognized on the electrocardiogram by fixed P-P and R-R intervals but variable P-R intervals. AV block is one cause of AV dissociation. *(Fuster, p. 860)*

16. **(E)** Nitroprusside is usually used in the setting of severe pulmonary congestion with adequate blood pressure. With significant hypotension, inotropic agents are generally administered prior to nitroprusside (or nitroglycerine). *(Fuster, pp. 1324–1325)*

17. **(A)** A ventricular septal defect is considered a relatively high risk lesion for infective endocarditis. Mitral valve prolapse with regurgitation, asymmetric septal hypertrophy, and pure mitral stenosis are considered intermediate risk. Atrial septal defects of the secundum type are considered low risk. *(Fuster, p. 2089)*

18. **(A)** The myxoma is a solitary globular or polypoid tumor varying in size from that of a cherry to a peach. About 75% are found in the left atrium, and most of the remainder in the right atrium. The clinical presentation is with one or more of the classical triad of constitution symptoms (fatigue, fever, anemia), embolic events, or obstruction of the valve orifice. *(Fuster, pp. 2179–2180)*

19. **(C)** Exercise electrocardiography represents an increasingly popular noninvasive method for early detection of latent ischemic heart

disease. As with other diagnostic tests, the exercise ECG is of most clinical value when the pretest probability of disease is moderate (ie, 30 to 70%). In men over 40 and women over 50 who plan to start vigorous exercise, use of exercise ECG is possibly, but not definitely, supported by the evidence (class IIb). *(Fuster, p. 471)*

20. **(D)** Contrast media used in cardiac catheterization may result in renal impairment. The group at highest risk includes diabetics with renal disease and those with pre-existing renal failure. Good hydration is essential. Other manifestations of contrast media include nausea and vomiting (common), and anaphylactoid reactions characterized by low-grade fever, hives, itching, angioedema, bronchospasm, and even shock. Side effects are reduced with the use of new low osmolality contrast media. *(Fuster, p. 493)*

21. **(E)** Pericarditis in clinical practice is commonly idiopathic and frequently assumed to be of possible viral origin. Coxsackieviruses are a common cause, but herpesviruses are not. Although TB, rheumatic fever, and myocardial infarction can cause pericarditis, they are unlikely in this case. *(Fuster, pp. 2063–2065)*

22. **(C)** Left-heart catheterization is a more accurate measurement, but involves a slightly increased risk. End-expiratory pulmonary artery diastolic pressure is very close (2 to 4 mm) to wedge pressure as well. A discordance between wedge pressure and pulmonary artery diastolic pressure suggests the presence of pulmonary hypertension. *(Fuster, p. 485)*

23. **(A)** This is characteristic of an atrial septal defect. Pulmonary blood flow is greater because of increased blood flow from the right atrium, which receives blood from the vena cava and left atrium. *(Fuster, p. 1851)*

24. **(B)** Angina or infarction in young patients should prompt the physician to consider congenital coronary artery anomaly or congeni-

tal coronary artery aneurysm. Acquired coronary artery aneurysm can be caused by atherosclerosis, trauma, angioplasty, atherectomy, vasculitis, mycotic emboli, Kawasaki syndrome, or arterial dissection. *(Fuster, pp. 1169, 1175)*

25. **(D)** This pulse is seen in aortic regurgitation. The pressure in diastole is usually 50 mm Hg or lower. This is known as a water-hammer or Corrigan's pulse. A bisferiens pulse may be present as well. Systolic blood pressure is elevated. *(Fuster, p. 1686)*

26. **(B)** Atrioventricular dissociation and paroxysmal atrial tachycardia with block are distinctive manifestations of digitalis toxicity. This arrhythmia is likely paroxysmal atrial tachycardia. Symptoms of digitalis toxicity include anorexia, nausea, fatigue, dizziness, and visual disturbances. The presence of hypokalemia increases the likelihood of digitalis toxicity. *(Fuster, pp. 819–820)*

27. **(C)** Commonly, no cause is found for constrictive pericarditis. Some patients do give a history of previous acute pericarditis. TB is now an uncommon cause. Cancer can cause constriction but is uncommon. Rheumatic fever does not cause pericarditis. *(Fuster, pp. 2072–2073)*

28. **(E)** Digitalis given in atrial flutter may cause atrial fibrillation, particularly if there is advanced heart disease. For acute management of atrial flutter, digoxin should be administered before other antiarrhythmias to prevent very rapid rates that might result if 1:1 AV conduction occurs. If hemodynamic instability is present, electrical cardioversion is the treatment of choice. *(Fuster, pp. 822–823)*

29. **(B)** Retention of fluid is complex and not due to any one factor; however, hormones may contribute. Growth hormone does not have fluid-retaining properties. The exact mechanisms that initiate renal conservation of salt and water are not precisely understood, but may include arterial volume receptors sensing a decrease in the *effective* arterial blood

volume. Aldosterone, renin, and vasopressin are generally increased in heart failure. *(Fuster, p. 664)*

30. **(A)** ST elevation persisting 2 weeks after an infarct, an abnormal pericardial impulse, and a bulge on the left ventricular border on x-ray are characteristic of an aneurysm. Ventricular aneurysms are most often a result of a large anterior infarct. The poor prognosis associated with these aneurysms is due to the associated left ventricular dysfunction, rather than to the aneurysm itself. *(Fuster, p. 1328)*

31. **(D)** In aortic stenosis, there is normal overall cardiac size, but dilatation of the proximal ascending aorta and blunt rounding of the lower left cardiac contour. Calcification of the valve is often difficult to determine on plain films. Although left atrial enlargement can occur, its presence on the chest x-ray should raise other diagnostic possibilities, such as mitral valve disease. *(Fuster, p. 1671)*

32. **(D)** This combination, although the total cholesterol is borderline, has a high HDL cholesterol, which is protective. Nevertheless, a level this high would likely require treatment. *(Fuster, p. 1137)*

33. **(B)** Besides coarctation of the aorta, aortic occlusive disease, dissection of the aorta, and abdominal aneurysm may lead to differential blood pressure in arms and legs. Coarctation is the third most common form of congenital cardiac disease. One third of patients will be hypertensive. The femoral pulses are weak, delayed, and even absent. *(Fuster, p. 1925)*

34. **(D)** He likely has left ventricular hypertrophy. Signs include left-axis deviation, high-voltage QRS complexes in V5 and V6, deep S in V1 and V2, and prolonged QRS in the left precordial leads. Age, orientation of the heart in the chest, and noncardiac factors make the ECG an imperfect tool for diagnosing or excluding left ventricular hypertrophy. The echocardiogram is more accurate and better for following progression or regression of left ventricular hypertrophy (LVH). *(Fuster, p. 301)*

35. **(E)** High urinary specific gravity, nocturia, and daytime oliguria occur in addition to albuminuria in uncomplicated, untreated CHF. *(Fuster, p. 679)*

36. **(C)** Thyroid disease may affect the heart muscle directly or there may be excessive sympathetic stimulation. Common symptoms of thyrotoxic heart disease include palpitations, exertional dyspnea, and worsening angina. Atrial fibrillation is particularly common in older individuals. *(Fuster, pp. 119, 826, 1237)*

37. **(B)** Cotton wool spots, hemorrhage, and papilledema are common. Fibrinoid necrosis occurs on the arterioles of many organs. Earlier manifestations of arteriosclerosis include thickening of the vessel wall. This is manifested by obscuration of the venous column at arterial crossings. *(Fuster, p. 1567)*

38. **(B)** Early atherosclerosis with tendon xanthomas, xanthelasma, and arcus senilis are characteristic of familial hypercholesterolemia. The disorder is inherited in an autosomal dominant manner. The mutant gene for the LDL receptor is located on chromosome 19. *(Fuster, p. 216)*

39. **(C)** Acute pericarditis is most often idiopathic and is typically self-limited (usually within 2 to 6 weeks). While small effusions are common, tamponade is unusual, as are heart failure and constriction. Other diseases causing pericarditis should be searched for, and may influence the prognosis. *(Fuster, p. 2077)*

40. **(D)** Orthostatic hypotension (systolic dropping by 20 mm or more) is particularly common in the elderly and in diabetics. Management includes avoidance of precipitating factors, simple adaptive maneuvers, volume expansion, and pharmacologic agents. *(Fuster, pp. 998–999)*

41. **(E)** In mitral valve prolapse, the first heart sound is usually preserved followed by a systolic click and late systolic murmur. The click is actually the most common finding. General

physical exam may reveal scoliosis, pectus excavatum, straightened thoracic spine, or narrow anteroposterior diameter of chest. *(Fuster, p. 1732)*

42. **(A)** The symptoms and signs are like any sudden paroxysmal tachycardia, but the ventricular rate is the clue, after carotid pressure, to the diagnosis of atrial flutter with 2:1 block. *(Fuster, p. 822)*

43. **(E)** The maneuvers listed increase the block and are useful for diagnosis, but not for converting the atrial flutter to a sinus rhythm. Often very low amounts of energy during cardioversion will convert atrial flutter. *(Fuster, p. 822)*

44. **(A)** Digitalis slows the ventricular rate and controls or prevents heart failure. Verapamil may be of help in both acute paroxysms of atrial flutter and chronic management. At times, catheter ablation of the flutter pathway is required in chronic atrial flutter. Surgical ablation is reserved for cases where other surgical interventions are required. *(Fuster, p. 823)*

45. **(E)** Tachycardia is not commonly associated with syphilitic heart disease. Coronary artery disease can cause flutter, but not commonly. The most common causes are congenital heart disease, mitral valve disorders, and cardiomyopathy. It is only rarely seen in normal subjects. The sudden change to half rate on vagal stimulation is diagnostic of atrial flutter with 2:1 block. *(Fuster, p. 820)*

46. **(E)** The basis of management is rate control by digoxin, beta blockers, or calcium channel blockers. The arrhythmia can be asymptomatic. Although the precise risk of stroke in chronic atrial flutter is unknown, current practice is to provide anticoagulation. *(Fuster, p. 823)*

47. **(C)** Pericarditis is the most likely diagnosis. The pain may be sternal or parasternal, and radiate to posterior or anterior cervical areas, to either trapezius, or to either shoulder. It may be indistinguishable from the pain of an acute myocardial infarction. *(Fuster, pp. 2064–2065)*

48. **(D)** Viruses include coxsackie B virus, echovirus, adenovirus, and infectious mononucleosis. The erythrocyte sedimentation rate is usually elevated, and an early leukocytosis is common. Cardiac enzymes are usually normal. Rising viral titers are required to confirm the exact causative virus. *(Fuster, pp. 2063, 2077)*

49. **(C)** Management of acute viral or idiopathic pericarditis includes analgesia (usually aspirin every 3 to 4 hours initially) and rest if the pain is severe. Occasionally, nonsteroidal anti-inflammatory drugs (NSAIDs) are required (eg, ibuprofen or indomethacin). Careful observation for increasing effusion and tamponade are essential. The classic findings of cardiac tamponade include arterial hypotension and pulsus paradoxus. *(Fuster, pp. 2065–2066, 2068–2069)*

50. **(B)** Pericardiocentesis would be the correct treatment. Often removal of even small amounts of fluid, such as 50 mL can result in considerable symptomatic and hemodynamic improvement. *(Fuster, pp. 2071–2072)*

51. **(C)** A water-bottle heart would probably be revealed. The association of clear lung fields with a large cardiac silhouette distinguishes pericardial effusion from heart failure. However, if tamponade is suspected, an echocardiogram is the first test that should be done. Any delay in diagnosis can be harmful. *(Fuster, pp. 336, 2070)*

52. **(C)** Essential hypertension is the most likely diagnosis. A secondary cause for hypertension is found in only 10% of patients, with 90% labeled as *essential*. Current recommendations for initial workup of a hypertensive patient include serum chemistry (glucose, potassium, creatinine), urinalysis, and electrocardiogram. *(Fuster, pp. 1565–1567)*

53. **(C)** Coarctation of the aorta is the diagnosis. There is a *reverse 3* deformity of the esopha-

gus, the belly of which represents the dilated aorta after the coarctation. The border of the descending aorta shows a medial indentation called the 3 or *tuck* sign, the belly of the 3 representing the poststenotic dilation and the upper portion by the dilated subclavian artery and small transverse aortic arch. *(Fuster, p. 1863)*

54. **(B)** Note the abnormal humped contour of the left ventricular border, with a curvilinear calcification following the abnormal cardiac contour. The presence of calcification in the ventricular wall and the abnormal left ventricular contour alert one to the consideration of a ventricular aneurysm. *(Fuster, pp. 326, 1328)*

55. **(B)** The cardiac rhythm is atrial flutter with 2:1 AV conduction. QRS complexes occur with perfect regularity at a rate of about 150/min. Their normal contour and duration indicate that ventricular activation occurs normally via the AV junction–His–Purkinje system. *(Fuster, p. 820)*

56. **(B)** The P-R interval of the first two complexes is normal at 0.20 seconds. The QRS duration is 0.16 seconds. The third P wave is nonconducted. This cycle recurs in the remainder of the strip. This is second-degree heart block of the Mobitz type II variety. Note the wide QRS. When this type of heart block develops, either de novo or in the course of an AMI, a cardiac pacemaker is usually recommended, as the incidence of complete heart block is high in this situation. *(Fuster, pp. 857–859)*

57. **(D)** The ST is depressed in leads II, III, aVF, and V4–6. These nonspecific abnormalities do not indicate significant coronary heart disease, especially in an apprehensive young patient. Further evaluations should be guided by clinical circumstances. *(Fuster, p. 288)*

58. **(E)** The underlying rhythm is regular sinus rhythm with a rate of 85 beats/min. The sinus rhythm is interrupted frequently by bursts of irregular ventricular, premature beats. Sinus

rhythm is uninterrupted as can be determined by plotting the P-P intervals, which are regular. The rhythm may be termed a *chaotic ventricular arrhythmia* or *ventricular tachycardia*. Its gross irregularity is unusual. Antiarrhythmic therapy is indicated. *(Fuster, p. 837)*

59. **(A)** No atrial activity is detected. The ventricular rate is slightly irregular. Beat number 4 is a ventricular premature contraction. The T waves are tall and markedly peaked. This type of T wave is characteristic of hyperkalemia, as is absence of visible atrial activity. The potassium level was 8.2 mmol/L. *(Fuster, pp. 302–303)*

60. **(C)** Sudden death, defined as death within 1 hour of onset of symptoms, is usually caused by cardiac disease in middle-aged and elderly patients, but in younger age groups noncardiac causes predominate. There is a bimodal distribution in the population, with the first peak before 6 months of age (sudden infant death syndrome). The most common coronary artery finding is extensive chronic coronary atherosclerosis, although acute syndromes do occur. *(Braunwald, pp. 228–229)*

61. **(B)** Although over 90% of hypertensives in the general population have essential hypertension, the referral bias of a hypertension clinic results in only 65 to 85% prevalence of essential hypertension. Only about 60% of hypertensives are very sensitive to salt. About 20% of hypertensives have low-renin essential hypertension. This is more common in blacks. Male sex, black race, youth, smoking, diabetes mellitus, excess alcohol ingestion, hypercholesterolemia, more severe hypertension, and evidence of end-organ damage are among the factors that suggest a poor prognosis. *(Braunwald, pp. 1414–1417)*

62. **(B, F, H, I)** In renal impairment, potassium-sparing diuretics can cause life-threatening hyperkalemia. The characteristic findings of hyperkalemia are a narrow-based, peaked T wave in conjunction with a widened QRS complex. Other causes of widened QRS com-

plexes do not coexist with a narrow-peak T wave. Also, the P-R interval prolongs and the P wave flattens with hyperkalemia. *(Fuster, pp. 302–303)*

63. **(D)** With severe hypercalcemia, the QT interval is markedly shortened. There is a correlation between the length of QT interval and the degree of hypercalcemia. *(Fuster, p. 304)*

64. **(C)** Hypokalemia results in prolongation of the Q-U interval. In severe cases, the ST segments become depressed. Quinidine, even in therapeutic doses, can cause similar ECG findings. This is felt to be a risk factor for ventricular arrhythmias, including Torsade de pointes. *(Fuster, p. 303)*

65. **(A, E, G, J)** Hypovolemic shock is characterized by a low cardiac output with normal or high systemic vascular resistance. The low right atrial filling pressure and low pulmonary artery wedge pressure reflect the inadequate venous return. *(Braunwald, p. 225)*

66. **(C, D, F, G, J, K)** This man has a right ventricular myocardial infarction. Primary right ventricular failure is characterized by a disproportionately high right atrial pressure with normal or high wedge pressure. The PA diastolic pressure is normal or elevated and the gradient between PA diastolic pressure and wedge pressure is usually increased. Systemic vascular resistance is usually normal. *(Fuster, p. 1320)*

67. **(A, D, E, H, I, K)** In septic shock, right atrial wedge pressures, cardiac output, and systemic vascular resistance are low. PA diastolic pressure is usually normal or high, therefore resulting in an increased gradient between PA diastolic and wedge pressures. *(Braunwald, p. 225)*

68. **(C, F, G, J, K)** Cardiogenic shock is characterized by high right atrial pressure (although it can be normal at times), high PA wedge pressure, high PA diastolic pressure, high systemic vascular resistance, and low cardiac output. *(Fuster, pp. 1324–1327)*

69. **(A, D, E)** In chronic, compensated mitral regurgitation, there is a holosystolic murmur, which starts with S_1 and extends to or past the aortic component of S_2. The S_1 is diminished, and there is increased splitting of S_2. This condition is often tolerated for years before symptoms develop. *(Fuster, p. 1713)*

70. **(B, C, F)** Coronary artery disease is the most common cause of acute mitral regurgitation in the United States. The murmur is often midsystolic early on, and a thrill may be present. The apex is usually hyperdynamic but actual forward stroke volume is usually diminished. The presentation is usually dominated by acute pulmonary edema and occurs most often 2 to 7 days post-MI. *(Fuster, p. 1326)*

71. **(A)** ECG changes in mitral stenosis are due to enlargement and hypertrophy of the left atrium and asynchronous atrial activation. The notched P wave is most prominent in lead II. In lead V1, the P wave has a negative terminal deflection. *(Fuster, p. 1702)*

72. **(B)** A prolonged P-R interval is the most frequent significant electrocardiographic abnormality in rheumatic fever. However, it is very nonspecific and seen in numerous other conditions. It is only a minor criterion for the diagnosis of acute rheumatic fever. *(Fuster, p. 1661)*

73. **(E)** In Wolff–Parkinson–White syndrome, the P-R interval is short, the QRS is widened, and there is slurring of the upstroke of the R wave. The shortened P-R interval reflects faster than normal conduction through an accessory pathway. The ventricular complex represents a fusion beat. The blurred upstroke of the QRS (delta wave) represents ventricular activation via the accessory pathway. The normal end portion of the QRS represents activation via the normal route through the AV node. *(Fuster, p. 816)*

74. **(D)** In hyperparathyroidism, hypercalcemia may prolong the QRS and shorten the ST and QT intervals. Serious arrhythmias rarely oc-

cur with hypercalcemia. Patients with hyper-parathyroidism might also have a higher prevalence of hypertension. *(Fuster, p. 304)*

75. **(C)** The ECG in severe aortic stenosis shows LVH, but is not perfectly sensitive and is not specific. Bundle branch blocks and ST-T changes can occur, but some patients have a normal ECG. *(Fuster, p. 1672)*

76. **(A)** Beta blockers are indicated in treatment of heart failure patents who are symptomatic despite ACE inhibition, even in older age. *(Fuster, p. 2349)*

77. **(C)** Both can potentially result in hypotension and left ventricular failure in patients with left ventricular dysfunction. Unlike beta blockers, the various calcium channel blockers have varying effects on cardiac function. Some, such as amlodipine, do not usually cause CHF. *(Fuster, pp. 1577–1588)*

78. **(B)** In chronic atrial flutter, control of ventricular rate is the goal of therapy. Beta blockers, Ca^{++} channel blockers, and digoxin are drugs commonly used. *(Fuster, p. 823)*

79. **(B)** Verapamil appears to mediate its effect by interfering with movement of calcium through the so-called slow channel. These slow channels predominantly allow calcium to enter, in contrast to the fast channels where sodium enters. Various classes of calcium channel blockers have differential effects on these slow channels, explaining their differential clinical effects. *(Fuster, p. 807)*

80. **(A, E, I, J)** Hydralazine has a greater dilator effect on arterioles than veins, the opposite for nitrates. Combined therapy with hydralazine and nitrates has been shown to reduce mortality in patients with heart failure, but not to reduce hospitalization for heart failure. Reflex tachycardia with hydralazine is common in patients with hypertension, but less so in heart failure. Tachycardia may precipitate angina. Calcium channel blockers are not generally used in CHF, because of their negative inotropic effect. However, amlodipine can be used for concurrent treatment of angina or hypertension. *(Fuster, p. 697)*

81. **(B)** Enalapril may exert its effect by inhibiting formation of angiotensin II. This lowers systemic vascular resistance. In addition, ACE inhibitors have a natriuretic effect by inhibition of aldosterone secretion. They have been shown to improve mortality and decrease hospitalization in patients with CHF. *(Fuster, pp. 693–695)*

82. **(F)** Hydralazine and enalapril increase cardiac output by decreasing impedance to left ventricular ejection. Digoxin is a direct inotropic agent, but is usually reserved for patients who are symptomatic after treatment with ACE inhibitors and diuretics. It can be used for rate control in atrial fibrillation, although beta blockers might be preferred. *(Fuster, p. 705)*

83. **(E)** Long-acting nifedipine has been a useful adjunct to the treatment of primary pulmonary hypertension, but great care must be used as even low doses of vasodilators can cause untoward reactions in patients with pulmonary hypertension. Lung transplants have provided a major therapeutic modality for managing severe pulmonary hypertension. ACE inhibitors and hydralazine have been tried, but are not effective. *(Fuster, pp. 1619–1620)*

84. **(D)** There are numerous potential mechanisms that might explain the beneficial effects of beta blockers in left ventricular dysfunction, and post–myocardial infarction. The benefit is additive to that provided by ACE inhibitors. *(Fuster, pp. 697–700)*

85. **(C)** A hyperkinetic pulse occurs in the setting of an elevated stroke volume (anemia, fever, anxiety) or an abnormally rapid runoff from the arterial system (patent ductus arteriosus, arteriovenous fistula). *(Fuster, p. 224)*

86. **(E)** A dicrotic pulse has a peak in systole and another in diastole. It occurs in patients with very low stroke volume, especially dilated cardiomyopathy. *(Fuster, p. 225)*

87. **(D)** The bisferiens pulse, two systolic peaks, occurs in hypertrophic cardiomyopathy and aortic regurgitation. In aortic regurgitation, the bisferiens pulse can occur both in the presence or absence of aortic stenosis. *(Fuster, pp. 224–225)*

88. **(A)** The pulsus tardus of aortic stenosis is the result of mechanical obstruction to left ventricular ejection and often has an accompanying thrill. The characteristic feel of the pulse is caused by a delayed systolic peak. *(Fuster, p. 225)*

89. **(B)** Pulsus paradoxus, a drop of greater than 10 mm Hg in systolic blood pressure during inspiration, is caused by pericardial tamponade, airway obstruction, or superior vena cava obstruction. At times, the peripheral pulse may disappear completely during inspiration. *(Fuster, pp. 225–226)*

90. **(E)** Tricuspid regurgitation increases the size of the V wave. When tricuspid regurgitation becomes severe, the combination of a prominent V wave and obliteration of the X descent results in a single, large, positive systolic wave. *(Fuster, p. 229)*

91. **(D)** Right atrial myxoma, or tricuspid stenosis, will slow the Y descent by obstructing right ventricular filling. The Y descent of the JVP is produced mainly by the tricuspid valve opening and the subsequent rapid inflow of blood into the right ventricle. *(Fuster, p. 229)*

92. **(C)** Right ventricular infarction and constrictive pericarditis frequently result in an increase in jugular venous pressure during inspiration (Kussmaul's sign). Severe right-sided failure can also be a cause. *(Fuster, pp. 228–229)*

93. **(F)** Right-sided heart failure is the most common cause of a positive abdominojugular reflux (normal JVP at rest, increases during 10 seconds of firm midabdominal compression, and only drops when pressure is released). *(Fuster, p. 227)*

94. **(A)** Large A waves occur with increased resistance to filling (tricuspid stenosis, pulmonary hypertension) or when the right atrium contracts against a tricuspid valve closed by right ventricular systole (Cannon A waves) in complete heart block or other arrhythmias. *(Fuster, p. 229)*

95. **(B, E)** With standing, most murmurs diminish. The two exceptions are hypertrophic cardiomyopathy, which becomes louder, and mitral valve prolapse, which becomes longer and louder. *(Fuster, p. 1732; Braunwald, p. 1258)*

96. **(A, C, D, F)** With the Valsalva maneuver, most murmurs will decrease. The exceptions are the murmurs of hypertrophic cardiomyopathy and mitral valve prolapse, which increase. After release of the Valsalva maneuver, right-sided murmurs tend to return to baseline more rapidly. *(Braunwald, p. 1258)*

97. **(B)** The murmur of hypertrophic cardiomyopathy often decreases with submaximal isometric exercise (handgrip). Murmurs across normal or obstructed valves will be increased. Handgrip can also accentuate an S_3 or S_4. *(Braunwald, p. 1258)*

98. **(A, B)** HCM often has a bisferiens pulse. It can also be found in pure aortic regurgitation or combined aortic regurgitation and aortic stenosis. *(Fuster, pp. 224–225)*

99. **(C)** This maneuver will increase the murmurs of mitral regurgitation, ventricular septal defect, and aortic regurgitation. Other murmurs are not affected. *(Braunwald, p. 1258)*

100. **(B)** Constrictive pericarditis is characterized by a prominent Y descent of the neck veins and low voltage on ECG. The presence of a positive Kussmaul's sign helps differentiate the syndrome from cor pulmonale and restrictive cardiomyopathies. *(Braunwald, p. 1367)*

101. **(A)** Cardiac tamponade can occur with as little as 200 mL of fluid if the accumulation is rapid. Physical exam reveals a pulsus paradoxus (a greater than 10 mm Hg inspiratory

decline in systolic arterial pressure), a prominent X descent of the jugular veins, but no Kussmaul's sign. The ECG may show low voltage. *(Braunwald, p. 1367)*

102. **(D)** RVMI is characterized by high neck veins, ECG abnormalities, and often a right-sided S_3. The low cardiac output associated with RVMI can often be treated by volume expansion. Although a third of patients with inferoposterior infarctions have some degree of right ventricular necrosis, extensive RVMI is uncommon. *(Braunwald, p. 1367)*

103. **(A)** Electrical alternans (a beat-to-beat alternation in one or more component of the ECG signal) can occur in pericardial effusion and numerous other conditions. Total electrical alternans (P-QRS-T) and sinus tachycardia is relatively specific for pericardial effusion (often with tamponade). *(Braunwald, p. 1367)*

104. **(B)** A pericardial knock is characteristic of constrictive pericarditis. It is in fact an early S_3, occurring 0.06 to 0.12 seconds after aortic closure. S_1 and S_2 are frequently distant. *(Braunwald, p. 1367)*

105. **(C)** The combination of absent pulsus and absent Kussmaul's sign with prominent X descent favors a restrictive cardiomyopathy. Unlike constrictive pericarditis, restrictive cardiomyopathies frequently present with an enlarged heart, orthopnea, left ventricular hypertrophy, and bundle branch blocks. *(Braunwald, p. 1367)*

106. **(E)** The cardiac lesions of gastrointestinal carcinoids are almost exclusively in the right side of the heart and occur only when there are hepatic metastases. Fibrous plaques are found on the endothelium of the cardiac chambers, valves, and great vessels. These plaques can distort cardiac valves; tricuspid regurgitation and pulmonic stenosis are the most common valvular problems. *(Braunwald, p. 1376)*

107. **(H)** The proximal aortitis of seronegative arthritis (ankylosing spondylitis, Reiter syndrome, psoriatic arthritis, or associated with inflammatory bowel disease) can result in aortic regurgitation and AV block. *(Braunwald, p. 1376)*

108. **(F)** Focal myocardial necrosis and inflammatory cell infiltration caused by high circulating levels of catecholamines are seen in about 50% of patients who die with pheochromocytoma. Hypertension can further impair left ventricular function. *(Braunwald, p. 1376)*

109. **(C)** The Means–Lerman scratch, a systolic scratchy sound heard at the left second intercostal space during expiration, is thought to result from the rubbing of the hyperdynamic pericardium against the pleura. Palpitations, atrial fibrillation, hypertension, angina, and heart failure are more common cardiac manifestations of hyperthyroidism. *(Braunwald, p. 1375)*

110. **(A)** Diabetes mellitus can result in a restrictive cardiomyopathy in the absence of large-vessel coronary artery disease. Histology reveals increased collagen, glycoprotein, triglycerides, and cholesterol in the myocardial interstitium. Abnormalities may be present in small intramural arteries. *(Braunwald, p. 1374)*

111. **(F)** Estrogens are effective in decreasing low-density lipoprotein (LDL) levels in postmenopausal women. They have been associated with endometrial cancer, and can also raise very low-density lipoprotein (VLDL) levels. They are not first line drugs for elevated cholesterol, and in fact the cardioprotective effect evident in epidemiological studies has not been verified in clinical trials. *(Braunwald, p. 1384)*

112. **(A)** Fibric acid derivatives decrease VLDL but have been associated with gallstones and myopathy. They act by decreasing VLDL synthesis and enhancing lipoprotein lipase action. They have been shown to decrease risk from ischemic heart disease. *(Braunwald, pp. 2254–2255)*

113. **(C)** The minimal absorption and lack of systemic toxicity of the resins make them good

choices for use in children with familial hypercholesterolemia and for primary prevention in young adults. They act by promoting sterol excretion and increasing LDL receptor-mediated removal. However, gastrointestinal side effects make compliance difficult. (Braunwald, pp. 2254–2256)

114. **(D)** The HMG-CoA reductase inhibitors block cholesterol synthesis and increase LDL receptor-mediated catabolism of LDL. They are very effective in lowering LDL with minimal side effects. Gastrointestinal (GI) symptoms and myopathy have been reported, however. They are usually the drug of choice in lowering cholesterol. (Braunwald, pp. 2254–2256)

115. **(E)** Probucol lowers levels of HDL, an important antirisk factor for atherosclerosis. Its mechanism of action is unknown, and it has not yet been definitely shown to decrease the risk from ischemic heart disease. It can also cause diarrhea. (Braunwald, pp. 2254–2255)

116. **(D, F)** Recent randomized trials (eg, Scandinavian Simvastatin Survival Study) have shown the benefits of *statin* treatment post-MI. The CARE trial (Cholesterol and Recurrent Events) suggests this conclusion is valid for those with normal cholesterol levels as well. The evidence for the benefits of estrogen is epidemiological but has yet to be verified in clinical trials. (Braunwald, p. 2254)

117. **(G)** ACE inhibitors have no adverse effects on glucose or lipid metabolism and may ac-

tually minimize the development of diabetic nephropathy by reducing renal vascular resistance and renal perfusion pressure. (Braunwald, pp. 1425–1428)

118. **(A)** Thiazides have been a cornerstone in most trials of antihypertensive therapy. Their adverse metabolic consequences include renal potassium loss leading to hypokalemia, hyperuricemia from uric acid retention, carbohydrate intolerance, and hyperlipidemia. (Braunwald, pp. 1421–1423)

119. **(G)** Although contraindicated in bilateral stenosis, ACE inhibitors are the drug of choice in unilateral renal artery stenosis. When ACE inhibitors are used in patients with impaired renal function, renal function should be monitored twice a week for the first 3 weeks. (Braunwald, pp. 1422–1423)

120. **(A)** Thiazides seem to work particularly well in blacks and the elderly. Younger individuals and whites respond well to beta blockers, ACE inhibitors, and calcium channel antagonists. (Braunwald, pp. 1415, 1428)

121. **(H)** Calcium channel blockers, particularly nifedipine, can cause edema. Nifedipine can also cause tachycardia, flushing, GI disturbances, hyperkalemia, and headache. Constipation can be a troublesome side effect. Some calcium channel blockers have a negative inotropic effect and should be used with caution in patients with left ventricular dysfunction. (Braunwald, p. 1424)

CHAPTER 2
Skin
Questions

DIRECTIONS (Questions 122 through 126): Each set of matching questions in this section consists of a list of lettered options followed by several numbered items. For each numbered item, select the appropriate lettered option(s). Each lettered option may be selected once, more than once, or not at all. EACH ITEM WILL STATE THE NUMBER OF OPTIONS TO SELECT. CHOOSE EXACTLY THIS NUMBER.

Questions 122 and 123

(A) psoriasis
(B) eczema
(C) hypersensitivity reactions
(D) lichen planus
(E) toxic erythemas
(F) lichen planus
(G) multiple purple dermal plaques
(H) melanotic nodules
(I) maculopapular rash
(J) serum-filled bullae

122. A 19-year-old man develops new lesions at the sites of skin trauma (SELECT TWO)

123. A 32-year-old man with human immunodeficiency virus (HIV) infection develops skin tumors (SELECT ONE)

Questions 124 through 126

(A) rarely involves border of scalp
(B) discoloration of upper eyelids
(C) skin atrophy
(D) never a permanent effect on skin
(E) potentially aggravated by available first aid

(F) drop-shaped lesions
(G) exacerbated by exposure to light
(H) worse on weekends
(I) high likelihood of malingering
(J) associated with squamous cell cancer
(K) extensive large plaques
(L) pitting of the nails
(M) lesions at various stages (progression of lesions)

124. A diagnosis of psoriasis, never previously treated, is made on a 22-year-old man. Findings may include (SELECT THREE)

125. A 63-year-old woman develops skin lesions and difficulty getting out of a chair. Evaluation might reveal (SELECT THREE)

126. A 43-year-old woman develops a rash on her arms after starting a new job in a factory. Findings might include (SELECT ONE)

DIRECTIONS (Questions 127 through 143): Each of the numbered items or incomplete statements in this section is followed by answers or by completions of the statement. Select the ONE lettered answer or completion that is BEST in each case.

127. A 19-year-old woman with asthma develops an eczematous-type rash. The best treatment includes

(A) psychoanalysis
(B) warm clothing
(C) dry environment
(D) environmental manipulation
(E) vigorous exercise

128. Keratoacanthoma is best characterized by

(A) rapid growth
(B) distinct pathology
(C) usual occurrence on the trunk
(D) a malignant potential
(E) a dark brown color

129. An 85-year-old woman has large blistering lesions on the abdomen and thighs that come and go without therapy. Nikolsky's sign is negative. She most likely has

(A) pemphigus vulgaris
(B) dermatitis herpetiformis
(C) bullous pemphigoid
(D) herpes gestationis
(E) erythema multiforme

130. A 69-year-old woman develops dark, velvety pigmentation in her axillae. She should be studied for

(A) a visceral carcinoma
(B) lymphoma
(C) diabetes mellitus
(D) sarcoidosis
(E) an allergy

131. A 22-year-old woman develops an acute contact dermatitis. Treatment during the bullous, oozing stage should include

(A) wet dressings
(B) systemic corticosteroids
(C) topical anesthetics
(D) systemic antibiotics
(E) antihistamines

132. Characteristics of ringworm of the scalp as compared with other dermatophytoses include a(n)

(A) more frequent occurrence in childhood
(B) high degree of contagiousness
(C) ability to invade the dermis
(D) sensitivity to penicillin
(E) ability to spread to other organs

133. A 27-year-old man develops warts on his hand. A correct statement concerning these skin lesions would be that they

(A) are viral in etiology
(B) may be premalignant lesions
(C) are found mainly in patients with lymphoma
(D) are contagious in children only
(E) may be treated with griseofulvin

134. A 27-year-old man develops a painless sore on his penis. A confirmatory serologic test may remain negative for up to

(A) 1 week
(B) 2 weeks
(C) 1 month
(D) 3 months
(E) 6 months

135. A 27-year-old woman has a 1-year history of loosely formed bowel movements associated with some blood and abdominal pain. The most likely skin disorder she will develop as a consequence is

(A) erythema multiforme
(B) erythema migrans
(C) erythema nodosum
(D) cutaneous lymphoma
(E) necrobiosis lipoidica

136. Mycosis fungoides is best described as a

(A) fungal infection of the epidermis
(B) benign skin lesion
(C) cutaneous lymphoma
(D) dermatitis
(E) form of eczema

137. A 58-year-old man complains of an enlarged, pitted nose. The most likely cause is

(A) acne vulgaris
(B) pemphigus
(C) acne rosacea
(D) psoriasis
(E) seborrheic dermatitis

138. An 81-year-old man presents with pallor, glossitis, cheilitis, and vitiligo. The likely diagnosis is

(A) sickle cell anemia
(B) cold agglutinin syndrome
(C) methemoglobinemia
(D) pernicious anemia
(E) polycythemia

Questions 139 through 143

139. A 70-year-old man develops multiple pruritic skin lesions and bullae mostly in the axillae and around the medial aspects of his groin and thighs. There are some lesions on his forearms and on his lower legs (first appeared in this location), and moderately painful oral lesions. Nikolsky's sign is negative. There is no eye involvement. The most likely diagnosis is

(A) dermatitis herpetiformis (DH)
(B) pemphigus vulgaris
(C) bullous pemphigoid
(D) cicatricial pemphigoid
(E) epidermolysis bullosa (EB)

140. Biopsy of his skin will reveal

(A) nonspecific changes
(B) immunoglobulin A (IgA) deposits
(C) lesions within the epidermis (acantholysis)
(D) basement membrane lesions
(E) IgM deposits

141. The usual treatment for severe forms of this disorder is

(A) plasmapheresis
(B) low-dose prednisone (10–20 mg/day)
(C) high-dose prednisone (50–100 mg/day)
(D) azathioprine 150 mg/day
(E) dapsone (100–150 mg/day)

142. The usual age of onset for pemphigus vulgaris (PV) is

(A) under 10 years of age
(B) 10 to 20 years of age
(C) 20 to 40 years of age
(D) 40 to 60 years of age
(E) 60 to 80 years of age

143. The most likely drug to cause pemphigus vulgaris is

(A) captopril
(B) D-penicillamine
(C) sulfonamides
(D) hydralazine
(E) quinidine

DIRECTIONS (Questions 144 through 150): Each set of matching questions in this section consists of a list of lettered options followed by several numbered items. For each numbered item, select the appropriate lettered option(s). Each lettered option may be selected once, more than once, or not at all. EACH ITEM WILL STATE THE NUMBER OF OPTIONS TO SELECT. CHOOSE EXACTLY THIS NUMBER.

Questions 144 and 145

(A) other areas of skin pigmentation
(B) associated with adenocarcinoma
(C) autosomal dominant inheritance
(D) insulin resistance
(E) viral etiology
(F) adenocarcinoma
(G) neural tumors most frequently appear during old age
(H) multiple neural tumors
(I) local therapy not indicated

144. A young child is found to have axillary freckling. Other characteristics include (SELECT THREE)

145. Grayish brown, thickened skin develops in the axillae of a 68-year-old woman. Other findings may include (SELECT FOUR)

Questions 146 through 150

    (A) basal cell cancer

    (B) basal cell nevus syndrome (BCNS)

    (C) melanoma

    (D) actinic keratosis

    (E) keratoacanthoma

    (F) seborrheic keratosis

    (G) lipoma

    (H) mongolian spot

    (I) spider angioma

    (J) glomus tumor

    (K) squamous cell cancer

Match the following descriptions with the correct diagnosis above.

146. Malignant, but does not metastasize beyond the skin (SELECT ONE)

147. Malignant and may metastasize beyond the skin (SELECT TWO)

148. May be cured with x-ray therapy (SELECT TWO)

149. More common in Asian children than Caucasian children (SELECT ONE)

150. May develop in long-standing scars (SELECT ONE)

DIRECTIONS (Questions 151 through 163): Each of the numbered items or incomplete statements in this section is followed by answers or by completions of the statement. Select the ONE lettered answer or completion that is BEST in each case.

151. The skin lesion pictured in Figure 2–1, from a 60-year-old man, suggests a diagnosis of

    (A) erythema nodosum

    (B) acanthosis nigricans

    (C) herpes zoster

    (D) alopecia variegata

    (E) bullous pemphigoid

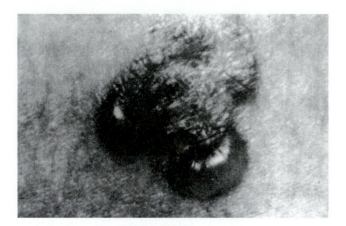

Figure 2–1.

152. Benefit to patients with severe acne is usually obtained with

    (A) dietary controls

    (B) radiotherapy

    (C) ultraviolet light

    (D) tetracycline

    (E) Isotretinoin

Questions 153 through 157

A 70-year-old man is seen in the emergency department with a generalized scaling eruption of the skin. The itching is very severe.

153. This disorder

    (A) is usually secondary to a systemic disorder

    (B) is usually benign and self-limiting

    (C) usually requires systemic therapy

    (D) usually has a malignant etiology

    (E) is usually worsened by oral steroids

154. Physical examination reveals diffuse lymphadenopathy. This finding points to

(A) a viral infect on
(B) pyoderma
(C) lymphoma
(D) leukemia
(E) nothing specific

155. Blood examination and histology both reveal unusually large monocytoid cells. The most likely diagnosis is

(A) leukemia
(B) visceral B-cell lymphoma
(C) primary cutaneous T-cell lymphoma
(D) viral infection (usually Epstein–Barr)
(E) paraneoplastic syndrome secondary to lung cancer

156. Prognosis for this syndrome is

(A) rapidly downhill
(B) determined by the type of medical care
(C) rarely fatal
(D) remissions and exacerbations, but with eventual progression to a fatal outcome
(E) eventual complete recovery, regardless of treatment

157. The treatment of this syndrome requires

(A) antibiotics
(B) antiviral medication
(C) aggressive systemic chemotherapy to ensure cure
(D) symptomatic treatment
(E) early use of high-dose systemic steroids

158. Which of the following features indicates a more negative prognosis for patients with malignant melanoma?

(A) female sex
(B) location on the leg
(C) dark pigmentation of the lesion
(D) nodularity of the lesion
(E) level A invasion

159. Zinc deficiency associated with inadequate nutrition in malabsorption syndromes may lead to

(A) ichthyosis
(B) acrodermatitis enteropathica
(C) Paget's disease
(D) candidiasis
(E) herpes simplex

160. A patient develops tender nodules on her shins with an erythematous base. These lesions are usually associated with

(A) aspergillosis
(B) children younger than 5 years
(C) males more than females
(D) malignant disease only
(E) streptococcal infection

161. A patch differs from a macule because

(A) it is more easily palpable
(B) a patch is erythematous
(C) a patch can contain fluid
(D) the etiology is very different
(E) it is larger

162. A 19-year-old man has a rash in the groin. A potassium hydroxide (KOH) preparation

(A) is done on skin obtained via a punch biopsy
(B) is useful in diagnosing herpesvirus infections
(C) is used in skin testing for allergies
(D) is prepared from skin scrapings
(E) will turn color in the presence of fungal elements

163. A 7-year-old boy develops crusting lesions in the axillary area. This syndrome is

(A) caused by fungi of the *Microsporum* species
(B) caused exclusively by staphylococcal infections
(C) characterized by premalignant changes
(D) treated by improved hygiene
(E) characterized by papulosquamous lesions

DIRECTIONS (Questions 164 through 174): Each set of matching questions in this section consists of a list of lettered options followed by several numbered items. For each numbered item, select the appropriate lettered option(s). Each lettered option may be selected once, more than once, or not at all. EACH ITEM WILL STATE THE NUMBER OF OPTIONS TO SELECT. CHOOSE EXACTLY THIS NUMBER.

Questions 164 through 169

    (A) generalized vitiligo

    (B) localized vitiligo

    (C) telangiectasia

    (D) erythroderma

    (E) papulosquamous lesions of palms and soles

    (F) scarring alopecia

    (G) yellow-colored papules

    (H) acanthosis nigricans

164. Tuberculoid leprosy (SELECT ONE)

165. Scleroderma (SELECT ONE)

166. Sulfa drugs (SELECT ONE)

167. Hyperlipoproteinemia (SELECT ONE)

168. Secondary syphilis (SELECT ONE)

169. Obesity (SELECT ONE)

Questions 170 through 174

    (A) dystrophic nail changes

    (B) may mottle teeth

    (C) black pigmentation of face

    (D) erythema nodosum

    (E) morbilliform eruption in patients with acquired immune deficiency syndrome (AIDS)

    (F) gingival hyperplasia

    (G) reactions in patients with nasal polyps

170. Bleomycin (SELECT ONE)

171. Chloroquine (SELECT ONE)

172. Birth control pills (SELECT ONE)

173. Tetracycline (SELECT ONE)

174. Sulfamethoxazole and trimethoprim (SELECT TWO)

Answers and Explanations

122. **(A, D)** Koebner's phenomenon is typically seen in psoriasis. The kind of injury eliciting the phenomenon is usually mechanical, but ultraviolet light or allergic damage to the skin may be provocative. Koebner's phenomenon can also occur in lichen planus, lichen nitidus, keratosis follicularis, and pemphigoid. The Koebner phenomenon has been used to study early skin changes in these diseases. *(Fitzpatrick, pp. 51, 114)*

123. **(G)** Kaposi's sarcoma often manifests as multiple blue dermal plaques. Lesions have two prominent features: accumulation of spindle cells and presence of vascular elements. Classical Kaposi's sarcoma is an indolent disease of later life and is much more common in men than women. Kaposi's sarcoma in association with HIV infection is a much more aggressive disorder. *(Fitzpatrick, pp. 526–527)*

124. **(F, K, L)** Psoriasis does not present a progression of lesions unless therapy is applied. Lesions vary in size and configuration from patient to patient and in the same patient from time to time and vary from drop-shaped lesions to large plaques. Nail changes are characteristic. *(Fitzpatrick, pp. 51–53)*

125. **(B, C, G)** In dermatomyositis, the dermatitis may be the most striking feature of the illness or so minor as to be easily overlooked. The classic manifestation is a purplish-red heliotrope erythema of the eyelids, upper cheeks, forehead, and temples, often with edema of eyelids and periorbital tissue. Telangiectasia and skin atrophy can occur. The typical hand changes involve scaly, bluish-red plaques around the base of the nails and backs of the joints of the fingers. These are most frequently found in elderly patients and are called Gottron's papules. There is an association with malignancy in those over 55 years of age. *(Fitzpatrick, p. 349)*

126. **(E)** The history should not reveal worsening eruption during the weekend. Allergy, acne, diabetes, psoriasis, xeroderma, or seborrheic dermatitis may all be mistaken for occupational disorders. The list of possible occupational skin hazards is long. At times, a site visit to the workplace is required to confirm the diagnosis. First aid in the workplace often involves sensitizing agents that worsen the situation. Skin problems can be severe and permanent. Relatively few patients are malingerers. *(Fitzpatrick, p. 24)*

127. **(D)** A change of environment is among the best treatments for atopic dermatitis. The patient should be kept in as dust free an environment as possible and should not wear rough garments. Maintenance of adequate humidity is also important. *(Fitzpatrick, p. 34)*

128. **(A)** This tumor as a rule occurs on exposed, hairy skin. It grows rapidly but involutes slowly, occasionally up to 1 year. It is more common in white-skinned males. The lesion starts as a small, rounded, flesh-colored or reddish papule. It grows rapidly and may reach 10 to 20 mm in a few weeks. There are telangiectasias just below the surface and the center contains a horny plug or is covered by a crust concealing a keratin-filled crater. His-

tology can be difficult to differentiate from squamous cell cancer. *(Fitzpatrick, p. 196)*

129. **(C)** There are antibodies to skin basement membrane, but unlike pemphigus, antibody levels do not correlate with disease activity. Bullous pemphigoid is most common in the elderly, and the disease often starts with urticaria-like and pruritic erythematous lesions before classic blisters occur. Unlike pemphigus, mucosal lesions are minimal or absent. *(Fitzpatrick, pp. 94, 98)*

130. **(A)** Patients with acanthosis nigricans should be studied for a visceral carcinoma. Other dermatoses associated with malignancy include dermatomyositis, flushing, acquired ichthyosis, and thrombophlebitis migrans. *(Fitzpatrick, pp. 82, 493)*

131. **(A)** Ointments are not used, but wet dressings are applied several times a day, using Burow's solution or boric acid, and baths are also included in the treatment. The key aspect of care is prevention. When contamination does occur, washing the affected area is the first mode of treatment. Oral corticosteroids are only used in severe cases. In less severe cases topical class I glucocorticoid preparations can be helpful. *(Fitzpatrick, p. 22)*

132. **(A)** Ringworm of the skin is most common in children because of their intimacy with animals and other children. The lesions are round or oval scaly patches. Secondary bacterial infection is common with certain fungi. *(Fitzpatrick, p. 700)*

133. **(A)** Verrucae are viral in etiology. The human papillomavirus is a deoxyribonucleic acid (DNA)-containing virus of the papovavirus group that includes animal tumor viruses. Although most warts are not felt to be premalignant, there is evidence to show that genital warts are correlated with malignancy. *(Fitzpatrick, p. 750)*

134. **(C)** This is likely a case of primary syphilis. The serology may remain negative for a period up to 1 month after the infection is con-

tracted. The serologic test for syphilis usually is positive within 1 week after the chancre appears. With therapy the chancre heals rapidly, but will heal in 4 to 6 weeks even without treatment. Genital chancres are usually painless unless superinfected, but extragenital chancres (eg, fingers) can be quite painful. *(Fitzpatrick, pp. 890–892)*

135. **(C)** About 15% of patients with ulcerative colitis will develop skin manifestations. Typical lesions include erythema nodosum, pyoderma gangrenosum (painless, but can heal with scarring), aphthous ulcers, and ocular inflammation (episcleritis, iritis, uveitis). The activity of the skin manifestations typically parallels the severity of the colonic disease. *(Braunwald, pp. 1686–1687)*

136. **(C)** Mycosis fungoides is best described as a cutaneous T-cell lymphoma. Lesions may remain confined to the skin for years, and internal organ involvement occurs when the disease advances into late stages. It is a disorder involving T lymphocytes. Treatment is usually palliative rather than curative. *(Fitzpatrick, pp. 535–536)*

137. **(C)** Rhinophyma is a complication of acne rosacea. It can be treated surgically by shaving off the excessive tissue with a scalpel, but regrowth occurs in time. There is very little evidence to support the association between alcoholism and rhinophyma. *(Fitzpatrick, pp. 9–10)*

138. **(D)** Jaundice results from hemolysis, and glossitis and cheilitis from the vitamin deficiency affecting rapidly turning over tissues. Patients may complain of a burning tongue, and examination reveals atrophy of papillae, a deep red mucosa, and a "cobblestone" appearance. Vitamin B_{12} administration rapidly relieves these symptoms. The vitiligo is caused by an associated autoimmune disorder. *(Braunwald, p. 677)*

139. **(C)** The description and age range (60 to 80) is typical of bullous pemphigoid. Pemphigus vulgaris is usually asociated with a positive

Nikolsky sign (pressure on blister leads to lateral extension), and very severe oral lesions. Cicatricial pemphigoid is also a disease of the elderly, but is rare and usually involves the eyes as well. EB is an inherited disorder that usually presents in earlier life. DH does not usually affect mucous membranes, and the lesions are grouped in clusters. However, it can mimic early bullous pemphigoid, and biopsy is needed for confirmation. *(Fitzpatrick, pp. 84–103)*

140. **(D)** In bullous pemphigoid, biopsy reveals IgG deposits in the basement membrane area. In pemphigus vulgaris, the immune deposition and damage is within the lower zone of the epidermis. IgA deposits are seen in DH. *(Fitzpatrick, pp. 94–98)*

141. **(C)** Severe cases require systemic steroids, often with the addition of azathioprine. Dapsone is useful in mild cases, and occasionally in very mild cases (or for local recurrences) topical glucocoticoid therapy will suffice. Permanent remission is frequent, and continued therapy would not be required. *(Fitzpatrick, p. 100)*

142. **(D)** PV is most common from 40 to 60 years of age, whereas bullous pemphigoid is seen most frequetly after the age of 80. Dermatitis herpetiformis is most common in the age group from 30 to 40, but has a wide age range. *(Fitzpatrick, pp. 94, 98, 102).*

143. **(B)** Captopril and other drugs can cause PV, but D-penicillamine is the most likely to cause the disease. Drug-induced PV usually, but not invariably, remits when the offending agent is withdrawn. *(Fitzpatrick, p. 96)*

144. **(A, C, H)** Neurofibromatosis is inherited in an autosomal manner. Incomplete forms are frequent. The skin manifestations include café au lait spots (more than six required for diagnosis), axillary freckles, cutaneous neurofibromas, and pigmented iris hamartomas (Liech nodules). There are numerous other manifestations as well including neural tumors. *(Fitzpatrick, p. 440)*

145. **(A, B, D, I)** Early recognition of acanthosis nigricans warrants a thorough search for underlying pathology such as malignancy or insulin resistance. The earliest changes are usually pigmentation, dryness, and roughness of the skin. The skin is gray-brown or black, palpably thickened, and covered by small papillomatous elevations, which give it a velvety texture. The most common sites are axillae, back, neck, anogenital region, and the groin. *(Fitzpatrick, p. 82)*

146. **(B)** Basal cell tumors have a substantial capacity for local destruction but metastasize very rarely. *(Fitzpatrick, p. 261)*

147. **(C, K)** Both squamous cell cancer and melanoma can spread beyond the skin. Only about 3 to 4% of squamous cell cancers metastasize, but metastasis is quite common in melanoma. Melanoma is the most dangerous primary skin cancer. *(Fitzpatrick, pp. 257, 299)*

148. **(A, K)** In both squamous and basal cell carcinomas, early detection may lead to cure by surgical removal. Radiotherapy may be curative, but is usually reserved for cases where surgery is not feasible, or likely to be disfiguring. *(Fitzpatrick, pp. 259, 265)*

149. **(H)** Mongolian spots are congenital gray-blue macular lesions, characteristically located on the lumbosacral area, although they can occur anywhere on the skin. They are almost always (99 to 100%) in infants of Asiatic or Amerindian origin, although reports in black, and rarely, white infants have occurred. They usually disappear in early childhood, and generally the lesions are solitary. *(Fitzpatrick, p. 171)*

150. **(K)** Squamous cell carcinoma of the skin can arise in areas of inflammation such as burn scars, chronic ulcers, radiation dermatitis, and chronic cutaneous lupus erythematosis. Other early lesions include solar keratoses, cutaneous horns, arsenical keratoses, and Bowen's disease. *(Fitzpatrick, pp. 257–258)*

151. **(E)** Bullous pemphigoid is most common in older adults. It is not as severe as pemphigus vulgaris, and histology reveals an absence of acantholysis and immunofluorescence reveals specific antibodies in the basement membrane area. *(Fitzpatrick, p. 98)*

152. **(E)** Tetracyclines are commonly used in the treatment of moderate acne, but may be associated with risk of dental discoloration or photosensitivity. Isotretinoin is the most effective drug for severe acne, but is teratogenic and may cause lipid abnormalities, hepatoxicity and night blindness. It cannot be combined with tetracycline because of the risk of pseudotumor cerebri. *(Fitzpatrick, p. 6)*

153. **(C)** Exfoliative dermatitis is a rare skin condition, but because of its severity, patients with this syndrome are often admitted to a hospital. The syndrome can be primary, appearing in otherwise healthy individuals, or secondary to malignancy, contact dermatitis, drugs, or other dermatologic diseases (eg, psoriasis). Even mild cases require systemic treatment for the severe itching. Antihistamines are usually the first choice. *(Fitzpatrick, pp. 152–154)*

154. **(E)** Most cases of exfoliative dermatitis will have widespread lymphadenopathy, whether they are primary or secondary forms. Biopsy will usually reveal nonspecific changes and is only warranted if there is a suspicion of lymphoma. *(Fitzpatrick, p. 154)*

155. **(C)** These large cells are typical of Sézary syndrome. This is frequently an early presentation of mycosis fungoides or cutaneous T-cell lymphoma. There may be a relationship to Epstein–Barr virus (and human T-lymphotropic virus [HTLV] I and II), but it is not universal. *(Fitzpatrick, pp. 535, 542)*

156. **(D)** The typical course of mycosis fungoides is an initial erythematous stage (which might become diffuse and cause an exfoliative dermatitis as in this case), a plaque stage, and a tumor stage. The course is usually progressive through these stages, but all stages can be bypassed. The early stages may progress slowly with remissions or exacerbations. The disease can be rapidly progressive, particularly when the tumor stage is reached. The disease is invariably fatal. *(Fitzpatrick, pp. 536–537)*

157. **(D)** There is no curative therapy, and most experts provide treatment only when symptoms occur. Therapy includes topical treatments such as tar cream plus ultraviolet light or local nitrogen mustard and systemic treatment with steroids and radiation therapy. Chemotherapy regimens are used but not with great success. *(Fitzpatrick, p. 533)*

158. **(D)** Nodular melanoma is invasive from the start. Women do better than men; trunk lesions and depigmented lesions carry a worse prognosis. Prognosis is directly related to depth of the lesion. *(Fitzpatrick, pp. 289, 305)*

159. **(B)** It is a persistent dermatitis around the mouth, with acral involvement that begins as vesicles but is soon crusted. The syndrome can rarely be inherited as an autosomal recessive. The inherited form in infants is also treated with zinc. It has been described after prolonged parenteral alimentation and chronic alcoholism. *(Fitzpatrick, p. 430)*

160. **(E)** Erythema nodosum is a hypersensitivity vasculitis associated with many infections and numerous diseases and is more common in females. The lesions are rare in children. It is a nodular erythematous eruption, usually on the extensor aspects of the legs, less commonly on the thighs and forearms. It regresses by bruiselike color changes in 3 to 6 weeks without scarring. *(Fitzpatrick, pp. 144–145)*

161. **(E)** A macule is a flat, colored lesion not raised above the surface of the surrounding skin. It is less than 1 cm in diameter. A patch differs from a macule only in size, being greater than 1 cm in diameter. *(Braunwald, p. 306)*

162. **(D)** A KOH preparation is useful when performed on scaling skin lesions when a fungal etiology is suspected. The scraped scales are

placed on a microscope slide, treated with one or two drops of KOH solution, and examined for hyphae, pseudohyphae, or budding yeast. *(Braunwald, p. 307)*

163. **(D)** Impetigo is a superficial bacterial infection of skin caused by group A beta-hemolytic streptococci or *Staphylococcus aureus.* It is characterized by superficial pustules that rupture, resulting in a honey-colored crust. The bullous variant is more likely staphylococcal in origin. Treatment requires improving hygiene and soaking the crust, as well as oral antibiotics. *(Fitzpatrick, pp. 586–590)*

164. **(B)** Localized areas of vitiligo can be seen in numerous primary skin disorders. It can also be caused by systemic disorders such as sarcoidosis and tuberculoid leprosy. In the latter disorder, there is associated anesthesia, anhidrosis, and alopecia of the lesions. Biopsy of the palpable border will reveal granulomas. *(Braunwald, p. 319)*

165. **(C)** Scleroderma is characterized by typical fibrotic and vascular lesions. These lesions may be periungual telangiectasia that are found in lupus erythematosus and dermatomyositis. Another form of telangiectasia, mat telangiectasia, is seen only in scleroderma. These lesions are broad macules 2 to 7 mm in diameter. They are found on the face, oral mucosa, and hands. The nailbeds of scleroderma patients often reveal loss of capillary loops with dilatation of the remaining loops when examined under magnification. *(Braunwald, p. 319)*

166. **(D)** Drug reactions most frequently result in papulosquamous reactions or diffuse erythroderma. Sulfa drugs frequently cause erythroderma. Other drugs commonly implicated include penicillins, gold, allopurinol, captopril, phenytoin, and carbamazepine. Fever, eosinophilia, and interstitial nephritis frequently accompany the erythroderma. *(Braunwald, p. 316)*

167. **(G)** Hyperlipoproteinemia is frequently associated with xanthomas, yellow-colored cutaneous papules or plaques. Xanthomas associated with hypertriglyceridemia are frequently eruptive; these yellow papules have an erythematous halo and are most frequently found on exterior surfaces of the extremities and buttocks. *(Braunwald, pp. 326–327)*

168. **(E)** Secondary syphilis often involves the palms and soles. Associated findings that help make the diagnosis include annular plaques on the face, nonscarring alopecia, condylomata, mucous patches, lymphadenopathy, malaise, fever, headache, and myalgia. *(Fitzpatrick, p. 895)*

169. **(H)** Obesity is the most common cause of acanthosis nigricans, a velvety, localized hyperpigmentation. Other causes include gastrointestinal malignancy and endocrinopathy such as acromegaly, Cushing syndrome, Stein–Leventhal syndrome, or insulin-resistant diabetes. *(Fitzpatrick, p. 82)*

170. **(A)** Cancer chemotherapy most frequently involves rapidly proliferating elements of the skin, resulting in stomatitis and alopecia. Bleomycin, hydroxyurea, and 5-fluorouracil can cause dystrophic nail changes. Other skin manifestations of cancer drugs include sterile cellulitis, phlebitis, ulceration of pressure areas, urticaria, angioedema, and exfoliative dermatitis. The underlying malignancy often makes diagnoses of skin disease more difficult. *(Braunwald, p. 340)*

171. **(C)** Chloroquine is used for certain skin diseases such as lupus and polymorphous light eruption, but can also cause skin reactions and exacerbate porphyria cutanea tarda. Black pigmentation can involve the face, mucous membrane, and pretibial and subungual areas. *(Braunwald, p. 341)*

172. **(D)** Birth control pills, sulfonamides, and penicillins are common drugs that can cause erythema nodosum. This is a panniculitis characterized by tender, subcutaneous, erythematous nodules characteristically found on the anterior portion of the legs. *(Braunwald, p. 433; Fitzpatrick, pp. 144–145)*

173. **(B)** The only common skin reaction with tetracyclines is photosensitivity. However, the drug is contraindicated in children under 8 years of age because of the risk of discoloring permanent teeth. *(Braunwald, p. 879)*

174. **(D, E)** The combination of sulfamethoxazole and trimethoprim causes two distinct cutaneous reactions: an urticarial eruption in the first few days of therapy and a morbilliform eruption occurring a week or more after therapy has begun. This latter reaction is particularly common in patients with AIDS. Sulfonamides cause numerous skin lesions, including erythema nodosum. *(Braunwald, pp. 340, 433, 879)*

CHAPTER 3

Endocrinology
Questions

DIRECTIONS (Questions 175 through 204): Each of the numbered items or incomplete statements in this section is followed by answers or by completions of the statement. Select the ONE lettered answer or completion that is BEST in each case.

175. A 42-year-old woman is found to have an elevated thyroid-stimulating hormone (TSH). The most likely cause is

    (A) trauma
    (B) radioactive iodine ingestion
    (C) primary hypothyroidism
    (D) parathyroid surgery
    (E) antithyroid chemicals

176. A 53-year-old man with gout is likely to have renal disease manifested by

    (A) nephrotic syndrome
    (B) isosthenuria and moderate albuminuria
    (C) acute renal failure
    (D) acute tubular necrosis
    (E) malignant hypertension

177. The most common presentation of anterior pituitary hyposecretion in a 26-year-old woman is

    (A) occurrence of myxedema
    (B) decreased melanin pigmentation
    (C) emaciation and cachexia
    (D) loss of axillary and pubic hairs
    (E) amenorrhea

178. A 19-year-old phenotypic female with primary amenorrhea and absent body hair is found to have a Y chromosome. This disorder is caused by

    (A) a membrane receptor defect
    (B) excess hormone production
    (C) an intracellular receptor defect
    (D) decreased hormone production
    (E) abnormal hormone production

179. A 17-year-old woman has cutaneous manifestations because of protoporphyria. The best treatment would be

    (A) phenobarbital
    (B) corticosteroids
    (C) high-carbohydrate diet
    (D) beta-carotene
    (E) chlorpromazine

180. In a 23-year-old woman, follicle-stimulating hormone (FSH) would be likely to

    (A) cause ovulation
    (B) encourage progesterone secretion
    (C) cause the secretory phase of the uterine mucosa
    (D) inhibit estrogen secretion
    (E) encourage maturation of the follicle

181. A healthy 42-year-old woman is found on routine blood testing to have a calcium level of 12 mg/dL. Other findings might include

    (A) osteoblastic lesions of bone
    (B) polycythemia
    (C) prolonged QT interval on electrocardiogram (ECG)
    (D) orthostatic hypotension
    (E) cystic bone tumors

182. A 32-year-old woman is feeling unwell. Her serum calcium level is low, suggesting hypoparathyroidism. The most likely cause is

   (A) idiopathic
   (B) familial
   (C) postradiation
   (D) end-organ resistance
   (E) surgical removal

183. A 27-year-old man has a low serum sodium and high serum potassium. Physical exam reveals skin pigmentation. A further finding would be that

   (A) the skin is shiny and pale
   (B) a diabetic glucose tolerance is characteristic
   (C) water diuresis is impaired
   (D) the urinary steroids are high
   (E) the serum calcium is elevated

184. A 17-year-old man is 5'7" tall and weighs 370 pounds. No medical cause for this "essential obesity" is found. He can be expected to have

   (A) normal mortality risk
   (B) hypothyroidism
   (C) low P_{CO_2} values
   (D) hypertriglyceridemia
   (E) hyperadrenocorticalism

185. Two family members, both nondrinkers, have extremely high ferritin levels. This condition is characterized by

   (A) diabetes mellitus (DM) as the most frequent presentation
   (B) arrhythmias as the most common cardiac manifestation
   (C) phlebotomy improving the arthropathy
   (D) arthritis involving the hands
   (E) pigmentation of the skin by iron

186. A 35-year-old man has had recurrent attacks of abdominal pain and proximal motor neuropathy since puberty. The attacks are associated with elevated porphobilinogen levels. He should avoid

   (A) chlorpromazine
   (B) barbiturates
   (C) a high-calcium diet
   (D) narcotics
   (E) steroids

187. A 43-year-old man weighs 85 kg and is 1.8 meters tall. This body build is associated with

   (A) DM
   (B) hyperlipoproteinemia
   (C) abnormal growth hormone response
   (D) atherosclerosis
   (E) no increased risk for mortality

188. The 2-year-old daughter of a Jewish couple whose parents immigrated from Russia develops progressive loss of motor skills and macular pallor on ophthalmic exam. This disorder is also associated with

   (A) glycogen storage
   (B) ganglioside accumulation
   (C) organomegaly
   (D) corneal opacity
   (E) autosomal dominant inheritance

189. A 63-year-old man develops macroglossia, nephrotic syndrome, and hepatomegaly. Serum immunoelectrophoresis reveals a monoclonal immunoglobulin. The characteristic neurologic finding is

   (A) peripheral motor and sensory neuropathy
   (B) spinal cord compression in the lumbar region
   (C) spinal cord compression in the thoracic region
   (D) a peripheral neuropathy associated with cerebral manifestations
   (E) a Guillain–Barré-type syndrome

190. A 30-year-old man presents with recurrent flushing. Elevated urinary 5-hydroxyindole-acetic acid suggests the diagnosis of

(A) phenylketonuria

(B) alkaptonuria

(C) malignant melanoma

(D) carcinoid syndrome

(E) disseminated carcinomatosis

191. A 40-year-old man has lipid investigations suggesting familial hyperbetalipoproteinemia (type II hyperlipoproteinemia). This is characterized by

(A) milky serum

(B) severe diabetes

(C) aggravation with ingestion of polyunsaturated fats

(D) an increased incidence of coronary artery disease (CAD)

(E) high serum triglycerides

192. An 8-year-old boy is found to have absence of beta-lipoproteins. He is also likely to have

(A) autonomic neuropathy

(B) crenated red blood cells (acanthocytosis)

(C) obesity

(D) elevated cholesterol

(E) cataracts

193. An adult patient with hepatosplenomegaly and large reticulated cells in the bone marrow containing glucocerebrosides can be diagnosed as having

(A) metachromatic leukodystrophy

(B) Gaucher's disease

(C) reticulum cell sarcoma associated with diabetes

(D) glycogen storage disease

(E) familial hyperchylomicronemia

194. Glycogen storage diseases

(A) do not affect the liver

(B) may cause xanthomas

(C) are always autosomal dominant

(D) are due to a single enzyme defect

(E) are corrected by surgery

195. A 33-year-old man passes a kidney stone that is predominantly cystine in composition. This disorder is characterized by

(A) mental retardation

(B) homocystinuria

(C) hexagonal crystals in the urine

(D) malnutrition due to urine loss of cystine

(E) symptomatic intestinal malabsorption

196. A 50-year-old develops hypomagnesemia. The most common cause in the United States is

(A) alcoholism

(B) chronic malabsorption

(C) DM

(D) kwashiorkor

(E) hypervitaminosis E

197. The syndrome of hepatomegaly, splenomegaly, leukopenia, anemia, periosteal changes, sparse and coarse hair, and increased serum lipids occurs in chronic

(A) vitamin D intoxication

(B) vitamin D deficiency

(C) vitamin A deficiency

(D) vitamin A intoxication

(E) acarotenemia

198. The patient whose hands are shown in Figure 3–1 is mentally retarded with a short, stocky build. What is the most likely diagnosis?

(A) achondroplastic dwarf
(B) Down syndrome
(C) Klinefelter syndrome
(D) pseudohypoparathyroidism
(E) Turner syndrome

200. A 28-year-old woman with diabetes has leg lesions as shown in Figure 3–2. What is the most likely diagnosis?

(A) eruptive xanthomas
(B) necrobiosis lipoidica diabeticorum
(C) gangrene
(D) staphylococcal infection
(E) erythema nodosum

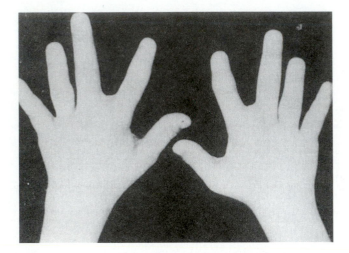

Figure 3–1.

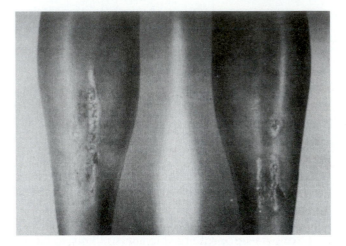

Figure 3–2.

199. Which of the following laboratory values is the patient in Figure 3–1 likely to show?

(A) hypercalcemia, hypophosphatemia
(B) hypocalcemia, low parathormone (PTH)
(C) hypocalcemia, high PTH
(D) hypocalcemia, hypophosphatemia
(E) hyperphosphatemia, low PTH

201. Allopurinol is useful in the prevention of gout because of which of the following mechanisms of action?

(A) inhibition of xanthine oxidase
(B) solubilization of uric acid
(C) reactivity with hypoxanthine
(D) anti-inflammatory effect on joint tissue
(E) increased renal tubular secretion of uric acid

202. A 53-year-old woman with chronic renal failure develops hyperphosphatemia. Clinically, this may result in

(A) lethargy
(B) neuromuscular irritability
(C) anorexia
(D) tachyarrhythmias
(E) hyperkalemia

203. A 22-year-old man with arm span greater than height, subluxed lenses, flattened corneas, and dilation of the aortic ring is most likely to have

    (A) Ehlers–Danlos syndrome
    (B) Marfan syndrome
    (C) Werner syndrome
    (D) Laurence–Moon–Biedl syndrome
    (E) Hunter syndrome

204. A 33-year-old man is passing more urine than usual. Which of the following drugs is the likely culprit?

    (A) lithium
    (B) cyclophosphamide
    (C) barbiturates
    (D) nicotine
    (E) morphine

DIRECTIONS (Questions 205 through 209): The group of matching questions in this section consists of a list of lettered options followed by several numbered items. For each numbered item, select the appropriate lettered option(s). Each lettered option may be selected once, more than once, or not at all. EACH ITEM WILL STATE THE NUMBER OF OPTIONS TO SELECT. CHOOSE EXACTLY THIS NUMBER.

Questions 205 through 209

    (A) palmar plane xanthomas
    (B) triglycerides greater than 1000
    (C) subcutaneous extensor tendon xanthomas
    (D) low serum cholesterol
    (E) normal cholesterol levels
    (F) xanthelasma after age 50 only

205. Hyperchylomicronemia (SELECT ONE)

206. Hyperbetalipoproteinemia (SELECT ONE)

207. Type III hyperlipoproteinemia (SELECT ONE)

208. Hyperprebetalipoproteinemia (SELECT ONE)

209. Hypertriglyceridemia (SELECT ONE)

DIRECTIONS (Questions 210 through 217): Each of the numbered items or incomplete statements in this section is followed by answers or by completions of the statement. Select the ONE lettered answer or completion that is BEST in each case.

Questions 210 through 213

210. A 20-year-old woman, otherwise well, has a long history of passing large amounts of urine. Urinalysis reveals no abnormalities, except that the urine is dilute. She weighs 60 kg, and her 24-hour urine output is over 4 liters. The most likely diagnosis is

    (A) DM
    (B) psychogenic polydipsia
    (C) diabetes insipidus (DI)
    (D) contracted bladder
    (E) solute diureses

211. This disorder is most commonly caused by a problem in the

    (A) adrenal cortex
    (B) kidneys
    (C) posterior pituitary
    (D) anterior pituitary
    (E) cerebral cortex

212. The most likely finding on cerebral magnetic resonance imaging (MRI) would be

    (A) hypothalamic tumor
    (B) hyperintense signals in the cerebral cortex
    (C) agenesis of the corpus callosum
    (D) lack of hyperintense signals from the posterior pituitary
    (E) communicating hydrocephalus

213. Lithium can cause this syndrome by

    (A) impairing glucose absorption at the cellular level
    (B) decreasing production of vasopressin
    (C) increasing production of vasopressin
    (D) causing a solute diuresis
    (E) impairing vasopressin action at the tubular level

Questions 214 through 217

214. A 62-year-old man is seen in the office. Routine blood testing reveals an elevated low-density lipoprotein (LDL) cholesterol. The most common cause of this in the United States would be

   (A) an autosomal dominant disease
   (B) an X-linked recessive disease
   (C) a polygenic disease
   (D) a poor diet
   (E) DM

215. The dietary abnormality most associated with elevated cholesterol levels is

   (A) inadequate fiber
   (B) excess calories resulting in obesity
   (C) excess dietary cholesterol
   (D) excess total fat intake
   (E) excess transfatty acid intake

216. The most common cause of genetic dyslipidemia is

   (A) familial combined hyperlipidemia
   (B) familial hypercholesterolemia
   (C) familial defective Apo B
   (D) Apo C-II deficiency
   (E) lipoprotein lipase deficiency

217. Which of the following statements concerning treatment of familial hypercholesterolemia is correct?

   (A) Dietary therapy is usually sufficient.
   (B) Cholestyramine is as effective as hepatic hydroxymethylglutaryl-coenzyme A (HMG-CoA) reductase inhibitors (statins).
   (C) Ninety percent of patients can be controlled with a statin.
   (D) A statin is the only type of medication suitable for monotherapy.
   (E) Combined therapy is frequently required.

DIRECTIONS (Questions 218 and 219): The group of matching questions in this section consists of a list of lettered options followed by several numbered items. For each numbered item, select the appropriate lettered option(s). Each lettered option may be selected once, more than once, or not at all. EACH ITEM WILL STATE THE NUMBER OF OPTIONS TO SELECT. CHOOSE EXACTLY THIS NUMBER.

   (A) renal calculi
   (B) decreased renal excretion of phosphorus
   (C) osteogenic sarcoma
   (D) decreased gastrointestinal (GI) absorption of calcium
   (E) secondary hyperparathyroidism
   (F) decreased renal excretion of calcium
   (G) hypocalcemia
   (H) hypophosphatemia
   (I) lytic lesions of bone

218. A 63-year-old asymptomatic woman is investigated for a high bone alkaline phosphatase and high urinary excretion of hydroxyproline. Complications include (SELECT TWO)

219. A 20-year-old man with vitamin D deficiency could develop (SELECT THREE)

DIRECTIONS (Questions 220 through 249): Each of the numbered items or incomplete statements in this section is followed by answers or by completions of the statement. Select the ONE lettered answer or completion that is BEST in each case.

220. A 19-year-old woman develops weight loss, goiter, and tremor. Which of the following cardiac changes is most likely to occur?

   (A) atrial fibrillation
   (B) systolic murmurs
   (C) bradycardia
   (D) decrease in heart size
   (E) pericardial effusion

221. For a 40-year-old woman with an enlarged thyroid, needle biopsy is most commonly used if the suspected diagnosis is

(A) chronic thyroiditis
(B) thyroid storm
(C) nontoxic multinodular goiter
(D) subacute thyroiditis
(E) malignant neoplasms

222. A 42-year-old man is found to have a high ferritin level during evaluation for elevated liver enzymes. The most likely sign of disease is

(A) insulin-dependent diabetes mellitus (IDDM)
(B) impaired renal function
(C) arthropathy
(D) hypogonadism
(E) skin pigmentation

223. The release of vasopressin is controlled by

(A) toxicity of the blood perfusing the liver
(B) phosphate levels in the renal plasma
(C) cerebrospinal fluid pressure
(D) calcium levels in the cerebral inflow
(E) volume receptors in the left atrium

224. A 23-year-old woman develops lightheaded episodes associated with hunger and low blood sugar. The differential diagnosis includes

(A) excess growth hormone
(B) Cushing's disease
(C) thyrotoxicosis
(D) tumor of the pancreatic beta cells
(E) gastrin deficiency

225. Amyloid deposition in primary amyloidosis is likely to cause symptoms in which of the following tissues?

(A) heart
(B) red cells
(C) thyroid
(D) pancreas
(E) liver

226. Glucagon can be best described as a hormone that is

(A) secreted by the alpha cells of the pancreas
(B) a carbohydrate in structure
(C) effective in lowering blood sugar levels
(D) antigenically similar to insulin
(E) effective in decreasing cyclic adenosine monophosphate (cAMP) in target cells

227. The most common manifestation of multiple endocrine neoplasia, type I (MEN I) is

(A) Zollinger–Ellison syndrome
(B) an adrenal adenoma
(C) primary hyperparathyroidism
(D) acromegaly
(E) testicular cancer

228. Administration of estrogen to a postmenopausal woman most likely results in

(A) protection from coronary artery disease
(B) a decreased likelihood of Alzheimer's disease
(C) thinning of the vaginal mucosa
(D) changes in urogenital epithelium
(E) hirsutism

229. A 7-year-old girl develops pubic and axillary hair. The tumors causing this

(A) can be benign or malignant
(B) are associated with hypertension
(C) are common in girls with early breast development
(D) are associated with an increase in the size of the clitoris
(E) are associated with hypothyroidism

230. A 43-year-old woman develops spadelike hands, coarsened facial features, and a gap between her incisors. In this syndrome, the most likely effect on muscles is

(A) enlargement
(B) spasm
(C) increased strength
(D) myositis
(E) rhythmic contraction

231. A 7-year-old boy has demineralized bones with pseudofractures. Physiologic doses of vitamin D do not result in improvement. This syndrome is associated with

    (A) hyperphosphatemia
    (B) low 1,25 (OH)$_2$ vitamin D levels
    (C) alopecia
    (D) osteoporosis
    (E) mental retardation

232. An 18-year-old girl is 5'8" tall and weighs 68 pounds. Risk of death is associated with

    (A) renal failure
    (B) ventricular tachyarrhythmias
    (C) DM
    (D) hyperthermia
    (E) pernicious anemia

233. A 53-year-old man develops severe podagra. The most likely associated condition is

    (A) pernicious anemia
    (B) DI
    (C) Alzheimer's disease
    (D) anorexia
    (E) renal disease

234. The most common nonskeletal manifestation of osteomalacia is

    (A) hyperphosphatemia
    (B) hypoparathyroidism
    (C) proximal myopathy
    (D) hypercalcemia
    (E) nephrocalcinosis

235. The early manifestations of hepatorenal syndrome include

    (A) intrarenal vasodilatation
    (B) sodium retention
    (C) potassium retention
    (D) severe jaundice
    (E) polyuria

236. In phenylketonuria, the best management includes

    (A) a gluten-free diet from age 6 months to age 12 years
    (B) supplemental insulin
    (C) enteral feeding
    (D) tyrosine supplements
    (E) a low-carbohydrate diet

237. A 21-year-old woman on no medications develops rigidity and tremor. The most likely associated finding is

    (A) renal failure
    (B) cirrhosis of the liver
    (C) elevated ceruloplasmin
    (D) sensory loss
    (E) increased plasma copper

238. Insulin acts at the cellular receptor level by

    (A) stimulating tyrosine kinase
    (B) binding to ion channels
    (C) binding to intracellular erb A receptors
    (D) stimulating guanylate cyclase
    (E) activating G-proteins

239. The metabolic effects of insulin on adipose tissue are most likely to include

    (A) decrease of glucose transport
    (B) decrease in glucose phosphorylation
    (C) decrease in lipolysis
    (D) decrease in lipoprotein lipase
    (E) enhancement of glucagon effect

240. A 32-year-old woman is suspected of having thyroid storm. What is the likely precipitating event?

    (A) propylthiouracil administration
    (B) high-dose prednisone therapy
    (C) beta-adrenergic blockade
    (D) pneumococcal pneumonia
    (E) salicylate administration

241. A 15-year-old youth has not gone through puberty. This is most likely due to

    (A) inadequate diet
    (B) normal variation
    (C) pituitary tumor

(D) Leydig cell dysfunction

(E) drug side effects

242. A woman is most likely to respond to tamoxifen treatment of metastatic carcinoma of the breast in which circumstance?

(A) metastases confined to liver

(B) patient more than 5 years premenopausal

(C) androgen receptors on the tumor cell membrane

(D) tumor has progesterone receptors

(E) metastases confined to brain

243. A woman's risk of breast cancer is increased by

(A) castration before age 40 years

(B) late first pregnancy

(C) long-term nursing

(D) history of breast cancer in an aunt

(E) multiparity

244. Which of the following statements is correct?

(A) Resting metabolic rate (RMR) is identical in men and women when corrected for weight and height.

(B) Virtually all nitrogen loss is through the urine in the form of urea.

(C) Increasing the proportion of protein in the diet increases the efficiency of protein production in the body.

(D) Generally, physical activity accounts for only 15% of total energy expenditure over most conditions.

(E) Recommended levels of adult protein ingestion should be decreased by 30% for the very elderly.

245. Figure 3–3 is the x-ray of a 35-year-old woman with chronic renal disease complaining of pain in the hand after dialysis. What is your diagnosis?

(A) scleroderma

(B) gout

(C) hyperparathyroidism

(D) pseudogout

(E) Paget's disease

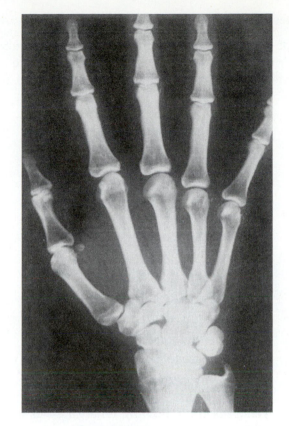

Figure 3–3.

246. The case work-up shown in Table 3–1 is of a 35-year-old woman presenting with hypertension, central obesity, and skin striae. The most likely diagnosis is

(A) adrenal hyperplasia secondary to hypothalamic dysfunction

(B) adrenal adenoma with complete autonomy

(C) exogenous steroids, iatrogenic

(D) pituitary tumor

(E) carcinoma of the adrenal

TABLE 3–1. CASE WORK-UP

	Normal	Patient
Plasma ACTH pg/mL	< 150	< 50
Plasma cortisol u/dL	17	35
Urine 17-OH mg/24 hr	2 to 10	25
Urine 17-Ks mg/24 hr	5 to 15	10
Urine 17-OH response to:		
ACTH IV	Increase × 5	No response
Dexamethasone 0.5 mg	< 3.0	No response
2.0 mg	< 3.0	No response
Metyrapone 750 mg	Increase × 2	No response

Questions 247 through 249

A 35-year-old obese woman complains of vulvar pruritus, recent weight loss in spite of a large appetite, and waking up frequently at night to urinate.

247. The most likely diagnosis is

(A) DM

(B) DI

(C) vaginitis and cystitis

(D) myxedema

(E) pheochromocytoma

248. The diagnosis is generally established by

(A) a urine osmolality

(B) an insulin tolerance test (ITT)

(C) a fasting blood sugar (FBS)

(D) a glucose tolerance test (GTT)

(E) TSH measurement

249. Which of the following renal diseases is this patient most likely to develop?

(A) acute glomerulonephritis

(B) obstructive uropathy

(C) glomerulosclerosis with mesangial thickening

(D) renal infarction

(E) polycystic kidneys

DIRECTIONS: (Questions 250 through 260): Each set of matching questions in this section consists of a list of lettered options followed by several numbered items. For each numbered item, select the appropriate lettered option(s). Each lettered option may be selected once, more than once, or not at all. EACH ITEM WILL STATE THE NUMBER OF OPTIONS TO SELECT. CHOOSE EXACTLY THIS NUMBER.

Questions 250 through 252

(A) microaneurysms

(B) vitreal hemorrhage

(C) dilated veins

(D) retinal detachment

(E) hemorrhage (dot and blot)

(F) open-angle glaucoma

(G) erythema multiforme

(H) pyoderma gangrenosum

(I) necrobiosis lipoidica

(J) candidiasis

Questions 250 through 252 apply to the patient in questions 247 through 249 (see column 1).

250. Which cutaneous manifestations may be found in this woman? (SELECT TWO)

251. These ophthalmoscopic findings would indicate "background" retinopathy. (SELECT THREE)

252. These ophthalmoscopic findings would indicate "proliferative" retinopathy. (SELECT TWO)

Questions 253 through 256

A 59-year-old man presents as an outpatient complaining of sexual dysfunction.

(A) loss of sexual desire

(B) failure of erection with absent nocturnal penile tumescence (NPT)

(C) absence of emission

(D) absence of orgasm with normal libido and erectile function

(E) failure of detumescence

253. Can be caused by high prolactin level (SELECT ONE)

254. Rarely indicates organic disease (SELECT ONE)

255. Can be caused by hematologic disease (SELECT ONE)

256. Can be caused by vascular disease (SELECT ONE)

Questions 257 through 260

A 24-year-old woman is referred for evaluation of hirsutism which she feels is cosmetically significant.

    (A) drugs
    (B) adrenal tumor
    (C) polycystic ovarian disease (PCOD)
    (D) adrenal hyperplasia
    (E) idiopathic hirsutism
    (F) ovarian tumor

257. Slight elevation of plasma testosterone and androstenedione (SELECT ONE)

258. Can be associated with anovulation, obesity, and amenorrhea (SELECT ONE)

259. May stimulate surrounding tissue to secrete androgens (SELECT ONE)

260. Often associated with elevated 17-hydroxyprogesterone levels (SELECT ONE)

DIRECTIONS (Questions 261 through 266): Each of the numbered items or incomplete statements in this section is followed by answers or by completions of the statement. Select the ONE lettered answer or completion that is BEST in each case.

Questions 261 through 264

261. A 15-year-old girl has been losing weight and exercising vigorously. Which of the following physical signs would suggest the diagnosis of anorexia nervosa?

    (A) salivary gland enlargement
    (B) coarse body hair
    (C) diarrhea
    (D) tachycardia
    (E) hypertension

262. A common laboratory abnormality would be

    (A) hypokalemia
    (B) hypochloremia
    (C) alkalosis

    (D) hypoglycemia
    (E) low blood urea nitrogen (BUN)

263. Serious cardiac arrhythmias are most likely found in the setting of

    (A) resting sinus tachycardia
    (B) low QRS voltage
    (C) hypotension
    (D) heart failure
    (E) prolonged QT interval

264. For this young woman, hospitalization should be considered at which of the following times?

    (A) when body weight is less than 90% of expected
    (B) when body weight is less than 75% of expected
    (C) when electrolyte disturbances occur
    (D) when body weight is less than 60% of expected
    (E) when vomiting is being induced

265. The dental abnormalities in bulimia nervosa are related to

    (A) self-induced physical trauma
    (B) self-induced vomiting
    (C) excess cortisol levels
    (D) osteoporotic changes
    (E) estrogen deficiency

266. Which of the following statements concerning the prognosis of anorexia nervosa (AN) and bulimia nervosa (BN) is correct?

    (A) Both have an excellent prognosis with mortality not different from age-matched controls.
    (B) AN has significant mortality (5% per decade), but BN does not.
    (C) BN has significant mortality (5% per decade), but AN does not.
    (D) Both diseases have a high recovery rate.
    (E) Both BN and AN have significant mortality (3 to 5% per decade).

DIRECTIONS: (Questions 267 through 272): Each set of matching questions in this section consists of a list of lettered options followed by several numbered items. For each numbered item, select the appropriate lettered option(s). Each lettered option may be selected once, more than once, or not at all. EACH ITEM WILL STATE THE NUMBER OF OPTIONS TO SELECT. CHOOSE EXACTLY THIS NUMBER.

Match the dietary manipulation to the appropriate clinical circumstance.

(A) DM

(B) obesity

(C) hypertension

(D) AN

(E) gastroesophageal reflux (GERD)

(F) postgastrectomy

(G) Parkinson's disease

(H) hepatic encephalopathy

(I) Crohn's disease

(J) osteoporosis

(K) celiac disease

(L) monoamine oxidase inhibitor (MAOI) therapy

(M) hyperlipidemia

267. Low fiber (SELECT ONE)

268. Tyramine controlled (SELECT ONE)

269. Low sodium (SELECT ONE)

270. Low simple sugar (SELECT ONE)

271. Low protein (SELECT ONE)

272. Avoid chocolate (SELECT ONE)

DIRECTIONS (Questions 273 through 277): Each lettered heading below describes an essential vitamin. Each numbered phrase describes a syndrome of vitamin deficiency or excess. For each numbered phrase, select the ONE lettered heading that is most closely associated with it. Each lettered heading may be selected once, more than once, or not at all.

(A) niacin

(B) thiamine

(C) pyridoxine

(D) vitamin C

(E) vitamin A

(F) vitamin E

(G) vitamin K

273. A 63-year-old bachelor develops perifollicular hemorrhage and splinter hemorrhages

274. Papilledema in a 26-year-old woman on megavitamin therapy

275. Flushing and pruritus secondary to histamine release in a man with hypercholesterolemia

276. High-output cardiac failure in an alcoholic

277. Dermatitis, dementia, diarrhea

Answers and Explanations

175. (C) Primary hypothyroidism is the most common cause of hypothyroidism in adults. Primary hypothyroidism is several times more common in women than in men and occurs most often between the ages of 40 and 60. Postablative hypothyroidism (radiation or surgery induced) is also very common. *(Felig, p. 316)*

176. (B) Diminished concentrating ability and proteinuria occur even when the glomerular filtration rate is near normal. The severity of renal involvement correlates with the duration and magnitude of serum uric acid elevation. Uric acid and monosodium urate deposit in the renal parenchyma. These deposits can cause intrarenal obstruction and elicit an inflammatory response as well. Hypertension, nephrolithiasis, and pyelonephritis can also contribute to the nephropathy of gout. *(Braunwald, p. 1608)*

177. (E) With pituitary hypofunctioning, gonadotropin deficiency is the most common early manifestation in both men and women. Growth hormone secretion is also impaired early on, but is less clinically apparent. *(Felig, p. 681)*

178. (C) Receptors for steroid hormones, thyroid hormones, and vitamin D are intracellular. Disease states due to abnormal intracellular receptors include androgen insensitivity; cortisol resistance; vitamin D–dependent rickets, type II; thyroid hormone resistance; and pseudohypoaldosteronism. There are several different types of cell membrane receptors. *(Braunwald, pp. 2021–2023, 2182)*

179. (D) Beta-carotene increases the patient's tolerance for sunlight, apparently by quenching active intermediates. Beta-carotene is an effective scavenger of free radicals. Although many affected individuals can tolerate sun exposure while taking beta-carotene, it has no effect on the basic metabolic defect in porphyrin–heme synthesis. *(Braunwald, p. 2267)*

180. (E) FSH is said to encourage maturation of the follicle in the human menstrual cycle. The cardinal hormonal change in phase one is a rise in FSH caused by a decrease in the level of estrogens and a waning activity of the corpus luteum. In men, FSH stimulates Sertoli cells, which have an important role in spermatogenesis. *(Felig, p. 178)*

181. (E) In hyperparathyroidism, bony lesions are lytic and can cause pain. The cortical surfaces are thinned and much of the bone is demineralized. The fibrotic bulging lesions within bone are termed "brown tumors." Fluid-filled cysts can also occur (osteitis fibrosa cystica). Anemia is common, and the QT interval can be shortened if the calcium is high enough. Hypertension is common. Most patients with hyperparathyroidism have a simple adenoma that functions autonomously, so that hormone is secreted with high calcium. In about 10 to 15% of cases, hyperplasia of all the parathyroid glands (chief cell hyperplasia) is the cause. Differentiation from adenoma is important to determine the correct surgical approach but is unfortunately very difficult. *(Felig, pp. 1114–1123)*

182. (E) Surgical removal is the most common cause of hypoparathyroidism. When the glands or their blood vessels have merely been damaged and not removed, tissue often regenerates. Hypoparathyroidism can frequently follow thyroid surgery. The incidence varies and depends on the extent of resection, the skill of the surgeon, and the degree of diligence in diagnosing hypocalcemia. *(Felig, p. 1141)*

183. (C) Water diuresis is impaired in adrenocortical insufficiency. Lack of aldosterone also favors the development of hyperkalemia and mild acidosis. The decreased circulating volume secondary to aldosterone deficiency is one of the factors resulting in elevated basal antidiuretic hormone (ADH) levels and thus hyponatremia. *(Felig, p. 436)*

184. (D) Hypertriglyceridemia may result in part from hyperinsulinism because insulin is one of the factors involved in lipoprotein secretion by the liver. With massive obesity, there is an increased prevalence of cardiovascular disease, hypertension, diabetes, pulmonary disorders, and gallstones. Young men with morbid obesity have a 12-fold higher mortality risk than the general population. Even in old age (65 to 74 years), the mortality is doubled in obese men. Cardiovascular disease is the most important factor. *(Felig, pp. 954–958)*

185. (D) The high ferritin suggests hemochromatosis. The arthritis is characterized by chondrocalcinosis, but, unlike idiopathic chondrocalcinosis, the hands are usually involved first. The arthropathy often progresses despite phlebotomy. Liver disease is usually the presenting feature. Skin pigmentation is predominantly by melanin. Heart failure is the most common cardiac problem. *(Braunwald, p. 2259)*

186. (B) In patients with acute intermittent porphyria, oral phenothiazines may be used for abdominal or muscle pains, and meperidine (Demerol) may also be used, but barbiturates should be avoided. Other unsafe medications include alcohol, sulfonamide, carbamazepine, valproic acid, and synthetic estrogens and progestogens. Most heterozygotes remain asymptomatic unless a precipitating factor such as a drug or weight loss is present. Poorly localized abdominal pain is the most common symptom. *(Braunwald, p. 2264)*

187. (E) One of the most efficient ways to define obesity is by body mass index (BMI), which is calculated by weight/(height)^2, calculated using kilograms for weight and meters for height. This man's BMI is between 23 and 24 kg/m^2 and confers no special risk. (The acceptable range is 20 to 25.) *(Braunwald, p. 479)*

188. (B) Glycogen storage is not characteristic of Tay–Sachs disease. Ganglioside accumulation can now be diagnosed by decreased hexosaminidase in peripheral leukocytes. Tay–Sachs is characterized as a lysosomal storage disease. Mental retardation, seizures, blindness, and a retinal cherry red spot are characteristic. It is most common in Ashkenazi Jews and is inherited in an autosomal recessive manner. *(Braunwald, p. 2277)*

189. (A) In addition to peripheral motor and sensory neuropathy, cardiac involvement, tongue enlargement, GI manifestations, and carpal tunnel syndrome are also seen in amyloidosis. The specific diagnosis requires tissue biopsy with presence of amyloid with specific stains. In primary amyloidosis and myeloma, the amyloid protein is of the AL type. In reactive amyloidosis the protein is of the AA type. *(Braunwald, pp. 1976–1978)*

190. (D) Carcinoid syndrome is characterized by increased levels of 5-hydroxyindolacetic acid. The syndrome occurs in relation to malignant tumors that have metastasized, usually with hepatic implants. Gastrointestinal carcinoids are most commonly found in the appendix. These are very slow growing, thus the 5-year survival rate is 99%. Many carcinoids are discovered as incidental findings on autopsy. *(Felig, pp. 1335–1337)*

191. (D) In type II hyperlipoproteinemia, there is an increased incidence of CAD, and hypercholesterolemia occurs along with tuberous xanthomas, arcus senilis, and atheromas. Most affected individuals are heterozygous for the mutant gene. The beta-lipoproteins accumulate because of impaired catabolism. It is expressed early in life, and has been found in cord blood samples. (Felig, pp. 1015–1019)

192. **(B)** In congenital absence of beta-lipoproteins, there is an inability to assemble or secrete apoprotein B containing lipoprotein from hepatocytes. Renal disease is not associated with this syndrome. The disease is caused by a rare autosomal recessive syndrome, so there is often no prior family history. Malnutrition, steatorrhea, ataxic neuropathy, and pigmentary retinal degeneration are other manifestations. Vitamin E has been used successfully for symptomatic therapy. (Felig, pp. 1034–1035)

193. **(B)** The diagnosis is Gaucher's disease. The glucocerebrosides are derived from lipid catabolites from the membranes of senescent leukocytes and erythrocytes. Although the juvenile form may have severe neurologic symptoms (mental retardation, spasticity, ataxia), the adult form usually has no neurologic symptoms. Like Tay–Sachs, it is a lysosomal storage disease with a predilection for Ashkenazi Jews. (Braunwald, p. 2280)

194. **(B)** Xanthomas may be caused by glycogen storage diseases because they cause hyperlipidemias. There are many types of glycogen storage diseases, each caused by a different enzymatic abnormality. The best-known types of glycogen storage disease are those that have hepatic–hypoglycemic pathophysiology (eg, von Gierke disease) or those that have muscle–energy pathophysiology (McArdle's disease). (Braunwald, pp. 2283–2285)

195. **(C)** Cystinuria is commonly associated with hexagonal crystals in the urine. Cystine, lysine, arginine, and ornithine are excreted in great excess by patients homozygous for the disease. The tissues manifesting the transport defect of cystinuria are the proximal renal tubule and the jejunal mucosa. It is inherited as an autosomal recessive trait. Cystine kidney stones are the major clinical manifestation. (Braunwald, p. 2313)

196. **(A)** Magnesium deficiency is most commonly due to alcoholism. Renal loss and malabsorption are also common causes. Magnesium deficiency is not seen in hypervitaminosis E. Causes of magnesium deficiency also include milk diets in infants, the diuretic phase of acute tubular necrosis, chronic diuretic therapy, acute pancreatitis, and inappropriate antidiuretic hormone. The symptoms of hypomagnesemia include anorexia, nausea, tremor, and mood alteration. Symptoms can also be caused by the associated hypocalcemia or hypokalemia. (Felig, pp. 1158–1159)

197. **(D)** Symptoms of vitamin A intoxication occur in infants or adults ingesting over 50,000 IU of vitamin A daily. The prognosis is good when vitamin A intake ceases. Rare occurrence of hypercalcemia with vitamin A intoxication have been reported. (Felig, pp. 1137–1138)

198. **(D)** The deformity of the hands is due to short metacarpals. Other deformities include short metatarsals, round facies, and thickening of the calvarium. The syndrome is caused by target organ unresponsiveness to PTH, and was the first hormone-resistance syndrome described. (Felig, pp. 1143–1145)

199. **(C)** The findings of hypocalcemia and hyperphosphatemia are the same as in hypoparathyroidism, but the serum PTH levels are appropriately increased. The normal urinary rise in cAMP does not occur when these patients are injected with exogenous (normal) PTH. (Felig, pp. 1143–1145)

200. **(B)** This lesion is more frequent in females and may antedate other clinical signs and symptoms of diabetes. The plaques are round, firm, and reddish-brown to yellow in color. They most commonly involve the legs but can also involve the hands, arms, abdomen, and head. (Braunwald, pp. 327, 2127)

201. **(A)** Allopurinol inhibits the enzyme xanthine oxidase, resulting in decreased uric acid production. Allopurinol is particularly useful in the treatment of uric acid nephrolithiasis in gouty individuals. Even if the gouty individual has calcium oxalate stones, allopurinol may be helpful. *(Felig, pp. 1233–1234)*

202. **(B)** Hyperphosphatemia rarely causes any symptoms directly. Its secondary effects on calcium can result in hypocalcemic tetany or metastatic calcification. The usual cause of hyperphosphatemia is uremia. *(Felig, pp. 1156–1157)*

203. **(B)** The severe form of Marfan syndrome is caused by a mutation in a single allele of the fibrillin gene (FBN1). The gene product is a major component of elastin-associated microfibrils. Long, thin extremities, ectopia lentis, and aortic aneurysms are the classical triad. Milder forms of the disease probably also occur but are hard to classify. Mutations in the FBN2 gene can also cause Marfan syndrome, but without aneurysms. *(Braunwald, pp. 2298–2299)*

204. **(A)** Nephrogenic DI can be caused by drugs, metabolic factors, vascular disease, ureteral obstruction, and genetic factors. *(Felig, p. 233)*

205. **(B)** In the familial type 1 form, the defect is believed to be a deficiency of lipoprotein lipase activity. It is a rare autosomal recessive syndrome and usually presents in childhood with typical eruptive xanthoma and abdominal pain secondary to acute pancreatitis. Secondary hyperchylomicronemia (diabetes, hypothyroidism, uremia) is a much more common syndrome. *(Felig, p. 1027)*

206. **(C)** Subcutaneous xanthomas begin to appear at about age 20 and may involve Achilles tendons, elbows, and tibial tuberosities. Familial hypercholesterolemia may be monogenic or polygenic in its inheritance. The disorder is common, and heterozygous familial hypercholesterolemia is felt to affect 1 in 500 individuals. It can be secondary to other diseases such as hypothyroidism, ne-

phrotic syndrome, or even porphyria. Xanthelasmas after the age of 50 are often not related to any dyslipidemia at all. *(Felig, p. 1016)*

207. **(A)** In the rare familial form, raised, yellow plaques appear on palms and fingers, and reddish-yellow xanthomas occur on the elbows. This disorder is felt to be secondary to accumulation of abnormal chylomicron and very low-density lipoprotein (VLDL) remnants. It is probably due to inherited homozygous defects in apo E-2 structure. *(Felig, pp. 1024–1025)*

208. **(E)** Triglycerides are over 150 and are raised by alcohol intake, estrogens, stress, insulin, and physical activity. Cholesterol levels are average or mildly elevated. High-density lipoprotein (HDL) is usually low. Dietary therapy and the maintenance of ideal weight is the cornerstone of therapy. *(Felig, pp. 1029–1030)*

209. **(B)** Hypertriglyceridemia is usually secondary to DM or drugs, rather than a genetic disorder. It can be a normal response to caloric excess or alcohol ingestion and is common in the third trimester of pregnancy. *(Felig, p. 1027)*

210. **(C)** In DM, there is an obligatory osmotic diuresis, but in DI there is lack of water resorption in the tubules. Both result in polyuria, but in DM, there will be substantial glucosuria as well. The large amount of urine output (usually greater than 50 mL/kg/day) is characteristic of polyuric states such as DI, not a bladder problem. Psychogenic polydipsia is commonly seen in patients with psychiatric problems on medications. *(Felig, p. 228)*

211. **(C)** Diabetes insipidus is most commonly caused by a primary deficit in the secretion of vasopressin by the posterior pituitary. It is usually caused by agenesis or destruction of vasopressin-producing neurons by either a developmental, acquired, genetic, or idiopathic disorder. *(Felig, p. 228)*

212. **(D)** Because DI is usually caused by destruction or agenesis of the posterior pituitary, its normal signaling is lost. Pituitary DI can also result from trauma, tumors (both primary and secondary), granulomas, infections, inflammatory diseases, chemical toxins, congenital malformations, and genetic disorders. Depending on the cause, the MRI may demonstrate other associated findings. *(Felig, p. 228)*

213. **(E)** Neprogenic diabetes insipidus is caused by a defect in the action of vasopressin on the renal tubules. This can be genetic, and variants include X-linked recessive, autosomal dominant, and autosomal recessive. Numerous drugs can cause the syndrome, as can many forms of renal disease. Hypercalcemia and hypokalemia can also cause the syndrome. *(Felig, p. 233)*

214. **(D)** In western societies, most dyslipidemias are secondary. The most common predisposing cause is diet, and the second common is DM. Hypothyroidism, renal disease, alcoholism, and AN are also associated with secondary dyslipidemias. Many drugs (eg, estrogen, glucocorticoids) can also cause secondary dyslipidemias. *(Felig, pp. 1009–1015)*

215. **(D)** The most important factors in diet-induced cholesterol elevation are the amount of total fat and saturated fat consumed. Cholesterol intake is next in importance. Obesity and caloric excess usually result in high triglyceride levels. *(Felig, p. 1010)*

216. **(A)** Familial combined hyperlipidemia has an incidence of 1 per 100. It is an autosomal dominant disorder and different affected family members may display different dyslipidemic phenotypes. Familial hypercholesterolemia (1/500) and familial defective Apo B (1/1000) are also common. The other two disorders (Apo C-II deficiency and lipoprotein lipase deficiency) are extremely rare. *(Felig, p. 1010)*

217. **(E)** In mild cases, dietary therapy may suffice, but the vast majority of patients require drug therapy. Statins are clearly the most effective medications available, but the major-

ity of patients will not have optimal cholesterol control, even with maximum doses of a statin. Homozygous patients always require combination therapy. *(Felig, pp. 1019–1021)*

218. **(A, C)** Renal calculi and osteogenic sarcoma are unusual complications of Paget's disease. Bony lesions are blastic and the sacrum and pelvis are most frequently involved, followed closely by the tibia and femur. Hypercalcemia can complicate immobilization. The etiology is unknown, but a viral agent has been postulated. Symptoms may be absent or severe (pain, deformity). *(Felig, pp. 1203–1207)*

219. **(B, G, H)** Many affected persons with vitamin D deficiency have no demonstrable abnormality except for hypophosphatemia. There is a decreased renal threshold for phosphate excretion. This is mediated by secondary hyperparathyroidism. This is caused by decreased calcium absorption with subsequent mild hypocalcemia. The filtered load of calcium in the kidneys is low, so, despite the hyperparathyroidism, renal excretion of calcium is low. *(Felig, pp. 1184–1187)*

220. **(A)** Atrial fibrillation and cardiomegaly are common cardiac manifestations, but are more common in the elderly. Other symptoms include palpitation, tachycardia, nervousness, sweating, and dyspnea. Sinus tachycardia is the most common cardiac manifestation. *(Felig, pp. 298, 1457)*

221. **(E)** Needle biopsy can be used in numerous diseases, but the main rationale is to differentiate benign from malignant nodules. The specimen must be read by an experienced cytologist. It is difficult to diagnose differentiated follicular carcinoma or to differentiate lymphoma from Hashimoto's thyroiditis. Papillary carcinoma is the easiest diagnosis to make by needle biopsy. *(Felig, pp. 364–365)*

222. **(E)** In hemochromatosis, arthropathy usually involves the second and third metacarpophalangeal joints, then knees, hips, and shoulders. It occurs in one quarter to one half of

patients. Diabetes occurs in 65% of patients and is more common in those with a family history of diabetes. Cardiac disease is the presenting symptom in 15% of patients, with heart failure being the usual manifestation. Hypogonadism may manifest as loss of libido, impotence, amenorrhea, testicular atrophy, and sparse body hair. Skin pigmentation is present in 90% of symptomatic patients at presentation, but renal involvement is not characteristic of the disease. *(Braunwald, p. 2259)*

223. **(E)** Regulation of vasopressin is by osmotic stimuli and nonosmotic stimuli such as volume and neural stimuli arising outside the hypothalamus. As little as 15% of cells remaining in the posterior hypothalamus are sufficient to prevent permanent DI. *(Felig, pp. 218–221)*

224. **(D)** Classification of hypoglycemia includes spontaneous causes such as reactive or fasting hypoglycemia and pharmacologic or toxic causes. The diagnosis of hypoglycemia is most certain when Whipple's triad is fulfilled: symptoms consistent with hypoglycemia, low plasma glucose, and relief of symptoms with elevation of plasma glucose to normal. *(Felig, p. 1357)*

225. **(A)** Cardiac failure and arrhythmias frequently occur in cardiac amyloid. The ECG reveals low voltage QRS complexes and conduction disturbances. Red cells are not involved, and involvement of the thyroid, liver, and pancreas is usually asymptomatic. The precursors of the AL amyloid protein found in primary amyloidosis and myeloma are kappa and lambda light chains. Serum amyloid A protein (SAA) is the precursor for the AA amyloid found in secondary amyloidosis. *(Braunwald, pp. 1976–1978)*

226. **(A)** Glucagon exerts a marked effect on carbohydrate, fat, and lipid metabolism, and increases cAMP in many tissues. Glucagonomas of the pancreas present with features such as mild DM, psychiatric disturbances, diarrhea, venous thromboses, and skin find-

ings (necrolytic migratory erythema). *(Felig, pp. 838–841, 1357–1358)*

227. **(C)** Primary hyperparathyroidism develops in over 87% of those with MEN I. Polyendocrine adenomatosis, type I, frequently includes islet cell tumors of the pancreas, leading to the Zollinger–Ellison syndrome, insulinomas, and glucagonomas. Inheritance is via an autosominal dominant pattern. Hypercalcemia does not usually occur until after the first decade. *(Felig, p. 1356)*

228. **(D)** Estrogens cause thickening of vaginal mucosa and can improve urogenital symptoms. The evidence for protection against coronary artery disease and dementia is epidemiological, and not yet confirmed by clinical trials. *(Braunwald, pp. 2166–2177)*

229. **(A)** This is the typical presentation of a feminizing adrenocortical tumor. Ultrasound can usually differentiate between benign and malignant tumors. Breast development alone is usually just premature thelarche and rarely needs investigation. Feminizing adrenocortical tumors can occur in boys and cause gynecomastia. *(Felig, pp. 448, 757)*

230. **(A)** Growth hormone excess in acromegaly produces hypertrophy of muscle. Initially, strength may be increased, but this is transient, and a third of patients will experience weakness, likely secondary to myopathy. *(Felig, p. 190)*

231. **(C)** Vitamin D–resistant rickets is a familial disorder with an X-linked recessive pattern treated with pharmacologic doses of vitamin D. Half the affected individuals have alopecia, and this tends to correlate with severity. Rickets and osteomalacia are characterized by impaired mineralization of bone. Osteoporosis is a disorder with a diminished amount of normally mineralized bone. *(Felig, p. 1186)*

232. **(B)** Risk of death in anorexia nervosa is also associated with hypothermia, suicide, or pneumonia with emaciation. Because of the

danger of ventricular tachyarrhythmias, patients should be followed with electrocardiograms. A prolonged Q-T interval is a sign of danger. In addition, severe weight loss can lead to both systolic and diastolic dysfunction of the ventricles. *(Braunwald, p. 489)*

233. **(E)** In gouty patients, nephrolithiasis and uric acid nephropathy may occur. The association of cardiovascular disease, hypertension, pyelonephritis, and hyperlipoproteinemia with gout contribute to the high prevalence of renal disease in these individuals. *(Braunwald, pp. 1608, 1994–1995)*

234. **(C)** Proximal muscle weakness can be insidious and may mimic primary muscle disease. In severe osteomalacia, there is bowing of the long bones, inward deformity of the long bones, and wide osteoid borders on bone surfaces. Hypocalcemia is characteristic of osteomalacia; however, secondary hyperparathyroidism often raises the serum calcium to low normal levels. The PTH-mediated increase in phosphate clearance often produces hypophosphatemia. *(Braunwald, pp. 2202–2204)*

235. **(B)** Hepatrenal syndrome frequently complicates hepatic failure. Although it can develop gradually, acute renal failure can also be precipitated by hemodynamic stresses (bleeding, diuresis). The earliest manifestations are intrarenal vasoconstriction and avid sodium retention. *(Braunwald, p. 1542)*

236. **(D)** In phenylketonuria, a low-phenylalanine diet with relentless attention to details of diet is required for a good outcome. The diet should be started by 3 weeks of age. Children of mothers with phenylketonuria can be affected if exposed to phenylalanine in utero. Therefore, women with the disorder should stay on a restricted diet until they complete childbearing. In phenylalanine hydroxylase deficiency, tyrosine becomes an essential amino acid and dietary supplements must be provided. *(Braunwald, p. 2305)*

237. **(B)** Wilson's disease includes cirrhosis of the liver, signs of basal ganglia disease, and a brownish-pigmented ring at the corneal margin. Ceruloplasm levels are low. The gene for Wilson's disease is located on the long arm of chromosome 13. In some cases, it is possible to identify carrier states and make prenatal diagnoses. The relationship between the abnormal gene and the metabolic defect (inability to regulate copper balance) is unclear. *(Braunwald, pp. 2274–2275)*

238. **(A)** Other stimulators of protein kinases include platelet-derived growth factor and epidermal growth factor. Tyrosine phosphorylation results from this interaction. Insulin-resistant states can be caused by prereceptor resistance (mutated insulin, anti-insulin antibodies) or receptor and postreceptor resistance. *(Braunwald, p. 2112)*

239. **(C)** The action of insulin involves all three major metabolic fuels (carbohydrate, protein, fat). It is active in liver, muscle, and adipose tissue. In each there are anticatabolic as well as anabolic effects. These tend to reinforce each other. *(Felig, p. 835)*

240. **(D)** Infection or other acute medical condition is the usual precipitant for thyroid storm. Radioactive iodine treatment or abrupt withdrawal of antithyroid medications are also implicated. The key diagnostic features are fever, tachycardia, and central nervous system dysfunction. *(Felig, pp. 309–310)*

241. **(B)** All the causes listed may delay puberty, but the most common cause by far is normal variation in growth pattern. There is often a family history of delayed puberty in parents or siblings. In these individuals, bone age often correlates better with the onset and progression of puberty than does chronological age. *(Felig, p. 678)*

242. **(D)** Approximately one third of unselected women with metastatic breast cancer will respond to tamoxifen. Presence of estrogen receptors (ER) or progesterone receptors (PR) improves the likelihood of response. If the tumor is both ER and PR positive, the response rate is 70%. *(Felig, p. 1441)*

243. **(B)** A generally increased risk of breast cancer is associated with nulliparity, late first pregnancy, and especially a history of maternal breast cancer. Prior history of breast cancer is of course a powerful risk factor. *(Felig, p. 1439)*

244. **(D)** Although the variation is great depending on occupation, hobbies, and so forth, generally only one third of energy is utilized for physical activity. Height is not used at all in calculating RMR, and RMR is higher in men than in women of identical weight. Amino acids ingested without other energy sources are inefficiently incorporated into protein. Current recommendations are to encourage full adult levels of protein, vitamins, and minerals in the elderly. *(Braunwald, p. 459)*

245. **(C)** The diagnosis is hyperparathyroidism. Calcium deposits are seen in the periarticular areas of the fourth and fifth metacarpophalangeal, third proximal interphalangeal, and fourth distal interphalangeal joints. There is slight soft tissue swelling, especially of the fourth and fifth metacarpophalangeal joints. Calcification in scleroderma is subcutaneous in location. In gout, if monosodium urate is deposited it could appear as a soft tissue mass. *(Felig, pp. 1115–1116, 1200–1201)*

246. **(B)** Autonomous adrenal tumors are adrenocorticotropic hormone (ACTH) insensitive and fail to demonstrate a brisk rise in urinary 17-hydroxycorticoids. Androgenic effects such as hirsutism are usually absent. In Cushing syndrome secondary to an autonomous adrenal tumor, onset is usually gradual, and hirsutism, other androgenic effects, and hyperpigmentation are absent. *(Felig, pp. 482–487)*

247. **(A)** Diabetes mellitus is a syndrome consisting of hyperglycemia, large vessel disease, microvascular disease, and neuropathy. The classic presenting symptoms are increased thirst, polyuria, polyphagia, and weight loss. In type 2 diabetes, the presentation can be more subtle and is often made when the patient is asymptomatic. *(Felig, p. 856)*

248. **(C)** The gold standard is still a fasting plasma glucose ≥ 7.0 mmol/L (126 mg/dL) on two separate occasions. Glucose tolerance tests are rarely required. With typical symptoms even an elevated random sugar is diagnostic. *(Felig, p. 857)*

249. **(C)** The patient is most likely to develop glomerulosclerosis. This can be diffuse or nodular (Kimmelstiel–Wilson nodules). Poor metabolic control is probably a major factor in the progression of diabetic nephropathy. *(Felig, pp. 900–901)*

250. **(I, J)** Pyoderma gangrenosum is not a cutaneous manifestation of diabetes. Perineal pruritus in a diabetic is almost always associated with *Candida albicans*. A severe external otitis can occur in older patients. It is caused by *Pseudomonas aeruginosa* and is characterized by ear pain, drainage, fever, and leukocytosis. Facial nerve paralysis can occur and is a poor prognostic sign. Necrobiosis lipoidica is a plaquelike lesion with a brown border and yellow center usually found on the anterior leg surface. *(Braunwald, pp. 1686–1687)*

251. **(A, C, E)** Background retinopathy is present in about 90% of diabetes after 25 to 30 years of disease. Microaneurysms, dilated veins, dot and blot hemorrhages, cotton-wool spots, and hard exudates are common findings. *(Felig, p. 898)*

252. **(B, D)** Proliferative retinopathy carries a high risk of vitreous hemorrhage, scarring, retinal detachment, and blindness. Proliferative retinopathy is associated with nephropathy and CAD and is associated with a poor prognosis, for life as well as for vision. *(Felig, pp. 898–899)*

253. **(B)** High prolactin level suppresses luteinizing hormone-releasing hormone (LHRH) and can result in low plasma gonadotropin and testosterone levels. It may not be obvious on physical examination. Therapy with a dopamine agonist may lower prolactin levels and reverse impotence. *(Braunwald, p. 293)*

254. (D) An absent orgasm when libido and erectile function are normal invariably indicates that organic disease is absent. Loss of desire can also be caused by psychological disturbance, but may indicate androgen deficiency or drug effect. (*Braunwald, pp. 293–294*)

255. (E) Failure of detumescence—priapism—can be caused by sickle cell anemia or chronic granulocytic leukemia. Priapism must be treated promptly to preserve future erectile functioning. (*Braunwald, p. 669*)

256. (B) Vascular disease, by itself or in conjunction with peripheral neuropathy in DM, is a common cause of erectile dysfunction. The lesions can be in large vessels (aortic occlusion, Leriche syndrome), small arteries, or even in the sinusoidal spaces. (*Braunwald, pp. 292–293*)

257. (E) Idiopathic hirsutism may simply represent an extreme of normal androgen production. It is diagnosed by demonstrating minimal elevation of androgens and exclusion of other causes. Management is primarily by cosmetic therapy, although drugs to suppress androgen production and/or androgen effects on the hair follicle can be used. (*Braunwald, pp. 298–300*)

258. (C) The most severe form of PCOD, Stein–Leventhal syndrome, is associated with chronic anovulation, hirsutism, enlarged cystic ovaries, obesity, and amenorrhea. The spectrum of disease, however, is quite wide, and some patients have only mild hirsutism. (*Braunwald, pp. 298–300*)

259. (F) Krukenberg tumors of the ovary stimulate surrounding ovarian stromal tissue to produce excess androgen. When onset of hair growth (with or without frank virilization) is very rapid, a neoplastic source of androgen is suggested. As well as ovarian tumors, the potential neoplasms include adenomas and carcinomas of the adrenal gland. (*Braunwald, pp. 298–300*)

260. (D) Attenuated forms of adrenal hyperplasia can present with hirsutism at puberty or in adulthood. Elevated levels of a precursor of cortisol biosynthesis such as 17-hydroxyprogesterone, 17-hydroxypregnenolone, or 11-deoxycortisol can present. ACTH infusion will increase the precursor level, and dexamethasone will suppress it. (*Braunwald, pp. 298–300*)

261. (A) Salivary gland enlargement occurs both in AN and BN. Other common findings in AN include constipation, bradycardia, hypotension, hypercarotinemia, and soft downy hair growth (lanugo). Menses are usually absent. (*Braunwald, p. 488*)

262. (D) Hypoglycemia and low estrogens and gonadotropins are frequently seen in AN. The BUN and creatinine may be elevated. Hypochloremia, hypokalemia, and alkalosis are frequently seen in BN. (*Braunwald, pp. 488–489*)

263. (E) Heart failure, if it occurs, usually is in the setting of refeeding. Low QRS voltages and STT changes are common. However, the presence of a prolonged QT interval is most suggestive of serious cardiac arrhythmias. (*Braunwald, p. 489*)

264. (B) Hospitalization should be considered when the body weight dips below 75% of expected. The goal is to achieve a weight of 90% of that expected. Vomiting is more characteristic of BN than AN. (*Braunwald, p. 489*)

265. (B) Recurrent vomiting and exposure of the teeth to stomach acid leads to loss of dental enamel and eventual chipping and erosion of the teeth. The vomiting may be manually induced, but eventually most patients with BN are able to trigger vomiting at will. (*Braunwald, p. 489*)

266. (B) AN has one of the highest mortality rates of any psychiatric illness at 5% per decade. The mortality for BN is very low, and 50% have a full recovery within 10 years. Only 25% have persistent symptoms of BN over many years, and the disease does not usually progress to AN. (*Braunwald, p. 489*)

267. **(I)** Low-fiber diets are frequently prescribed during flares of inflammatory bowel disease to reduce diarrhea and pain. There is no Level 1 evidence to support this practice. Similar diets are often prescribed for diverticulitis or other conditions associated with a narrowed or stenosed colon. It may be prescribed for patients with a new ostomy. When acute symptoms subside, however, restrictions concerning dietary fiber should be stopped. *(Braunwald, p. 473)*

268. **(L)** Limiting foods with high tyramine content for patients on MAOIs might prevent elevations of blood pressure. Such foods include old cheeses and red wine. *(Braunwald, p. 434)*

269. **(C)** Some patients with hypertension are salt sensitive, and will lower their blood pressure with salt restriction. Low-sodium diets are also recommended in patients with congestive heart failure (CHF), ascites, or chronic renal failure. *(Braunwald, p. 1420)*

270. **(F)** After gastrectomy, avoiding simple sugars and limiting liquids can ameliorate symptoms of dumping. Early dumping occurs within 30 minutes of eating and is characterized by vasomotor symptoms such as palpitations, tachycardia, lightheadedness, and diaphoresis. Late dumping includes similar symptoms plus dizziness, confusion, and even syncope. It occurs 1½ to 3 hours after eating. *(Braunwald, p. 1660)*

271. **(H)** The symptoms of hepatic encephalopathy are improved with protein restriction. It is presumed that this results in lower levels of serum ammonia, but other substances in the serum may be implicated. These include mercaptans, short-chain fatty acids, and phenol. Gamma-aminobutyric acid (GABA) levels in the brain are also increased. Restricting daytime protein intake in patients with Parkinson's disease may improve the efficacy of levodopa therapy. *(Braunwald, p. 471)*

272. **(E)** Chocolate, ethanol, caffeine, and tobacco decrease lower esophageal sphincter pres-

sure. Other effective treatments for GERD include low-fat diet, avoiding bedtime snacks, and elevating the head of the bed while sleeping. *(Braunwald, p. 240)*

273. **(D)** Scurvy is characterized by a tendency to hemorrhage and perifollicular hyperkeratotic papules in which hairs become fragmented and buried. Gums are involved only if teeth are present. It can occur in infants 6 to 12 months of age who are on processed milk formulas without citrus fruit or vegetable supplementation. The peak incidence in the United States is in poor and elderly people and alcoholics. It is frequently associated with other nutritional deficiencies (eg, folic acid). *(Braunwald, p. 464)*

274. **(E)** Excessive vitamin A ingestion can cause abdominal pain, nausea, vomiting, headache, dizziness, and papilledema. Deficiency of vitamin A can cause night blindness and progress to visual loss. It is common in children in developing countries and is a major cause of blindness. *(Braunwald, p. 466)*

275. **(A)** Pharmacologic doses of niacin for hypercholesterolemia may cause histamine release, which results in flushing, pruritus, and gastrointestinal disturbance. Asthma may be aggravated, acanthosis nigricans can occur, and in high doses elevation of uric acid and fasting blood sugar can occur. Hepatic toxicity, including cholestatic jaundice, has been described with large doses. *(Braunwald, p. 463)*

276. **(B)** Thiamine deficiency can cause high-output cardiac failure (wet beriberi) or neurologic symptoms (dry beriberi). In North America, thiamine deficiency occurs in alcoholics or those with chronic disease. In alcoholics, deficiency is secondary to low intake, impaired absorption and storage, and accelerated destruction. Genetic factors are important as clinical manifestations occur only in a small proportion of chronically malnourished individuals. Beriberi heart disease is characterized by peripheral vasodilatation, sodium and water retention, and high-output CHF. *(Braunwald, pp. 461–462)*

277. **(A)** Diarrhea, dementia, and dermatitis are the classic triad for pellagra (niacin deficiency). The diagnosis is based on clinical suspicion and response to therapy, and can be confirmed by demonstrating low levels of the urinary metabolites 2-methylnicotinamide and 2-pyridone. Small doses of niacin (10 mg/day) with adequate dietary tryptophan will cure pellagra secondary to nutritional deficiency. *(Braunwald, p. 463)*

CHAPTER 4

Gastroenterology
Questions

DIRECTIONS (Questions 278 through 287): Each set of matching questions in this section consists of a list of lettered options followed by several numbered items. For each numbered item, select the appropriate lettered option(s). Each lettered option may be selected once, more than once, or not at all. EACH ITEM WILL STATE THE NUMBER OF OPTIONS TO SELECT. CHOOSE EXACTLY THIS NUMBER.

Questions 278 through 283

A 48-year-old man presents with periumbilical pain made worse by eating and weight loss. A small bowel x-ray reveals an area of narrowing.

(A) polypoid adenoma
(B) leiomyoma
(C) lipoma
(D) adenocarcinoma
(E) primary gastrointestinal (GI) lymphoma
(F) carcinoid tumor

278. The most common endocrine tumor of the GI tract (SELECT ONE)

279. The most common primary malignancy of the small bowel (SELECT ONE)

280. One form can be treated with antibiotics (SELECT ONE)

281. The appendix is a very common site of involvement (SELECT ONE)

282. More common in patients with celiac disease (SELECT ONE)

283. The distal ileum is the most commonly involved part of the small bowel (SELECT TWO)

Questions 284 through 287

(A) celiac sprue
(B) mediated by hormones
(C) associated with decrease in pancreatic enzymes
(D) hyperthyroidism
(E) regional enteritis
(F) associated arthritis
(G) associated with skin pigmentation
(H) increase in pancreatic enzymes
(I) hypersensitivity reaction
(J) an infectious agent
(K) may present with iron deficiency
(L) associated with skin disease

284. A 29-year-old woman has recently developed milk intolerance. This may be secondary to (SELECT TWO)

285. A 19-year-old man has a long history of weight loss, abdominal distention, bloating, and diarrhea. Investigation reveals steatorrhea, and a small bowel biopsy reveals blunting and flattening of villi. This disease may be (SELECT FOUR)

286. A 53-year-old man presents with weight loss, low-grade fever, and peripheral lymphadenopathy. Steatorrhea is documented, and small bowel biopsy reveals para-aminosalicylic acid positive macrophages. This disease is associated with (SELECT TWO)

287. A 43-year-old woman has had a 10-year history of severe and recurrent peptic ulcer disease (PUD). She has chronic diarrhea, but not enough fat to make the diagnosis of steatorrhea. Evaluation for *Helicobacter pylori* infection is negative. This syndrome is (SELECT ONE)

DIRECTIONS (Questions 288 through 310): Each of the numbered items or incomplete statements in this section is followed by answers or by completions of the statement. Select the ONE lettered answer or completion that is BEST in each case.

288. A 79-year-old woman with severe constipation is found to have multiple diverticuli on colonoscopy. The most useful therapy would be

   (A) stool softeners
   (B) prophylactic surgery
   (C) phenolphthalein laxatives
   (D) increasing stool bulk
   (E) psychotherapy

289. A 71-year-old man develops progressive weight loss and dysphagia over a 3-month period. This disorder generally

   (A) is very responsive to chemotherapy
   (B) is more common in females
   (C) has a 5-year cure rate of 20%
   (D) may be either adenocarcinoma or squamous cell carcinoma
   (E) is characterized by significant complications from hemorrhage

290. A 23-year-old woman has weight loss and diarrhea. Routine lab tests suggest generalized malnutrition. The most definitive test for diagnosis of malabsorption is

   (A) xylose absorption
   (B) Schilling test
   (C) x-ray studies
   (D) stool fat quantitation
   (E) small intestinal biopsy

291. A 33-year-old man has never been vaccinated for hepatitis B. Serologic tests reveal negative hepatitis B surface antigen (HBsAg) and positive antibody to surface antigen. This is indicative of

   (A) previous hepatitis B infection
   (B) chronic active hepatitis
   (C) acute hepatitis B infection
   (D) poor prognosis
   (E) need for vaccine to hepatitis B

292. A 29-year-old woman is found on routine annual blood testing to have an increase in unconjugated bilirubin. There is no evidence of hemolysis, and liver tests are otherwise normal. The likely diagnosis is

   (A) Crigler–Najjar syndrome
   (B) Dubin–Johnson syndrome
   (C) Rotor syndrome
   (D) Gilbert syndrome
   (E) pregnanediol therapy

293. An 18-year-old woman was diagnosed 7 years earlier with precocious pseudopuberty secondary to ovarian tumor. Physical examination reveals oral and lingual dark pigmentation. The most likely diagnosis is

   (A) Peutz–Jeghers syndrome
   (B) Gardner syndrome
   (C) Lynch syndrome
   (D) juvenile polyposis
   (E) Turcot syndrome

294. A 63-year-old man has stools positive for occult blood. The most likely location of a bowel cancer is

   (A) cecum
   (B) sigmoid
   (C) transverse colon
   (D) appendix
   (E) ascending colon

295. A 74-year-old man underwent some type of peptic ulcer surgery years ago. He has symptoms that include abdominal pain and bloating about 30 to 40 minutes after eating, accompanied by nausea. If he vomits, the symptoms are relieved. These symptoms are likely caused by

(A)   early dumping syndrome

(B)   late dumping syndrome

(C)   bile reflux gastropathy

(D)   retained gastric antrum

(E)   afferent loop syndrome

296.   A 55-year-old man from China is known to have chronic liver disease secondary to hepatitis B infection. He has recently felt unwell, and his hemoglobin level has increased from 130 g/L 1 year ago to 195 g/L. The blood test most likely to be helpful is

(A)   alkaline phosphatase

(B)   alpha-fetoprotein (AFP)

(C)   aspartate transaminase (AST)

(D)   AST/ALT (alanine transaminase) ratio

(E)   unconjugated bilirubin

297.   A 63-year-old man with a long history of alcohol abuse presents with ascites. The ascitic fluid in uncomplicated cirrhosis would be expected to show

(A)   hemorrhage

(B)   protein greater than 25 g/L

(C)   bilirubin level twice that of serum

(D)   specific gravity less than 1.016

(E)   more than 1000 white cells per mm^3

298.   A 64-year-old woman has a dilated common bile duct secondary to stones. These stones

(A)   all originate in the gallbladder

(B)   always produce jaundice

(C)   produce constant level of jaundice

(D)   can be painless

(E)   indicate anomalies of the bile duct

299.   A 53-year-old man presents with diarrhea. He also complains of facial flushing lasting minutes at a time. Physical examination reveals facial telangiectasias and a heart murmur not present 2 years before. This murmur is accentuated by deep breathing. The most helpful test would be

(A)   urinary vanillylmandelic acid (VMA)

(B)   serum noradrenaline levels

(C)   barium enema

(D)   serum serotonin levels

(E)   urinary 5-hydroxyindolacetic acid (5-HIAA)

300.   A 29-year-old woman complains of dysphagia with both solids and liquids, worse when she is eating quickly or is anxious. Manometry reveals normal basal esophageal sphincter pressure with minimal change on swallowing. Management of this syndrome could include

(A)   beta-blocker therapy

(B)   partial esophagectomy

(C)   anticholinergic drugs

(D)   calcium channel blockers

(E)   dietary modification

301.   A 34-year-old woman complains bitterly of heartburn. Physical examination reveals healing lesions of the fingertips that she says were small ulcers. Esophageal manometry reveals a decrease in the expected amplitude of smooth muscle contraction. Lower esophageal sphincter tone is subnormal, but relaxes normally with swallowing. This syndrome is

(A)   characterized by systemic signs of inflammation

(B)   predominantly treated symptomatically

(C)   characterized by a poor prognosis

(D)   usually more frequent in men

(E)   characterized by death secondary to a renal crisis

302.   A 59-year-old man presents with abdominal pain, anorexia, and nausea. He has started to develop edema. Endoscopy reveals large gastric mucosal folds. The edema is secondary to

(A)   hypoalbuminemia secondary to malnutrition

(B)   hypoalbuminemia secondary to protein loss

(C)   impaired hepatic synthesis of albumen

(D)   humorally mediated cardiac disease

(E)   constrictive pericarditis

303. A 35-year-old white man presents with a long history of fulminant diarrhea and rectal bleeding (Fig. 4–1). What is the most likely diagnosis?

    (A) toxic megacolon

    (B) amoebic colitis

    (C) appendicitis

    (D) ischemic colitis

    (E) annular carcinoma

304. A 45-year-old man with a long history of alcoholic intake comes into the emergency room with upper gastrointestinal (UGI) bleeding (Fig. 4–2). What is the most likely diagnosis?

    (A) esophageal varices

    (B) esophageal carcinoma

    (C) foreign body

    (D) tertiary waves

    (E) Barrett's esophagus

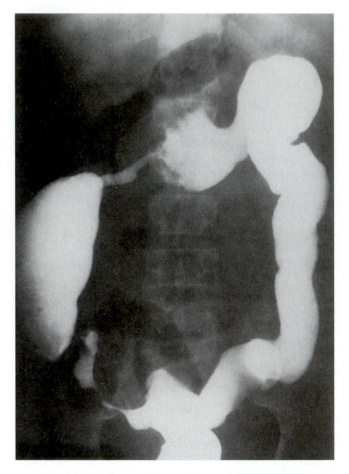

Figure 4–1.

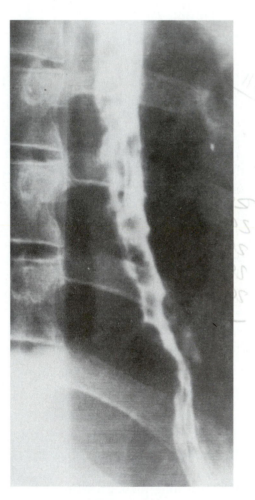

Figure 4–2.

305. A 40-year-old taxicab driver presents with worsening epigastric pain (Fig. 4–3). What is the most likely diagnosis?

(A) benign gastric ulcer
(B) malignant gastric ulcer
(C) duodenal ulcer
(D) normal
(E) hiatus hernia

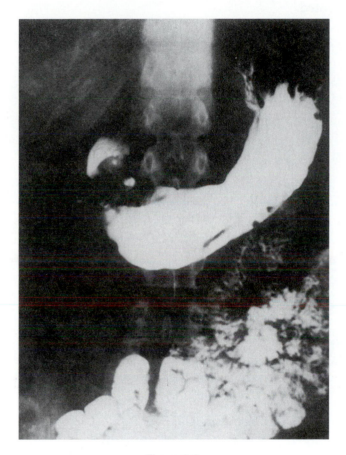

Figure 4–3.

306. Which statement concerning peptic ulcer disease is correct?

(A) Duodenal ulcer is seen more often in older people than is gastric ulcer.
(B) Clinically, gastric ulcers are more common than duodenal ulcers.
(C) Duodenal ulcers can frequently be malignant.
(D) Infection can cause both types of peptic ulcer.
(E) Peptic gastric ulcers are usually quite proximal in the stomach.

307. Which of the following is a risk factor for *H. pylori* infection?

(A) excess exposure to antibiotics
(B) female sex
(C) alpha$_1$-antitrypsin deficiency
(D) poverty
(E) proton pump inhibitor therapy

308. Which of the following is an established risk factor for nonsteroidal anti-inflammatory disease (NSAID)-induced gastric or duodenal ulceration?

(A) *H. pylori* infection
(B) cigarette smoking
(C) alcohol consumption
(D) glucocorticoids
(E) age under 30

309. NSAIDs promote ulceration by which mechanism?

(A) increasing acid production
(B) causing direct epithelial cell death
(C) promoting replication of *H. pylori*
(D) an antiplatelet effect
(E) inhibiting mucosal repair

310. The most appropriate treatment for a duodenal ulcer would likely be

(A) 6 to 8 weeks of omeprazole or ranitidine
(B) long-term acid suppression with omeprazole
(C) antibiotic therapy
(D) antibiotic therapy with omeprazole
(E) bismuth citrate therapy

DIRECTIONS (Questions 311 through 318): Each set of matching questions in this section consists of a list of lettered options followed by several numbered items. For each numbered item, select the appropriate lettered option(s). Each lettered option may be selected once, more than once, or not at all. EACH ITEM WILL STATE THE NUMBER OF OPTIONS TO SELECT. CHOOSE EXACTLY THIS NUMBER.

A 29-year-old man presents with an acute illness characterized by jaundice and abnormal liver enzymes, and viral hepatitis is suspected.

(A) hepatitis A virus
(B) hepatitis B virus
(C) hepatitis C virus
(D) hepatitis D virus
(E) hepatitis E virus

311. Symptoms could have been prevented by vaccination (SELECT THREE)

312. Likely spread via fecal–oral route (SELECT TWO)

313. Sexual transmission is common (SELECT TWO)

314. Most likely to lead to chronic infection (SELECT ONE)

315. Can respond to specific antiviral therapy (SELECT TWO)

316. Perinatal transmission is of major epidemiologic significance (SELECT ONE)

317. Passive immunotherapy can provide some protection (SELECT TWO)

318. Requires presence of another infectious agent before becoming clinically apparent (SELECT ONE)

DIRECTIONS (Questions 319 through 348): Each of the numbered items or incomplete statements in this section is followed by answers or by completions of the statement. Select the ONE lettered answer or completion that is BEST in each case.

Questions 319 through 322

A 53-year-old man presents to the emergency department with severe abdominal pain. His white count is 15,000/mL and amylase is markedly elevated.

319. Another common laboratory abnormality would be

(A) hypoglycemia
(B) hypercholesterolemia
(C) hyperglycemia
(D) hypercalcemia
(E) hypercarbia

320. In the United States, the most common predisposing factor for this disorder would be

(A) drugs
(B) gallbladder disease
(C) malignancy
(D) alcohol
(E) hypertriglyceridemia

321. In acquired immune deficiency syndrome (AIDS) patients, the disorder can be triggered by infection with

(A) toxoplasmosis
(B) *Mycobacterium avium* complex
(C) *Mycobacterium tuberculosis*
(D) *Pneumocystis carinii*
(E) herpesvirus

322. Interpretation of the most valuable blood test is confused in the presence of

(A) maturity-onset diabetes mellitus (DM)
(B) gastric ulcer
(C) renal failure
(D) sulfonamide therapy
(E) gastric carcinoma

Questions 323 and 324

A 43-year-old man feels vaguely unwell. Physical examination is unremarkable except for evidence of scleral icterus. The skin appears normal.

323. The jaundice is visible in the eyes but not the skin because of

(A) the high type II collagen content of scleral tissue
(B) the high elastin content of scleral tissue
(C) the high blood flow to the head with consequent increased bilirubin delivery
(D) secretion via the lacrimal glands
(E) the lighter color of the sclera

324. Blood work reveals predominantly unconjugated bilirubin. The most likely diagnosis is

(A) hemolysis
(B) gallstones
(C) alcoholic liver disease
(D) pancreatic carcinoma
(E) Dubin–Johnson syndrome

325. Which of the following is most likely to cause protein-losing enteropathy?

(A) scleroderma
(B) amyloidosis
(C) disaccharidase deficiency
(D) ischemic colitis
(E) Ménétrier's disease

326. A 28-year-old man presents with chronic diarrhea and arthritis. The most likely diagnosis is

(A) lymphoma of the bowel
(B) amyloid infiltration
(C) chronic pancreatitis
(D) ulcerative colitis
(E) tropical sprue

327. A 57-year-old man recently discharged from the hospital develops severe diarrhea and abdominal pain. Sigmoidoscopy reveals a granular friable mucosa. The most common cause of this syndrome is

(A) clindamycin therapy
(B) rotavirus
(C) *Clostridium perfringens* infection
(D) cephalosporin therapy
(E) bacterial invasion of the bowel wall

Questions 328 and 329

A 42-year-old woman presents with pruritus. She has otherwise been well, and laboratory evaluation reveals an alkaline phosphatase level of three times normal.

328. The next text that should be performed is

(A) international normalized ratio (INR) or prothrombin time
(B) antinuclear antibodies
(C) protein immunoelectrophoresis
(D) abdominal ultrasound
(E) antimitochondrial antibodies

329. Effective therapy will prevent

(A) end-stage liver disease
(B) visual problems
(C) hepatic fibrosis
(D) arthritic complications
(E) encephalopathy

330. A 53-year-old man has steatorrhea. The small bowel mucosa is most likely to be normal in which of the following syndromes?

(A) tropical sprue
(B) postgastrectomy steatorrhea
(C) Whipple's disease
(D) nontropical sprue
(E) abetalipoproteinemia

331. A 22-year-old man with inflammatory bowel disease is noted to have a "string sign" in the ileal area on barium enema. This sign is most often seen

(A) in the stenotic or nonstenotic phase of the disease
(B) in the stenotic phase only
(C) as a rigid, nondistensible phenomenon
(D) with gastric involvement
(E) with rectal involvement

332. A 59-year-old man presents with abdominal distention and a decrease in bowel movements. He has had previous abdominal surgery. The diagnosis of large bowel obstruction over small bowel would be favored by which of the following findings?

    (A) mild degree of pain
    (B) temperature 103.1°F
    (C) stepladder pattern on abdominal films
    (D) green vomitus
    (E) hiccups

Questions 333 through 337

333. A 57-year old man comes to the office with a complaint of food "sticking on the way down." Which of the following characteristics suggests a benign problem is causing the dysphagia?

    (A) severe weight loss in comparison to the degree of dysphagia
    (B) hoarseness following the onset of dysphagia
    (C) episodic dysphagia for several years
    (D) difficulty only with solids
    (E) hiccups

334. Which of the following characteristics suggests a Zenker's diverticulum?

    (A) severe weight loss
    (B) greater problems with liquids than solids
    (C) hoarseness
    (D) worse in semirecumbent position
    (E) aspiration unrelated to swallowing

335. If pain (odynophagia) on swallowing is a symptom, the most likely diagnosis would be

    (A) mid esophageal cancer
    (B) distal esophageal cancer
    (C) peptic stricture
    (D) candida infection
    (E) bacterial esophagitis

336. The patient points to his midthorax as a site where food is sticking. If there is a mechanical obstruction, this historical information suggests which location?

    (A) at the location the patient points to
    (B) at or above the location the patient points to
    (C) below the location the patient points to
    (D) at or below the location the patient points to
    (E) the historical information is unhelpful in suggesting a location

337. The patient describes severe chest pain associated with dysphagia. He has been seen twice in the emergency room, but cardiac disease has been excluded. This symptom is likely caused by

    (A) herpetic infection
    (B) a motor disorder
    (C) mid esophageal cancer
    (D) peptic stricture
    (E) external esophageal compression

338. A 16-year old girl has recently been referred to your family practice. She is a recent immigrant from southeast Asia and has been taking isoniazid (INH) and rifampin for uncomplicated tuberculosis. Routine blood tests are unremarkable except for an elevated direct bilirubin. Other liver tests are completely normal. The likely diagnosis is

    (A) hemolytic anemia
    (B) INH toxicity
    (C) Crigler–Najjar syndrome type I
    (D) rifampin toxicity
    (E) Rotor syndrome

339. Which of the following panel of lab tests would be characteristic in a patient with jaundice secondary to alcoholic hepatitis?

    (A) ratio of AST:ALT is 3:1 and the AST is 500 U/L
    (B) ratio of AST:ALT is 3:1 and the AST is 250 U/L
    (C) ratio of AST:ALT is 1:1 and the AST is 500 U/L
    (D) ratio of AST:ALT is 1:1 and the AST is 250 U/L
    (E) ratio of AST:ALT is 1:3 and the AST is 750

340. Which of the following medications causes predictable, dose-dependent hepatocellular injury?

    (A) morphine
    (B) isoniazid
    (C) gold
    (D) acetaminophen
    (E) acetylsalicyclic acid (ASA)

341. The toxicity of the above medication is mediated by

    (A) an allergic mechanism
    (B) an active metabolite
    (C) a reaction with hepatic glycogen stores
    (D) direct toxicity of the parent compound
    (E) circulating immune complexes

342. A specific antidote for this hepatotoxin would be

    (A) ethanol to compete with the parent drug for metabolism, therefore preventing formation of toxic metabolites
    (B) narcan to block its actions directly
    (C) intravenous prostacyclins to maintain cellular integrity
    (D) N-acetylcysteine to allow binding of the toxic metabolite
    (E) glucocorticoids to block the immune cascade

343. Blood-filled lesions in the liver (peliosis hepatis) are most likely to be seen with which of the following medications?

    (A) methyltestosterone
    (B) oral contraceptives
    (C) trimethoprim–sulfamethoxazole
    (D) chlorpromazine
    (E) erythromycin

Questions 344 through 346

344. A 16-year-old girl is referred to the office because of chronic diarrhea. Which of the following characteristics would suggest that this is a secretory diarrhea?

    (A) small volume stools
    (B) precipitated by eating
    (C) predominantly solid stool
    (D) painless
    (E) positive for occult blood

345. Physical examination reveals a healthy young woman who is 5'7" tall and weighs 97 pounds. The most likely cause of a secretory diarrhea in this young woman would be

    (A) surreptitious use of senna products
    (B) carcinoid tumor
    (C) ulcerative colitis
    (D) lactose deficiency
    (E) celiac disease

346. Further history reveals that this young woman does not take laxatives. However, in an effort to stay slim she eats very little other than sugar-free gum and sugarless candy. She in fact consumes a prodigious amount of both. It is possible that her diarrhea is caused by

    (A) direct stimulant effect of chemicals in the candies
    (B) lack of fiber in her diet
    (C) pancreatic insufficiency secondary to chronic protein-calorie malnutrition
    (D) secondary intestinal mucosal atrophy
    (E) nonabsorbed carbohydrates

Questions 347 and 348

347. A 52-year-old man has suffered with chronic diarrhea for several years, but has refused to see a doctor. He finally comes because he is having trouble driving at night because of difficulty seeing. Physical examination reveals a slender, pale, unwell-looking man. His diarrhea is likely caused by

   (A) malabsorption
   (B) osmotic diarrhea
   (C) secretory diarrhea
   (D) inflammatory bowel disease
   (E) colonic tumor

348. The definitive diagnosis in this man is likely to be made by

   (A) presence of fecal osmotic gap
   (B) D-xylose test
   (C) stool fat measurements
   (D) Schilling test
   (E) mucosal biopsy

DIRECTIONS (Questions 349 through 353): Each set of matching questions in this section consists of a list of lettered options followed by several numbered items. For each numbered item, select the appropriate lettered option(s). Each lettered option may be selected once, more than once, or not at all. EACH ITEM WILL STATE THE NUMBER OF OPTIONS TO SELECT. CHOOSE EXACTLY THIS NUMBER.

   (A) chronic gastritis type A
   (B) chronic gastritis type B
   (C) Ménétrier's disease
   (D) eosinophilic gastritis
   (E) granulomatous gastritis
   (F) gastritis following gastric surgery
   (G) acute erosive gastritis

349. Ischemia of the gastric mucosa implicated in the pathogenesis (SELECT ONE)

350. Associated with *H. pylori* infection (SELECT ONE)

351. Immune or autoimmune pathogenesis suspected (SELECT ONE)

352. Commonly associated with protein-losing enteropathy (SELECT ONE)

353. Bile reflux implicated in pathogenesis (SELECT ONE)

Answers and Explanations

278. **(F)** Carcinoid tumors account for up to 75% of all GI endocrine tumors. They are frequently multiple. Primary carcinoid tumors of the appendix are common but rarely metastasize. Those in the large colon may metastasize but do not function. Carcinoids are the most common GI endocrine tumors. They arise from neuroendocrine cells most commonly in the GI tract, pancreas, or bronchi. GI carcinoids cause abdominal pain, bleeding, or even obstruction (usually via intussusception). Carcinoid syndrome is characterized by flushing, diarrhea, and valvular heart disease. *(Braunwald, pp. 596–599)*

279. **(D)** Adenocarcinoma of the small bowel accounts for about 50% of malignant tumors of the small bowel. They are most commonly found in the distal duodenum and proximal jejeunum. Hemorrhage or obstruction are the most common presenting symptoms. X-ray findings can mimic chronic duodenal ulcer disease or Crohn's disease. *(Braunwald, p. 587)*

280. **(E)** There is one unique form of lymphoma called immunoproliferative small intestinal disease (IPSID) or Mediterranean lymphoma. It diffusely involves the small intestine and usually presents with diarrhea and steatorrhea. Oral antibiotics early in the disease provide some benefit, suggesting a possible infectious component to the disorder. Antibiotics and chemotherapy are frequently combined. *(Braunwald, p. 587)*

281. **(F)** Appendiceal tumors make up nearly half of all carcinoid tumors and are a frequent finding in routine appendectomy specimens. They are usually small, solitary, and benign. Even if they invade locally, they rarely metastasize. *(Braunwald, p. 596)*

282. **(E)** Primary small bowel lymphoma is more common in the settings of celiac disease, regional enteritis, congenital immune disorders, prior organ transplantation, autoimmune disorders, and AIDS. *(Braunwald, p. 587)*

283. **(C, F)** Lipomas and carcinoid tumors are most frequently found in the distal ileum. Adenocarcinomas are characteristically more proximal. The ileum has more lymphatic tissue than the rest of the small bowel so lymphoma is more common here than in the jejunum or duodenum. However, there is not as strong a predilection for the distal ileum as there is for lipomas and carcinoids. *(Braunwald, pp. 586–587)*

284. **(A, E)** Acquired lactase deficiency is very common in GI diseases with evidence of mucosal damage. Examples include celiac and tropical sprue, viral and bacterial infections, giardiasis, cystic fibrosis, ulcerative colitis, and regional enteritis. It is not caused by a hypersensitivity reaction. *(Braunwald, p. 167)*

285. **(A, C, K, L)** This syndrome is likely celiac sprue, but a clinical and histological improvement with a gluten-free diet would be required for confirmation. The decrease in pancreatic enzyme production is secondary to decreased intestinal secretion of hormones that stimulate the pancreas. Dermatitis herpetiformis might be related to celiac disease. Although gross malabsorption is the classical description of celiac sprue, it can present with isolated deficiencies such as iron deficiency anemia. *(Braunwald, pp. 1673–1675)*

286. **(F, J)** Whipple's disease is caused by infection with a gram-positive bacillus called *Tropheryma whippelii*. The disease, previously invariably fatal, can be controlled with long-term antibiotic therapy (at least one year), and some patients seem to be cured. Arthritis and CNS involvement are other manifestations of this rare disease. *(Braunwald, p. 1677)*

287. **(B)** Zollinger–Ellison syndrome is caused by a nonbeta islet cell tumor of the pancreas. It may be associated with the syndrome of multiple endocrine neoplasia, type I (MEN I). The syndrome should be suspected in patients with multiple ulcers, ulcers resistant to therapy, ulcers in unusual locations, strong family history of ulcers, unexplained diarrhea, or evidence of MEN I. *(Braunwald, pp. 1661–1662)*

288. **(D)** Diverticula are present in over 50% of octogenarians. Most patients remain asymptomatic. They are most common in the sigmoid colon and decrease in frequency in the proximal colon. The relative scarcity of diverticula in underdeveloped nations has led to the hypothesis that low-fiber diets result in decreased fecal bulk, narrowing of the colon, and an increased intraluminal pressure to move the small fecal mass. This results in thickening of the muscular coat and eventually herniations or diverticula of the mucosa at the points where nutrient arteries penetrate the muscularis. *(Braunwald, pp. 1695–1696)*

289. **(D)** This presentation is typical of esophageal cancer. Lesions in the upper two thirds of the esophagus are squamous, but in the distal esophagus most are adenocarcinomas. The adenocarcinomas develop more commonly from columnar epithelium in the distal esophagus (Barrett's esophagus). Adenocarcinomas of the esophagus have the biologic behavior of gastric cancers. The incidence of squamous cell cancer of the esophagus is de-creasing while adenocarcinoma is increasing. Currently, over 50% of esophageal cancer is adenocarcinoma. The 5-year survival for esophageal cancer is less than 5%. Combination therapy seems to be more effective than surgery alone. *(Braunwald, pp. 578–579)*

290. **(D)** Fat malabsorption demonstrated on stool collection for 72 hours is the gold standard, but does not indicate the exact cause. The Schilling test is useful in testing for vitamin B_{12} absorption. X-rays can be helpful in diagnosing underlying disorders, but are nonspecific. Small intestinal biopsy is useful in determining the cause of malabsorption. *(Braunwald, p. 1671)*

291. **(A)** The antibody can be demonstrated in 80 to 90% of patients, usually late in convalescence, and indicates relative or absolute immunity. In contrast, HBsAg occurs very early and disappears in less than 6 months. Persistence of HBsAg indicates chronic infection. The pattern in this patient is also seen postvaccination, and perhaps as a consequence of remote infection. *(Braunwald, p. 1731)*

292. **(D)** Gilbert syndrome may be associated with impaired hepatic uptake of bilirubin. It is caused by hereditary decrease in the activity of glucoronosyltransferase in the UGT1 family. More severe enzyme deficits are the cause of the two variants of Crigler–Najjar syndrome. *(Braunwald, pp. 1715–1719)*

293. **(A)** Intestinal polyposis is a possible indication of Peutz–Jeghers syndrome associated with dark brown spots on the lips and palate. There is characteristic distribution of pigment around lips, nose, eyes, and hands. Tumors of the ovary, breast, pancreas, and endometrium are associated with this syndrome. *(Braunwald, pp. 320, 586, 620)*

294. **(B)** Despite some decline, distal tumors are still the most common. The fact that up to 60% of tumors are located in the rectosigmoid is the rationale for screening via flexible, fiberoptic sigmoidoscopes. Occult blood

testing and colonoscopy are other possible screening techniques. *(Braunwald, p. 584)*

295. **(E)** This pattern of symptoms is characteristic of afferent loop syndrome. It is caused by distention and incomplete drainage of the afferent loop and requires surgical correction. Bacterial overgrowth of the afferent loop is more common. Its clinical presentation includes postprandial abdominal pain, bloating, and diarrhea. Fat and vitamin B_{12} malabsorption can occur. *(Braunwald, p. 1660)*

296. **(B)** Hepatoma is the most likely diagnosis in this man. In China, it is estimated that the lifetime risk of hepatoma in people with chronic hepatitis B is close to 40%. AFP elevations over 500 to 1000 mg/L in the absence of a colonic tumor (or pregnancy) suggest hepatoma. Paraneoplastic syndromes are not common but include erythrocytosis, hypercalcemia, and acquired porphyria. *(Braunwald, pp. 588–589)*

297. **(D)** Ascitic fluid in uncomplicated cirrhosis of the liver shows a specific gravity less than 1.016. Protein is less than 25 g/L, and the gross appearance is straw colored. In spontaneous bacterial peritonitis, the fluid may be cloudy and the number of white cells (neutrophils) increased. In uncomplicated ascites, the difference between plasma albumin and ascitic fluid albumin is greater than 1.1 g/dL. *(Braunwald, p. 261)*

298. **(D)** Common duct stones can be painless, or may give rise to severe pain, chills, and fever. The jaundice is generally conjugated hyperbilirubinemia. Partial obstruction of the common duct produces variable amounts of jaundice and is influenced by the presence of concurrent hepatocellular disease or cholangitis. Although most such stones originate in the gallbladder, hemolytic disorders and parasitic infections can result in primary bile duct stones. *(Braunwald, pp. 1780–1781)*

299. **(E)** The syndrome is characteristic of carcinoid of midgut origin. The cardiac lesions are more common on the right side (hence murmur accentuation on deep inspiration). Foregut carcinoids (bronchus, stomach, duodenum) frequently are associated with wheezing. The most important mediator of the carcinoid syndrome is serotonin. Serotonin is rapidly metabolized to 5-HIAA, which is rapidly cleared by the kidneys. The measurement of 5-HIAA in the urine is thus the most useful diagnostic test. Its specificity is enhanced by an appropriate diet before testing. *(Braunwald, pp. 597–598)*

300. **(D)** These findings are characteristic of achalasia. Anticholinergic medications and dietary changes do not provide much help. Successful therapies include nitroglycerine nifedipine (a calcium channel blocker), botulinum toxin injected endoscopically, balloon dilatation, and esophageal myotomy (not excision). *(Braunwald, pp. 1644–1645)*

301. **(B)** These findings are characteristic of scleroderma. If the disease is limited, the prognosis is not necessarily poor. The limited form is characterized by calcinosis, Raynaud's (often with distal ulceration), esophageal motility disorder, sclerodactyly, and telangiectasia. It has a female preponderance. Renal disease can be severe, but is not the most common cause of death. Esophageal symptoms should be treated aggressively. *(Braunwald, p. 1645)*

302. **(B)** The clinical description suggests Ménétrier's disease; however, biopsy is essential to rule out lymphoma or carcinoma. The edema is usually secondary to protein-losing enteropathy. Treatment consists of a high-protein diet, anticholinergic therapy, and H_2 blockers. In some cases, gastrectomy is required. *(Braunwald, p. 1665)*

303. **(E)** The carcinoma has occurred in a patient with ulcerative colitis. The barium enema shows a long, constricting lesion in the transverse colon, with the whole colon devoid of haustral markings. Some pressure effects are seen in the ileum due to metastases. The diagnosis of ulcerative colitis is made from the clinical symptoms and proctosigmoidoscopic examination of an abnormally inflamed

colonic mucosa. *(Braunwald, pp. 1682–1683, 1691–1692)*

304. **(A)** In esophageal varices, the esophageal folds are thick and tortuous, giving rise to a wormy or worm-eaten appearance. The radiographic picture would vary with the severity of the varices, as well as the distention of the esophagus. When varices are severe, they should be appreciated in any projection. The left anterior oblique projection is most ideal for its demonstration. *(Braunwald, pp. 1759–1760)*

305. **(A)** In benign gastric ulcer, an ulcer niche is present in the prepyloric area, with folds radiating to and extending up to the margin of the niche with a halo around it. The differentiation between benignity and malignancy may be difficult at times, but proper use of radiographic criteria could boost the accuracy to 98%. In the presence of an ulcer niche, a Hampton line, which is an ulcer collar, or a mound should be sought on a profile view. Endoscopy with biopsy is the gold standard of diagnosis. *(Braunwald, p. 1655)*

306. **(D)** *H. pylori* infection is the cause of most peptic ulcers, and the usual route of infection is via the water supply. Duodenal ulcer is clinically more common, although the prevalence on autopsy series is similar. Duodenal ulcer does not represent a malignant potential. Gastric ulcers are seen in an older population and can be malignant. Benign peptic gastric ulcers tend to be more distal. *(Braunwald, pp. 1651–1652)*

307. **(D)** Infection usually occurs early in life and is related to classic socioeconomic indicators such as poverty, domestic crowding, unsanitary living conditions, and unclean water. It is much more common in developing countries. *(Braunwald, p. 1652).*

308. **(D)** Concomitant steroid use increases the likelihood of ulceration, as does advanced age. *H. pylori* infection, smoking, and alcohol use are suspected, but not yet established, risk factors. *(Braunwald, p. 1654).*

309. **(E)** NSAIDs inhibit prostaglandins, which play an important role in maintaining gastroduodenal mucosal integrity and repair. *(Braunwald, p. 1653)*

310. **(D)** Eradication of *H. pylori* is the most effective treatment for duodenal ulcer disease. The most popular regimes include antibiotics and acid suppression medications. *(Braunwald, p. 1657)*

311. **(A, B, D)** Specific vaccines are available for hepatitis A and B. Hepatitis D is most frequently symptomatic in association with hepatitis B infection, so vaccination for hepatitis B will decrease the likelihood of symptomatic hepatitis D infection. *(Braunwald, pp. 1735–1736)*

312. **(A, E)** Both hepatitis A and E are usually spread by the fecal–oral route. Other forms of transmission are exceedingly uncommon. *(Braunwald, p. 1728)*

313. **(B, D)** Only hepatitis B and D are frequently spread by sexual transmission. It does not seem to occur with hepatitis E, and the evidence is equivocal for hepatitis A and C. *(Braunwald, p. 1728)*

314. **(C)** Chronic hepatitis C infection occurs in 80 to 90% of patients. About 50 to 70% will have evidence of chronic liver disease. In contrast, only 1 to 10% of adults infected with hepatitis B will go on to chronic infection. *(Braunwald, p. 1728)*

315. **(B, C)** Interferon has been used in both hepatitis B and C infection. The response is better in hepatitis B infection. Combination therapy with interferon and ribavirin is more effective in hepatitis C. *(Braunwald, pp. 1743, 1748)*

316. **(B)** In neonates, the transmission of hepatitis B results in a 90% probability of developing chronic infection. The ongoing infection (often resulting in hepatoma) is a major cause of morbidity and mortality in many parts of the world. *(Braunwald, p. 1728)*

317. **(A, B)** Immunoglobulin injection can provide prophylaxis against hepatitis A, and it is felt that hepatitis B immune globulin is protective for hepatitis B. *(Braunwald, p. 1728)*

318. **(D)** Hepatitis D is a defective ribonucleic acid (RNA) virus that requires the helper function of hepatitis B virus (or other hepadnavirus) for its replication and expression. *(Braunwald, p. 1723)*

319. **(C)** Hyperglycemia is very common in pancreatitis and is usually multifactorial in origin. Factors involved include decreased insulin release, increased glucagon release, and elevated adrenal glucocorticoids and catecholamines. *(Braunwald, p. 1794)*

320. **(D)** The most common causes of acute pancreatitis are alcohol, gallstones, metabolic factors, and drugs. In the United States, alcohol is the most common factor, but in England, gallstones are the number one cause. *(Braunwald, p. 1793)*

321. **(B)** Pancreatitis in AIDS patients can be caused by cytomegalovirus and cryptosporidium as well as *M. avium* complex. Drugs are another cause of AIDS-related pancreatitis. *(Braunwald, p. 1796)*

322. **(C)** Amylase accumulates in the setting of renal failure and thus becomes a less valuable diagnostic test. Numerous other conditions involving the pancreas, the gut, and the salivary glands can raise amylase levels. Sulfonamides cause pancreatitis; therefore, an elevated amylase is not confusing, but rather a useful test for pancreatitis in patients taking the drug. Morphine can elevate amylase levels in the absence of pancreatitis. *(Braunwald, p. 1790)*

323. **(B)** The sclera are high in elastin content, which has an affinity for bilirubin. Therefore, jaundice is usually detected here first. Fluorescent lighting makes recognition more difficult. In some individuals, dark skin color makes jaundice more difficult to detect. *(Braunwald, p. 255)*

324. **(A)** Hemolysis results in predominantly unconjugated bilirubin. Unconjugated hyperbilirubinemia is caused by overproduction, decreased uptake, or decreased conjugation. *(Braunwald, pp. 256–257)*

325. **(E)** Ménétrier's disease, an uncommon disease involving the stomach, is characterized by large gastric folds. Intravenous administration of radioactive-labeled albumin may show up to a 40% loss in the GI tract in protein-losing enteropathy but is not available for routine clinical use. Treatment of protein-losing enteropathy is usually directed at the underlying condition. *(Braunwald, p. 1678)*

326. **(D)** Joint involvement in inflammatory bowel disease may involve sacroilitis or specific large joint peripheral arthritis. The latter type of arthritis parallels the course of the bowel disease. The sacroilitis (spondylitic) variety follows an independent course. *(Braunwald, p. 1687)*

327. **(D)** This likely represents diarrhea secondary to *Clostridium difficile* infection. It is mediated by toxins, not direct bacterial invasion. Cephalosporins, because they are so widely used are the most common cause of the disease. On a per case basis, however, clindamycin is the most likely antibiotic to cause the disease. *(Braunwald, p. 923)*

328. **(E)** The patient with primary biliary cirrhosis is typically a middle-aged woman with itching. Patients are often asymptomatic and diagnosed only on routine blood work. The cause of primary biliary cirrhosis is unknown, but a disordered immune response may be involved. A positive antimitochondrial antibody test is found in over 90% of symptomatic patients. *(Braunwald, p. 1757)*

329. **(B)** There is no known effective therapy to prevent progression of liver disease in primary biliary cirrhosis (PBC). Ursodeoxycholic acid seems effective in providing at least symptomatic improvement. Replacement of fat-soluble vitamins (eg, vitamin A to prevent night blindness) is an important part of therapy. *(Braunwald, p. 1758)*

330. **(B)** Postgastrectomy steatorrhea does not result from mucosal abnormality. The mucosa is also normal in pancreatic steatorrhea. Postgastrectomy maldigestion and malabsorption is caused by rapid gastric emptying, reduced dispersion of food in the stomach, reduced luminal levels of bile, rapid transit of food, and impaired pancreatic secretory response. *(Braunwald, pp. 1660–1661, 1673)*

331. **(A)** The string sign represents long areas of circumferential inflammation and fibrosis. In addition to the string sign, abnormal puddling of barium and fistulous tracts are other helpful x-ray signs of ileitis. Other radiologic findings in Crohn's disease include skip lesions, rectal sparing, small ulcerations, and fistulas. *(Braunwald, pp. 1683–1684)*

332. **(A)** Colonic obstruction usually causes less pain and less vomiting than small bowel obstruction. Fever is usually absent in both. The stepladder pattern is characteristic of small bowel obstruction, as are hiccups. *(Braunwald, pp. 1703–1704)*

333. **(C)** Episodic dysphagia to solids of several years' duration suggests a benign disease and is characteristic of a lower esophageal ring. Motor dysphagia presents with dysphagia to solids and liquids. Dysphagia due to obstruction starts with solids and can progress to liquids as well. Hoarseness following the onset of dysphagia can be caused by an esophageal cancer extending to involve the recurrent laryngeal nerve or because of laryngitis secondary to gastroesophageal reflux. Severe weight loss suggests malignancy, and hiccups are a rare occurrence in distal problems of the esophagus. *(Braunwald, p. 234)*

334. **(E)** Aspiration unrelated to swallowing is seen in a Zenker's diverticulum, achalasia, or gastroesophageal reflex. *(Braunwald, p. 234)*

335. **(D)** Painful swallowing can be caused by candida or herpes infection or pill-induced esophagitis. Patients with immunodeficiency states (eg, AIDS) may have herpetic, candidal, or cytomegalovirus (CMV) esophagitis, as well as tumors (lymphoma, Kaposi's sarcoma). *(Braunwald, p. 235)*

336. **(D)** The history is helpful. The site of obstruction is usually at or below where the patient says the sticking occurs. *(Braunwald, p. 234)*

337. **(B)** Severe chest pain is characteristic of diffuse esophageal spasm and related motor disorders. *(Braunwald, p. 235)*

338. **(E)** Rotor syndrome is one of the two rare inherited disorders causing elevations in direct bilirubin. The other is Dubin–Johnson syndrome, and both have an excellent prognosis. Hemolytic anemia causes elevation in indirect bilirubin, and hematologic changes would be expected. INH causes elevation in liver enzymes, and although Rifampin can cause isolated hyperbilirubinemia, it is of the indirect kind. Crigler–Najjar type I is a severe disorder of neonates with elevated indirect bilirubin. *(Braunwald, pp. 256–257)*

339. **(B)** In alcoholic hepatitis, the AST:ALT ratio is usually greater than 2, and the level of AST is usually less than 300. When viral hepatitis or toxin-induced hepatitis cause jaundice, the AST:ALT ratio is usually 1 or less, and the transaminases are usually greater than 500. *(Braunwald, p. 258)*

340. **(D)** Acetaminophen reliably produces hepatocellular damage when taken in large doses. *(Braunwald, p. 258)*

341. **(B)** An active metabolite of acetaminophen is hepatotoxic. It is detoxified by binding to glutathione, and when hepatic glutathione stores are depleted, severe liver damage can occur. *(Braunwald, p. 1739)*

342. **(D)** N-acetylcysteine probably acts by providing a reservoir of sulfhydryl groups to bind the toxic metabolite of acetaminophen. Narcan is effective for narcotic overdose, and

ethanol is the antidote for methanol intoxication. *(Braunwald, p. 1739)*

343. **(A)** Anabolic steroids usually cause cholestasis and jaundice without inflammation. Sinusoidal dilatation and peliosis occur less frequently, and there have been deaths linked to peliosis. The other medications also cause various types of liver disease, but not peliosis. *(Braunwald, p. 1741)*

344. **(D)** Secretory diarrhea is caused by a derangement in fluid and electrolyte transport across the gut mucosa. The resultant diarrhea is watery, large volume, painless, and persists even when the patient fasts. *(Braunwald, p. 244)*

345. **(A)** Although carcinoid tumor can cause diarrhea, it is very uncommon. This young woman is very slender, suggesting an eating disorder, which is associated with laxative abuse. Abuse of stimulant laxatives such as senna can cause a secretory diarrhea. Magnesium-based laxatives will cause an osmotic diarrhea. *(Braunwald, pp. 244–245, 487)*

346. **(E)** Sugarless gums and candy often contain sorbitol, a sugar that is not absorbed in the gut. It thus produces an osmotic diarrhea if present in sufficient quantity. *(Braunwald, p. 245)*

347. **(A)** His anemia and general appearance are compatible with chronic inflammatory bowel disease as well, but his night blindness suggests vitamin A deficiency which is much more likely in a malabsorption syndrome. *(Braunwald, p. 1679)*

348. **(E)** The osmotic gap is a characteristic of osmotic diarrhea in particular. Stool fat, D-xylose testing, and Schilling tests help establish the diagnosis of malabsorption, but not the etiology. The most common cause of such diffuse malabsorption, celiac disease, has a characteristic biopsy pattern with short or absent villi. Confirmation of the disease requires response to a gluten-free diet. *(Braunwald, pp. 1673–1674)*

349. **(G)** Acute erosive gastritis is most commonly seen in critically ill hospitalized patients. Ischemia of the gastric mucosa with breakdown of the normal protective barriers of the stomach is a key factor in the syndrome. *(Braunwald, p. 1663)*

350. **(B)** Type B chronic gastritis is the more common cause of chronic gastritis. It becomes more common with advancing age and is uniformly associated with *H. pylori* infection. Eradication of *H. pylori* produces histologic improvement, but is not routinely recommended unless peptic ulcer or mucosa-associated lymphoid tissue (MALT) lymphoma occurs. *(Braunwald, p. 1664)*

351. **(A)** Type A chronic gastritis may lead to pernicious anemia. Antibodies to parietal cells and to intrinsic factor are frequently seen in the sera, suggesting an immune or autoimmune pathogenesis. *(Braunwald, pp. 1663–1664)*

352. **(C)** Ménétrier's disease is not a true gastritis, as inflammation is not present on histologic examination. It is characterized by large, tortuous gastric mucosal folds and usually presents with abdominal pain. Protein-losing enteropathy often develops, resulting in hypoalbuminemia and edema. *(Braunwald, p. 1665)*

353. **(F)** Gastric surgery seems to accelerate the development of asymptomatic gastritis with progressive parietal cell loss. However, some patients develop bile reflux gastritis with symptoms of pain, nausea, and vomiting. *(Braunwald, p. 1660)*

CHAPTER 5

Hematology
Questions

DIRECTIONS (Questions 354 through 359): Each of the numbered items or incomplete statements in this section is followed by answers or by completions of the statement. Select the ONE lettered answer or completion that is BEST in each case.

354. During the winter months, a 65-year-old man presents with livedo reticularis and purple fingertips. Other symptoms include arthralgia and weakness. Renal impairment is present on laboratory testing. The most likely diagnosis is

    (A) cold agglutinin disease
    (B) Henoch–Schönlein purpura
    (C) antiphospholipid antibody syndrome
    (D) cryoglobulinemia
    (E) cholesterol embolic disease

355. The syndrome in the above question is caused by

    (A) breakdown of erythrocytes
    (B) medium vessel vasculitis
    (C) aggregation of abnormal platelets
    (D) temperature-dependent antibodies
    (E) cold-precipitable proteins

356. A 34-year-old man develops acute myeloblastic leukemia (AML). This disease is generally characterized by

    (A) peak incidence in childhood
    (B) high leukocyte alkaline phosphatase
    (C) Philadelphia chromosome
    (D) Auer bodies in blast cells
    (E) response to vincristine and prednisone

357. A 62-year-old man is found to have a left upper quadrant (LUQ) abdominal mass, and lab tests reveal a total white blood count of 50,000. This includes granulocytes at all stages of development. Cytogenic studies are likely to reveal

    (A) deletion of chromosome 14
    (B) reciprocal translocation of 9 and 22
    (C) translocation of the renal artery stenosis (RAS) oncogene
    (D) trisomy 21
    (E) translocation of 8 to 14

358. A patient with aplastic anemia receives a bone marrow transplant from a human lymphocyte antigen (HLA)-matched sister. The most likely complication will be

    (A) graft-versus-host disease
    (B) graft failure
    (C) radiation sickness
    (D) development of leukemia
    (E) secondary skin cancer

359. A 19-year-old man has had recurrent hemarthrosis. The symptoms of hemophilia A are associated with

    (A) normal immunoreactive factor VIII
    (B) normal functional factor VIII
    (C) decreased immunoreactive factor VIII
    (D) prolonged bleeding time
    (E) platelet function abnormality

DIRECTIONS (Questions 360 through 366): Each set of matching questions in this section consists of a list of lettered options followed by several numbered items. For each numbered item, select the appropriate lettered option(s). Each lettered option may be selected once, more than once, or not at all. EACH ITEM WILL STATE THE NUMBER OF OPTIONS TO SELECT. CHOOSE EXACTLY THIS NUMBER.

Questions 360 and 361

(A) secondary hyperthyroidism

(B) rectal cancer

(C) antibodies to Epstein–Barr virus

(D) heterophil antibodies

(E) hypernephroma

(F) rheumatoid factor

(G) normal liver enzymes

(H) cerebellar hemangioma

(I) glioblastoma multiforme

(J) antibodies to sheep red cells

360. A 63-year-old man is found to have an elevated hemoglobin of 20.5, normal white blood count, and normal platelet count. There is no palpable spleen. This syndrome might be secondary to (SELECT TWO)

361. A 19-year-old college student develops a severe sore throat, cervical lymphadenopathy, and atypical lymphocytes on blood film. Other characteristics of this syndrome include (SELECT THREE)

Questions 362 and 363

(A) increased target cells

(B) bone pain

(C) osteoblastic bone lesions

(D) increased spleen size

(E) her fertility is impaired

(F) Bence Jones proteinuria

(G) increased osmotic fragility

(H) type III cryoglobulin

(I) marrow hyperplasia

(J) increased plasma cells in bone marrow

362. A 19-year-old woman is found to be homozygous for hemoglobin C (SELECT THREE)

363. A 74-year-old woman with anemia is found to have an immunoglobulin G (IgG) spike on serum protein electrophoresis (SELECT THREE)

Questions 364 through 366

(A) decreased red cell survival

(B) thalassemia

(C) postsplenectomy

(D) increased numbers of reticulocytes

(E) thiamine deficiency

(F) acute hemorrhage

(G) low fecal urobilinogen

(H) pyridoxine deficiency

(I) immediate postoperative period

(J) acute lymphocytic leukemia

(K) iron deficiency

(L) increased urine urobilinogen

364. A 49-year-old woman is suspected of having hemolysis, which could be associated with (SELECT THREE)

365. A 69-year-old man is found to have a hypochromic microcytic anemia. This could be associated with (SELECT THREE)

366. A 72-year-old woman has a platelet count of 1,200,000. This can be associated with (SELECT FOUR)

DIRECTIONS (Questions 367 through 379): Each of the numbered items or incomplete statements in this section is followed by answers or by completions of the statement. Select the ONE lettered answer or completion that is BEST in each case.

367. A 7-year-old boy with homozygous betathalassemia requires frequent transfusions. The regimen should also include

(A) oral calcium supplements

(B) fresh frozen plasma

(C) desferrioxamine

(D) penicillamine

(E) cryoprecipitate

368. A 67-year-old man has platelets over 1 million. The diagnosis of essential thrombocythemia rather than reactive thrombocytosis would be favored by the presence of

(A) increased megakaryocyte number

(B) increased total platelet mass

(C) increased platelet turnover

(D) normal platelet survival

(E) thromboembolism and hemorrhage

369. A 19-year-old man is found to have a decreased eosinophil count. Which of the following is the most likely cause?

(A) asthma

(B) contact dermatitis

(C) yeast infection

(D) mycobacterial infection

(E) prednisone administration

370. A 68-year-old man with aplastic anemia has had fever with transfusions. Filtered blood can be used to reduce the likelihood of fever by limiting the transfusion of

(A) non-A, non-B hepatitis

(B) acquired immune deficiency syndrome (AIDS)

(C) malaria

(D) leukocytes

(E) reticulocytes

371. An infant is found to have sickle cell disease. Which of the following is most likely?

(A) reduced adult height

(B) splenomegaly postpuberty

(C) low reticulocyte count

(D) shortened erythrocyte life span

(E) symptoms improved in patients with low hemoglobin (Hb) F concentrations

372. A 59-year-old man taking ticlopidine for recurrent transient ischemic attacks (TIAs) is most likely to have hemolysis from

(A) thermal injury

(B) isoantibodies

(C) autoantibodies

(D) red cell fragmentation

(E) hemoglobinopathy

373. A 23-year-old woman has a decrease in plasma antithrombin III levels. Her most likely clinical presentation will be with

(A) aspirin sensitivity

(B) heparin resistance

(C) warfarin (Coumadin) resistance

(D) platelet dysfunction

(E) disseminated intravascular coagulation

374. A 4-month-old infant is anemic. The most likely cause for this is

(A) inadequate diet

(B) hemolysis

(C) late clamping of cord

(D) malabsorption

(E) folate deficiency

375. The presence of increased levels of 2,3-BPG in the red cell is associated with

(A) hemolytic anemia due to sulfa drugs

(B) increased oxygen affinity

(C) decreased oxygen affinity

(D) loss of red cell energy

(E) multiple congenital abnormalities

376. A 63-year-old man has group AB blood. He requires an emergency transfusion. Which of the following statements is correct?

(A) He is a universal recipient.

(B) He has anti-A and anti-B in his serum.

(C) If a cross-match is not available, group O, Rh-positive red blood cells are universal.

(D) If insufficient AB blood is available, type A can be used.

(E) If insufficient AB blood is available, type B can be used.

377. Figure 5–1A and B are the x-rays of a 60-year-old white man with pain in the right chest. What is the most likely diagnosis?

(A) aneurysmal bone cyst

(B) multiple myeloma

(C) lymphosarcoma

(D) prostatic metastases

(E) hyperparathyroidism

378. Figure 5–2 is an x-ray of a 30-year-old black woman with recurrent abdominal pain and pallor. What is the most likely diagnosis?

(A) sickle-cell anemia

(B) thalassemia

(C) acute lymphoblastic leukemia

(D) promyelocytic leukemia

(E) multiple myeloma

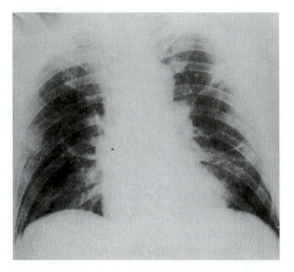

Figure 5–1A.

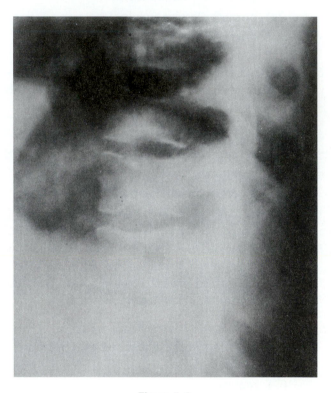

Figure 5–2.

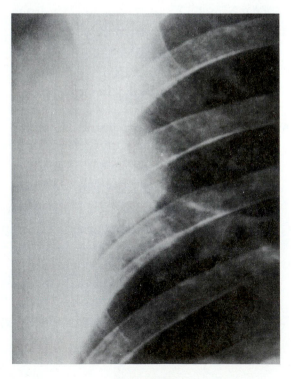

Figure 5–1B.

379. The case workup shown in Table 5–1 is that of a 30-year-old woman presenting with a hemoglobin of 6.0 g/100 mL. The most likely diagnosis is

(A) iron deficiency

(B) congenital spherocytosis

(C) liver failure and hemolysis

(D) splenomegaly and hemolysis

(E) autoimmune hemolytic anemia

TABLE 5–1. CASE WORKUP

Blood film	Polychromatophilia, some spherocytes
Bilirubin	2 mg/100 mL total
	0.3 mg/100 mL direct
Haptoglobin	10 mg/100 mL
Lactate dehydrogenase	200 IU/L
Urine bilirubin	Negative

DIRECTIONS (Questions 380 through 389): Each set of matching questions in this section consists of a list of lettered options followed by several numbered items. For each numbered item, select the appropriate lettered option(s). Each lettered option may be selected once, more than once, or not at all. EACH ITEM WILL STATE THE NUMBER OF OPTIONS TO SELECT. CHOOSE EXACTLY THIS NUMBER.

Questions 380 through 381

(A) aspirin

(B) naproxen

(C) tirofiban

(D) trimethoprim-sulfamethoxazole

(E) clopidogrel

(F) fish oils

(G) systemic lupus

(H) uremia

Match the mechanism of prolonged bleeding time below with the most likely cause above.

380. Impairs fibrinogen binding to its receptor (SELECT ONE)

381. Depletes platelet arachidonic acid (SELECT ONE)

Questions 382 through 386

(A) beta-thalassemia major

(B) HbH disease

(C) sickle-cell disease

(D) HbC disease

(E) HbM disease

382. Hemoglobin turns into a firm gel when hypoxic (SELECT ONE)

383. A mild hemolytic anemia with intra-erythrocytic crystals seen on fixed blood smears (SELECT ONE)

384. May result from defect in processing of globin messenger ribonucleic acid (RNA) (SELECT ONE)

385. Decreased alpha-chain production leads to four-beta-chain tetramer formation (SELECT ONE)

386. Bone infarction can occur that may be difficult to distinguish from osteomyelitis (SELECT ONE)

Questions 387 through 389

(A) loss of Achilles tendon reflex

(B) increased perioperative morbidity

(C) renal concentration defect

(D) helmet cells and schistocytes are common

(E) occurs most commonly in the first trimester

(F) constipation

(G) cardiac arrhythmias

(H) increased HbH

(I) responds to folic acid

(J) more common in epileptics

(K) paresthesias

387. A 63-year-old woman with lymphoma has been treated with vincristine for many months (SELECT THREE)

388. A 19-year-old girl is positive for sickle-cell trait (SELECT ONE)

389. A 24-year-old pregnant woman is found to be anemic (SELECT TWO)

DIRECTIONS (Questions 390 through 412): Each of the numbered items or incomplete statements in this section is followed by answers or by completions of the statement. Select the ONE lettered answer or completion that is BEST in each case.

390. A 32-year-old woman has had a previous child with beta-thalassemia. She has just been confirmed as being 6 weeks pregnant. Prenatal diagnosis would be best accomplished by

   (A) fetal ultrasound at 12 weeks
   (B) cord blood electrophoresis
   (C) chorionic villus sampling
   (D) buccal mucosal cytology of both parents
   (E) electrophoresis of amniotic fluid

391. Hemolytic disease of the newborn (erythroblastosis fetalis) due to Rh incompatibility is usually associated with

   (A) a positive direct Coombs' test using the mother's red blood cells
   (B) toxemia of pregnancy
   (C) a negative direct Coombs' test using the baby's red blood cells
   (D) simultaneous ABO incompatibility
   (E) a more severe course than hemolysis secondary to ABO compatibility

392. A 63-year-old woman is found to have hairy cell leukemia. The preferred treatment is

   (A) cytosine arabinoside
   (B) alpha-interferon
   (C) cladribine
   (D) interleukin-3 (IL-3)
   (E) retinoic acid

393. A 22-year-old long-distance runner is found to be mildly anemic. He is asymptomatic. His stool is intermittently positive for occult blood. Which intervention is most likely to result in return of the hemoglobin to normal?

   (A) using more supportive footwear
   (B) iron replacement
   (C) folate replacement
   (D) altering his exercise program
   (E) investigating and treating gastrointestinal (GI) pathology

394. A 22-year-old medical student donates his blood to a lab experiment and he is discovered to have persistent HbF. He feels well. This syndrome is a(n)

   (A) cause of sickling red cells
   (B) disease of infants only
   (C) variant of thalassemia major
   (D) anemia exacerbated by fava beans
   (E) benign genetic abnormality

395. A 19-year-old man had his spleen removed a year ago after a motorcycle accident. His blood film is likely to show

   (A) increase in macrophages
   (B) leukopenia
   (C) polycythemia
   (D) Pappenheimer bodies
   (E) red cells with nuclear fragments

396. A 69-year-old trauma victim is transfused with type O "universal donor" cells. A possible danger in this practice may be

   (A) type O donors have a higher incidence of hepatitis C virus
   (B) type O donors have a shorter survival time when transfused than do other cell types
   (C) at times, type B blood may be mistyped as type O
   (D) type O donors may have high titers of anti-A and anti-B in their plasma
   (E) conversion of the recipient to type O blood

397. A young child presents with petechiae and bone pain. Blood film reveals neutropenia and leukemic lymphoblasts. The most important adverse prognostic factor is

   (A) age of 7
   (B) male gender
   (C) splenomegaly
   (D) total platelet count
   (E) systemic symptoms

Questions 398 through 402

A 50-year-old white woman presents with a 3-week history of tiredness and pallor. A family member has noted some yellowness of her eyes, but she denies darkening of the urine. Physical examination reveals only slight jaundice. Laboratory data include an Hb of 9 g, reticulocyte count of 12%, a bilirubin in the serum of 2 mg/dL indirect reacting, and some microspherocytes on peripheral smear.

398. The most likely cause of this woman's anemia is

 (A) blood loss externally
 (B) decreased red cell production
 (C) ineffective erythropoiesis
 (D) intravascular hemolysis
 (E) extravascular hemolysis

399. Spherocytosis may be commonly found with which of the following?

 (A) multiple long-bone fracture
 (B) hereditary elliptocytosis
 (C) Coombs'-positive hemolytic anemia
 (D) glucose-6-phosphate dehydrogenase (G6PD) deficiency
 (E) leukemia

400. Which of the following may be expected in this case?

 (A) increased haptoglobin level
 (B) increased bilirubin in the urine
 (C) increased urobilinogen in the stool
 (D) increased myoglobin in the blood
 (E) increased hemopexin in the blood

401. Bone marrow examination is most likely to show

 (A) megaloblastic changes
 (B) giant metamyelocytes
 (C) increased erythroid-to-myeloid ratio
 (D) increased lymphocytes
 (E) shift to left of the myeloid series

402. Autoimmune causation of this condition would be confirmed by

 (A) positive antinuclear antibody (ANA)
 (B) positive rheumatoid factor
 (C) polyclonal gammopathy
 (D) presence of Heinz bodies
 (E) positive Coombs' test

Questions 403 through 407

A 57-year-old man with a history of chronic alcohol ingestion is admitted to the hospital with acute alcoholic intoxication and lobar pneumonia. Physical examination reveals pallor; a large, tender liver; and consolidation of the right lower lobe. Laboratory data include an Hb of 7 g, white blood count (WBC) of 4000, and platelet count of 85,000.

403. The most likely factor for the anemia is

 (A) hemolysis
 (B) hemobilia
 (C) vitamin B_{12} deficiency
 (D) toxic marrow suppression
 (E) hemoglobinopathy

404. The most likely vitamin deficiency related to the pancytopenia is

 (A) B_{12}
 (B) folate
 (C) pyridoxine
 (D) thiamine
 (E) riboflavin

405. Toxic marrow suppression is most likely to affect

 (A) developing erythrocytes and myelocytes
 (B) mature polymorphonuclear leukocytes
 (C) mature red cells
 (D) mature platelets
 (E) eosinophils

406. Examination of the peripheral smear might show

 (A) a dimorphic pattern
 (B) basophilia
 (C) red cell fragments
 (D) increased platelet adhesiveness
 (E) atypical lymphocytes

407. A deficiency of coagulation factors in this patient would most likely include factors

(A) V and VIII
(B) VIII, IX, XI, and XII
(C) XIII
(D) II, V, VII, and X
(E) I, V, and VIII

Questions 408 through 412

An 18-year-old man of Italian extraction is found to have a hypochromic microcytic anemia of 10% g. In addition, there is a fair degree of anisocytosis, poikilocytosis, and targeting on smear. The WBC is 9500, the platelet count is 240,000, and the reticulocyte count is 7%. The spleen is palpated 5 cm below the left costal margin.

408. The most likely diagnosis is

(A) sickle-cell trait
(B) thalassemia minor
(C) HbS-C disease
(D) sideroblastic anemia
(E) hereditary spherocytosis

409. Which of the following would be most helpful in distinguishing this case from one of pure iron deficiency anemia?

(A) peripheral blood smear
(B) osmotic fragility test
(C) Ham test
(D) Hb electrophoresis on paper
(E) serum ferritin determination

410. One would expect to find which of the following in this man?

(A) an increased amount of fetal or HbA_2
(B) increased osmotic fragility of the red cells
(C) absent bone marrow iron
(D) increased macroglobulins in the serum
(E) small amounts of HbS

411. The present treatment of choice for this man is

(A) splenectomy
(B) removal of the abnormal Hb pigment
(C) purely supportive
(D) plasmapheresis
(E) intramuscular iron

412. A 28-year-old man originally from West Africa is found on routine exam to have splenomegaly. His hemoglobin is 9.5 g/dL and blood film examination reveals target cells. The likely abnormal hemoglobin is

(A) HbM
(B) HbS
(C) Hb Zurich
(D) HbC
(E) Hb Barts

DIRECTIONS (Questions 413 through 426): Each set of matching questions in this section consists of a list of lettered options followed by several numbered items. For each numbered item, select the appropriate lettered option(s). Each lettered option may be selected once, more than once, or not at all. EACH ITEM WILL STATE THE NUMBER OF OPTIONS TO SELECT. CHOOSE EXACTLY THIS NUMBER.

Questions 413 through 417

A 42-year-old man is feeling chronically fatigued. His hemoglobin is 11.5 g/dL and the blood film is hypochromic and microcytic

(A) iron deficiency anemia
(B) beta-thalassemia trait
(C) anemia of chronic disease
(D) sideroblastic anemia

413. Serum iron increased, total iron-binding capacity (TIBC) normal, ferritin increased, HbA_2 normal (SELECT ONE)

414. Serum iron normal, TIBC normal, ferritin normal, HbA_2 elevated (SELECT ONE)

415. Serum iron decreased, TIBC increased, ferritin decreased, HbA$_2$ normal (SELECT ONE)

416. Serum iron decreased, TIBC decreased, serum ferritin increased, HbA$_2$ normal (SELECT ONE)

417. Generally requires a bone marrow aspiration for definitive diagnosis (SELECT ONE)

Questions 418 through 422

(A) spherocytes
(B) schistocytes
(C) sickle cells
(D) burr cells
(E) agglutinated cells
(F) Heinz bodies

418. Found in severe liver disease (SELECT ONE)

419. Represent precipitated Hb (SELECT ONE)

420. Caused by loss of red cell membrane (SELECT ONE)

421. Caused by polymerization of an abnormal Hb (SELECT ONE)

422. Caused by trauma to red cell membranes (SELECT ONE)

Questions 423 through 426

(A) most common inherited bleeding disorder
(B) factor VIII is implicated in the pathogenesis of the disease
(C) prolonged bleeding time
(D) normal bleeding time
(E) inherited on the X chromosome
(F) can be caused by an infection
(G) bleeding caused by vessel wall damage

423. Von Willebrand's disease (SELECT THREE)

424. Hemophilia A (SELECT THREE)

425. Hemophilia B (SELECT TWO)

426. Thrombotic thrombocyclopenic purpura (TTP) (SELECT TWO)

Answers and Explanations

354. **(D)** The symptoms are typical of cryoglobulinemia. Cold agglutinin disease would present with hemolytic anemia. The other syndromes would not generally be temperature sensitive. *(Beutler, p. 1611)*

355. **(E)** The syndrome is caused by cold-precipitable proteins (cryoglobulins) that are found in plasma or serum. These cryoproteins can be single component (immunoglobulin G, M, or A [IgG, IgM, IgA]) or mixed (usually IgG molecules complexed with IgM molecules having anti-IgG reactivity). The single component cryoglobulins can be type I (no antibody activity against other immunoglobulins) or type II (antibody activity against other immunoglobulins). Mixed cryoglobulinemia is called type III. *(Beutler, p. 1611)*

356. **(D)** Auer bodies are slender, pink, staining rods containing lysozyme and are exclusively seen in AML. Although similar to normal azurophilic granules in content and staining properties, they are distinguished by their gigantic size. Special stains can enhance the detection of Auer bodies. They are only seen in a minority of cases. *(Beutler, p. 1050)*

357. **(B)** This is a case of chronic myelogenous leukemia. The reciprocal translocation involves the long arms of 22 and 9, and results in translocation of the ABL proto-oncogene from chromosome 9 adjacent to a portion of the BCR gene on chromosome 22. The resultant abnormal chromosome 22 is known as the Philadelphia (Ph^1) chromosome. *(Beutler, pp. 117–118)*

358. **(A)** Graft-versus-host disease is a frequent complication of hematopoietic cell transplantation. It is caused by a reaction of immunologically competent donor derived T cells that react with recipient tissue antigens. It can be acute or chronic. Numerous treatment regimens involving methotrexate, glucocorticoids, cyclosporine, and other drugs are used in treatment. *(Beutler, pp. 229–231)*

359. **(A)** Antibodies to factor VIII may detect normal quantities in hemophilia A, but function of the molecule is abnormal. The activated partial thromboplastin time (APTT) is prolonged, and the prothrombin consumption test is abnormal. The prothrombin time, thrombin clotting time, and bleeding time are usually normal. *(Beutler, pp. 1639, 1646)*

360. **(E, H)** Hypernephroma, cerebellar hemangiomas, hepatoma, and giant uterine myomas are the tumors associated with secondary polycythemia. Endocrine disorders, hypoxia, and high-affinity hemoglobins can also cause secondary polycythemia. *(Beutler, pp. 690–692)*

361. **(C, D, J)** Presence of rheumatoid factor is not characteristic of infectious mononucleosis. Heterophil antibodies react against sheep red cells and are not absorbed out by guinea pig kidney. In 90% of cases, liver enzymes are elevated. Examination of the blood film reveals a lymphocytosis with atypical lymphocytes. *(Beutler, p. 1013)*

362. **(A, D, I)** Homozygous C red cells are often target-shaped with "extra" membrane to make them more resistant to osmotic fragility. However, cells containing principally HbC are more rigid than normal and their fragmentation in the circulation may result in microspherocytes. Intracellular crystals and oxygenated HbC can be seen. The spleen is invariably enlarged. Women can become pregnant and tolerate the pregnancy well. *(Beutler, pp. 570, 594–595)*

363. **(B, F, J)** Bone lesions in myeloma are destructive, but the alkaline phosphatase is usually normal, indicating little blastic activity. Osteolysis, when combined with immobilization, can lead to hypercalcemia. It is usually mediated by osteoclast activating factor from neoplastic myeloma cells in the adjacent marrow. Bone pain can be severe. Bence Jones proteinuria and myeloma cells in the marrow are typical. If cryoglobulinemia occurs, it is type I. *(Beutler, pp. 1279–1287)*

364. **(A, D, L)** Hemolytic anemias are not associated with erythroid hypoplasia of the marrow. Erythroid hyperplasia is present except during infections or insults that lead to aregenerative crises. As a result, there is usually an increased number of reticulocytes and elevated fecal and urinary urobilinogen. Decreased red blood cell (RBC) survival is a hallmark of the disease. *(Beutler, pp. 438, 641–642)*

365. **(B, H, K)** Microcytic hypochromic anemias are caused by disorders of iron, globin, heme, or porphyrin metabolism and are not seen in thiamine deficiency. Thiamine has been implicated in a rare megaloblastic anemia in children. The biochemistry is not understood. The small cells in spherocytosis are not hypochromic. *(Beutler, pp. 454, 565, 722–723)*

366. **(C, D, F, K)** Postsplenectomy thrombocytosis usually resolves within 2 months. Both acute blood loss and chronic iron deficiency can increase platelets. Hemolytic anemia is associated with both increased reticulocytes and thrombocytosis. Thromboembolic or hemorrhagic phenomena are more common in essential thrombocytosis rather than secondary causes. *(Beutler, pp. 1542–1543)*

367. **(C)** Iron chelation with desferrioxamine will reduce the toxicity from iron overload if given regularly in high doses. The most lethal toxicity of iron load is iron infiltration of the myocardium, with resultant dysfunction and death. *(Beutler, p. 571)*

368. **(E)** Reactive thrombocytosis is usually transitory, without thromboembolism, hemorrhage, splenomegaly, or leukocytosis. Causes of secondary thrombocytosis include chronic inflammatory disorders (eg, rheumatoid arthritis), acute inflammatory disease, acute or chronic blood loss, and malignancy. Recovery from thrombocytopenia ("rebound") can also result in very high platelets. A common cause is withdrawal from alcohol. *(Beutler, pp. 1542–1543)*

369. **(E)** Steroids cause decreased numbers of eosinophils to circulate, so that eosinophilia may be seen in Addison's disease, for example. Beta blockers may cause eosinophilia by blocking beta-adrenergic eosinopenia. Atopic and nonatopic chronic asthma are frequently associated with mild eosinophilia. Numerous allergic diseases, allergic rhinitis, atopic dermatitis, and urticaria can also cause eosinophilia. Parasites are the most common worldwide cause of eosinophilia, but other infections rarely cause it. *(Beutler, pp. 790–791, 794)*

370. **(D)** Febrile reactions to leukocytes may be severe and cause hypotension, especially in repeatedly transfused patients. Antibodies to platelets can also develop. Usually, at least seven transfusions are required to induce sensitization. *(Beutler, p. 1886)*

371. **(D)** Because sickle cell anemia is a chronic hemolytic anemia, the reticulocyte is chronically elevated, except in aplastic crises, and erythrocyte life span is shortened. Infection is the most common precipitant of an aplastic crisis, particularly those caused by parvovirus B19. Adult height is normal and, although splenomegaly is prominent in childhood, fibrosis supervenes by adulthood, resulting in a normal or small spleen. The

milder expression of sickle cell disease in Saudi Arabia is not well understood, but might be related to the alpha-thalassemia gene. *(Beutler, pp. 583, 586)*

372. **(D)** The antiplatelet drug ticlopidine has been associated with TTP. The microangiopathic anemia of TTP is characterized by red cell fragments, and a low haptoglobin level and elevated lactic dehydrogenase (LDH). Plasma and urinary hemoglobin levels may also be increased. *(Beutler, pp. 623–625)*

373. **(B)** Heparin appears to act as catalyst in the inactivation of thrombin and factors XA, IXA, XIA, and by antithrombin III. However, not all patients with thrombosis and heparin resistance have antithrombin III deficiency. *(Beutler, pp. 1703–1704)*

374. **(A)** Iron deficiency is the most common cause of anemia in infancy. Sixty percent of body iron concentration at birth is contained in circulating Hb. Milk is a poor source of iron, so the most common cause of iron deficiency in infancy is prolonged breast or bottle feeding. Cereals are high in iron content. *(Beutler, pp. 449–450)*

375. **(C)** The 2,3-BPG binds to the central cavity of the heme molecule and changes the configuration in favor of oxygen release. The other common factors that affect oxygen affinity are temperature and pH. The oxygen affinity of Hb is easily characterized by the P_{50}; the oxygen tension at which Hb is half saturated. *(Beutler, pp. 349–350)*

376. **(D)** Group AB has neither anti-A nor anti-B, as both A and B antigens are on the red cells. It is a rare blood group (only 2 to 3% of population); if large amounts of blood are required in an AB individual, A type blood can be used, as anti-B in the donor plasma rarely destroys AB cells. It would still be preferable to remove the plasma and use packed red cells. If donor O blood is used, significant hemolysis can occur unless donor plasma is removed. *(Beutler, pp. 1855–1856)*

377. **(B)** There is lytic destruction of the sixth rib with a pathologic fracture and an extrapleural mass. The most common manifestation of multiple myeloma is multiple, "punched-out" lesions in the flat and tubular bones. Some may appear as a discrete lytic lesion and remain as a solitary lesion. *(Beutler, pp. 1283–1285)*

378. **(A)** The diagnosis is sickle-cell anemia. There is a biconcave appearance or configuration of the vertebral bodies, giving rise to a "fish mouth" appearance. Some sclerotic changes are seen. *(Beutler, pp. 586–587)*

379. **(E)** Autoimmune hemolytic anemia is the most likely diagnosis. Spherocytosis is seen as well in burn victims, in microangiopathic hemolysis, and in congenital spherocytosis. *(Beutler, pp. 641–642)*

380. **(E)** Clopidogrel impairs the binding of fibrinogen to the GPIIb/IIIa platelet receptor. This results in a prolongation of bleeding time that is greater than that produced by acetylsalicylic acid (ASA). The effects last for 4 to 10 days after discontinuation. Clopidogrel is a prodrug that relies on an active metabolite for its effect, and might be more effective than ASA. The effect on bleeding time is additive to that of ASA. *(Beutler, pp. 1591–1592)*

381. **(F)** Fish oils cause a slight prolongation of the bleeding time. The mechanism is twofold: they reduce platelet arachidonic acid, and as well they compete with arachidonic acid for cyclo-oxygenase. Other foods that may effect platelet function include garlic, onions, and black tree fungus (found in Chinese cuisine). *(Beutler, p. 1766)*

382. **(C)** A number of factors influence the rate and degree of HbS aggregation, including concentration of S in the cell, cellular dehydration, and the length of time in deoxy conformation. *(Beutler, pp. 582–583)*

383. **(D)** The patients with homozygous HbC disease have mild hemolysis, splenomegaly, target cells, and HbC crystals. Unlike sickle-cell disease, the prognosis is favorable. *(Beutler, p. 595)*

384. **(A)** In one class of beta-thalassemia (beta-plus), there is a mutation that affects processing of the beta-globin messenger RNA precursor. *(Beutler, p. 582)*

385. **(B)** Hemoglobin H most commonly results from the compound heterozygous state for alpha-plus-thalassemia and either deletion or nondeletion alpha-plus-thalassemia. However, the phenotypic expression of the disease is quite variable. *(Beutler, pp. 559, 567, 572)*

386. **(C)** If the bone infarction occurs in proximity to a joint, an effusion can develop. The underlying pathology is a vaso-occlusive phenomenon. *(Beutler, pp. 586–587)*

387. **(A, F, K)** Neurotoxicity is the dose-limiting side effect of vincristine. Neurologic toxicity is usually the result of a cumulative dose and usually begins when the total dose exceeds 6 mg/m^2. Paresthesia of fingers and feet and loss of deep tendon reflexes are the usual initial manifestation. Continual administration may lead to severe motor weakness, particularly in the elderly. Constipation is the result of autonomic neuropathy. Syndrome of inappropriate diuretic hormone (SIADH) with hyponatremia can occur. *(Beutler, pp. 191–192)*

388. **(C)** The renal concentrating defect and positive sickle prep are constant, but occlusive phenomena and hematuria may occur under stress. In sickle-cell trait, more than half the hemoglobin is HbA. Thus, the cells are resistant to sickling until an oxygen tension of about 15 mm Hg. There is no evidence for increased perioperative morbidity. In general, sickle-cell trait adds little, if any, increase in morbidity and mortality to affected individuals. *(Beutler, pp. 587, 594)*

389. **(I, J)** The megaloblastic anemia of pregnancy is the most common of all folate deficient states. Dilutional anemia and iron deficiency also occur in pregnancy. In pregnancy, a low Hb concentration may simply be due to a disproportionate increase in plasma volume, rather than a true anemia. The exact hormonal mechanism is unknown. Folate levels fall during pregnancy; therefore, frank deficiency is most common in the third trimester. Anticonvulsants may impair folate absorption, and folate deficiency is associated with fetal neural tube defects. *(Beutler, pp. 428–429)*

390. **(C)** Chorionic villus sampling in the first trimester with deoxyribonucleic acid (DNA)-based diagnosis has a high degree of accuracy. Cord blood electrophoresis is suitable for screening high-risk infants at birth. *(Beutler, p. 573)*

391. **(E)** This condition is usually associated with a positive Coombs' test using the baby's RBCs and a positive indirect Coombs' test using the mother's serum. Prevention of Rh immunization by the administration of Rh antibody (via Rh immune globulin) has been an effective preventive measure for this disorder. ABO hemolytic disease of the newborn is clinically mild because the antigens are not fully expressed in utero. *(Beutler, pp. 666–668)*

392. **(C)** Purine analogues such as cladribine produce complete remissions in hairy cell leukemia. Recombinant alpha-interferon is not as effective. The disease is characterized by "hairy" cells in blood and bone marrow, splenomegaly, and pancytopenia. *(Beutler, pp. 1195–1199)*

393. **(D)** Supportive footwear will decrease the likelihood of "march" hemolysis, but this rarely causes anemia. Similarly, although 20% of long-distance runners have GI blood loss, this is rarely of a magnitude to explain anemia. Most elite athletes have increases in both plasma volume and red cell mass, but the increase in plasma volume is greater, resulting in a dilutional-type anemia. This is physiologically beneficial (increased O_2 transport with increased blood fluidity), so there is no reason to cease exercising to correct the Hb. *(Beutler, p. 627)*

394. **(E)** HbF is evenly distributed among red cells, unlike the increased F in other conditions. It is a heterogeneous condition, and can be classified into deletion and nondeletion forms. Clinically, it can have features similar to mild thalassemia. *(Beutler, p. 548)*

395. **(E)** The spleen normally functions to pit nuclei and their fragments from red cells. These nuclear fragments are called Howell–Jolly bodies. The spleen has immune functions and filter functions. It also enhances iron reutilization and acts as a reservoir and blood-volume regulator. In disease states, it can be a site of extramedullary hematopoiesis. *(Beutler, pp. 683–685)*

396. **(D)** Anti-A and anti-B in the donor plasma are usually absorbed in the recipient's tissues but have the capacity to harm recipient cells. *(Beutler, p. 1885)*

397. **(B)** In acute lymphoblastic leukemia (ALL), age under 1 or over 9, male gender, and, in adults, high white counts are all adverse prognostic indicators. The better prognosis for females remains in adults with ALL, but is less marked. It is the most common malignancy in children under age 15 in the United States, accounting for 25% of all cancers in white children. It is less common in black children. *(Beutler, pp. 1141–1143)*

398. **(E)** Extravascular hemolysis usually occurs in the liver, spleen, or other reticuloendothelial sites and liberates unconjugated bilirubin. Intrinsic causes of hemolytic anemia are usually inherited and are a result of abnormalities of membranes, red cell enzymes, globins, or heme. Extrinsic hemolysis is a result of mechanical forces, chemicals or microorganisms, antibodies, or sequestration in the monocyte–macrophage system. *(Beutler, p. 641)*

399. **(C)** Spherocytosis is not associated with G6PD deficiency, trauma, or leukemia. The typical changes in G6PD deficiency include the presence of Heinz bodies. The cell morphology is not usually changed unless hemolysis is very severe. In hereditary spherocytosis, the Coombs' test is negative. *(Beutler, p. 641)*

400. **(C)** Bilirubin is excreted in the bile and converted to urobilinogen by bacterial reduction in the bowel, and can be reabsorbed and excreted in the urine. There is no bilirubin in the urine because unconjugated bilirubin is not cleared by the kidney as it is tightly bound to plasma proteins. *(Beutler, pp. 641–642)*

401. **(C)** Bone marrow examination is most likely to show increased erythroid-to-myeloid ratio. Erythroid hyperplasia is common to all hemolytic anemias, and megaloblastic features may develop unless folate is supplied. *(Beutler, p. 642)*

402. **(E)** The diagnosis of autoimmune hemolytic anemia requires demonstration of immunoglobulin and/or complement in the patient's RBC. The broad-spectrum Coombs' test is an excellent screen. *(Beutler, p. 642)*

403. **(D)** Anemia is usually multifactorial in alcoholics and includes marrow suppression, GI bleeding, hemorrhagic diathesis, and nutritional deficiency. *(Beutler, p. 473)*

404. **(B)** Folate deficiency results from decreased intake and malabsorption. Body folate stores are meager and therefore easily depleted when intake is poor. Alcohol itself can depress folate levels acutely and also can cause pancytopenia directly. *(Beutler, p. 473)*

405. **(A)** Alcohol is directly toxic to dividing and maturing cells but may also affect neutrophil function. The hematologic effects of alcohol may be direct or indirect, via diet, infection, liver disease, and GI disease. The resulting hematologic abnormalities may be profound. *(Beutler, pp. 473–474)*

406. **(A)** Because both iron deficiency and folate deficiency are very common in alcoholics, a dimorphic blood film can be seen. Macrocytes, hypersegmented neutrophils, and hypochromic microcytes can be found on the same slide. *(Beutler, p. 473)*

407. **(D)** Coagulation factors II, V, VII, and X would most likely be deficient. These are some of the factors that are synthesized in the liver, but V is not dependent on vitamin K. *(Beutler, p. 1673)*

408. **(B)** Thalassemia minor usually represents a heterozygous state and is often asymptomatic. Symptoms may develop during periods of stress such as pregnancy or severe infection. Hemoglobin values are usually in the 9 to 11 g/dL range. The red cells are small and poorly hemoglobinized. *(Beutler, pp. 565–566)*

409. **(E)** A serum ferritin determination would be most helpful. Iron stores in thalassemia are normal or increased. Some of the increase may be secondary to injudicious iron therapy. *(Beutler, p. 565)*

410. **(A)** An increased amount of fetal or HbA_2 would be expected. As beta chains are decreased, the alpha chains combine with gamma and delta chains to make F and A_2. *(Beutler, pp. 566–567)*

411. **(C)** The present treatment of choice for thalassemia minor is purely supportive. Care is taken to watch for anemia during intercurrent illness, due to aregenerative crises. *(Beutler, p. 565)*

412. **(D)** HbC characteristically produces targeting in the peripheral blood and also hemoglobin crystals in the cells. HbC is found in 17 to 28% of West Africans. Splenomegaly is a fairly constant feature, but most patients are quite asymptomatic. *(Beutler, p. 565)*

413. **(D)** Sideroblastic anemia is associated with an increased serum iron and ferritin. TIBC is generally normal. HbA_2 is usually decreased. *(Braunwald, p. 663)*

414. **(B)** Beta-thalassemia trait is characterized by normal iron studies and an elevated HbA_2. *(Braunwald, p. 663)*

415. **(A)** Iron deficiency is characterized by low serum iron and ferritin and an increase in TIBC. HbA_2 is normal. *(Braunwald, p. 663)*

416. **(C)** Anemia of chronic disease is characterized by decreased serum iron and TIBC, an elevated ferritin, and normal HbA_2. *(Braunwald, p. 663)*

417. **(D)** Beta-thalassemia trait is diagnosed by demonstrating an elevated HbA_2, iron deficiency by iron studies and ferritin levels, and anemia of chronic disease by demonstrating a chronic disease. Sideroblastic anemia generally requires a bone marrow aspiration revealing ringed sideroblasts for diagnosis. *(Braunwald, p. 663)*

418. **(D)** Burr cells and stomatocytes are found in severe liver disease and might result from abnormal membrane lipids. *(Braunwald, p. 666)*

419. **(F)** Heinz bodies (precipitated Hb) are found in disorders with unstable Hb or after oxidant stress. *(Braunwald, p. 671)*

420. **(A)** Spherocytes are caused by loss of membrane, as in hereditary spherocytosis or autoimmune hemolytic anemia. *(Braunwald, p. 682)*

421. **(C)** Sickle-cell disease results in polymerization of HbS and the characteristic sickle cells. *(Braunwald, p. 669)*

422. **(B)** Schistocytes are caused by traumatic disruption of the red cell membrane (eg, microangiopathic syndromes). *(Braunwald, p. 689)*

423. **(A, B, C)** Von Willebrand's disease is the most common inherited bleeding disorder. The abnormal plasma glycoprotein, von Willebrand factor (vWF) has two major functions: facilitating platelet adhesion and serving as a carrier for factor VIII. The disease is heterogeneous in its manifestations but can be very severe (type III disease). Evaluation reveals a prolonged bleeding time and decreased factor VIII activity. *(Braunwald, pp. 747–749)*

424. **(B, D, E)** Hemophilia A results from a deficiency or dysfunction of the factor VIII molecule. It is a sex-linked disease affecting 1 in 10,000 males. The partial thromboplastin time (PTT) is prolonged, but the bleeding time is characteristically normal. *(Braunwald, p. 751)*

425. (D, E) Hemophilia B is clinically indistinguishable from hemophilia A and is also inherited via the X chromosome. The bleeding time is usually normal, but the PTT is usually elevated. Differentiation from hemophilia A requires factor assay. *(Braunwald, pp. 752–753)*

426. (D, G) TTP is a fulminant disorder that can be fatal. It has been associated with malignancy, pregnancy, metastatic cancer, and high-dose chemotherapy. Most often, the classical tests of hemostasis and platelet function are normal. The classical symptoms include fever, thrombocytopenia, microangiopathic hemolytic anemia, renal failure, and fluctuating neurologic defects. *(Braunwald, pp. 748–749)*

CHAPTER 6

Oncology
Questions

DIRECTIONS (Questions 427 through 452): Each of the numbered items or incomplete statements in this section is followed by answers or by completions of the statement. Select the ONE lettered answer or completion that is BEST in each case.

427. A 33-year-old man has blanching skin lesions and a history of sinopulmonary infections. There is no family history. The most likely diagnosis is

(A) neurofibromatosis
(B) tuberous sclerosis
(C) ataxia–telangiectasia
(D) von Hippel–Lindau syndrome
(E) Peutz–Jeghers syndrome

428. You are caring for a 33-year-old male immigrant from Taiwan who has positive hepatitis B virus (HBV) serology. Which of the following statements is correct?

(A) Previous HBV infection dramatically increases the risk of hepatocellular carcinoma (HCC).
(B) HCC occurs only in the setting of cirrhosis.
(C) Age of infection is not relevant to the likelihood of HCC.
(D) Cirrhosis and HCC are the most common causes of death for those with a hepatitis B surface antigen (HBsAg) chronic carrier state in endemic areas.
(E) The chronic carrier state of HBsAg increases the relative risk of HCC by 10-fold in endemic areas such as Taiwan.

429. A 42-year-old man received radiation exposure at a nuclear power plant in Eastern Europe. Which of the following statements is correct?

(A) Malignancies occur within 10 years of exposure.
(B) Leukemia has the shortest latency period of all malignancies.
(C) Large exposure is required to develop the most serious malignancies.
(D) Risk increases with advancing age at the time of exposure.
(E) Therapeutic radiation therapy given without chemotherapy does not increase the risk of a second malignancy.

430. Appropriate cancer screening for a 25-year-old woman would include

(A) mammography every 5 years
(B) Pap smear at least every 3 years
(C) stool for occult blood
(D) chest x-ray (CXR) every 3 years
(E) physical examination of the breast by a physician

431. A 25-year-old woman presents with intermittent double vision. A CXR reveals an anterior mediastinal mass. Further evaluation will include

(A) measurement of serum calcium
(B) magnetic resonance imaging (MRI) scan of the brain
(C) evaluation of T-cell function
(D) measurement of serum gamma globulins
(E) assessment of glucose tolerance

432. A 40-year-old nonsmoking woman with a history of moderate alcohol use presents with a 4-month history of weight loss and dysphagia. An important finding on physical examination related to this presentation would be

(A) pigmentation of the lips
(B) telangiectasia of the oropharynx
(C) lichen planus
(D) hyperkeratosis of the palms
(E) psoriasis vulgaris

433. Which of the following is a risk factor for carcinoma of the stomach in a 62-year-old man?

(A) high-fat diet
(B) high socioeconomic status
(C) high-protein diet
(D) high alcohol consumption
(E) low dietary vitamin A

434. A young man with leukemia is treated with methotrexate. This drug works by

(A) preventing absorption of folic acid
(B) inhibiting dihydrofolate reductase
(C) preventing formation of messenger ribonucleic acid (RNA)
(D) forming a cytotoxic metabolite
(E) preventing proper functioning of membrane adenosine triphosphatase (ATPase)

435. Which of the following statements is true regarding a 52-year-old man who develops abdominal pain and jaundice suggestive of cancer of the pancreas?

(A) Tumors of the pancreas are divided almost equally between those arising from the exocrine portion and those arising from the endocrine portion.
(B) Most endocrine tumors of the pancreas are malignant.
(C) The body of the pancreas is the most common site of malignancy.
(D) Ductal adenocarcinoma is the most common pancreatic cancer.
(E) Extension is through local invasion; metastases are a late manifestation.

436. A 73-year-old man was born in Taiwan and came to the United States 3 years ago. He is known to be HBsAg positive. Which of the following findings suggests the development of HCC?

(A) hepatomegaly
(B) hepatic bruits
(C) ascites
(D) jaundice
(E) all of the above

437. A 47-year-old man develops gastrointestinal (GI) bleeding, and a small bowel enema suggests a small bowel tumor. Which of the following statements concerning small bowel tumors is correct?

(A) Carcinoid tumors frequently present with flushing, watery diarrhea, and asthma.
(B) Malignant adenocarcinoma most frequently occurs in the duodenum.
(C) Malignant tumors bleed more frequently than benign tumors.
(D) Peutz–Jeghers syndrome is characterized only by benign hamartoma.
(E) Most primary gastrointestinal lymphomas are located in the ileum.

438. Which of the following factors improves the prognosis for carcinoma of the colon?

(A) age under 40
(B) male gender
(C) rectal bleeding
(D) small tumor size
(E) location in the rectum

439. Which of the following is correct for both carcinoma of the uterine cervix and carcinoma of the uterine endometrium?

(A) associated with diabetes mellitus and obesity
(B) most common in middle age
(C) associated with nulliparity

(D) common in Jews and Muslims

(E) associated with herpesvirus type 2 (HSV-2) infection

440. You are seeing a 62-year-old woman with a family history of breast cancer. A further increase in risk would be caused by

(A) early onset of menopause

(B) early onset of menarche

(C) late-life radiation exposure

(D) multiparity

(E) early full-term pregnancy

441. A 67-year-old former pipefitter develops an occupational cancer. The most likely presenting symptoms are

(A) hemoptysis

(B) pleuritic chest pain and cough

(C) dyspnea and nonpleuritic pain

(D) due to metastatic disease

(E) bony pain

442. A 23-year-old man's bone biopsy reveals sarcoma. Which of the following statements is correct?

(A) Distal bone sarcomas have a better prognosis.

(B) Lung metastases are a late sign.

(C) Local lymph node involvement is very common.

(D) Articular cartilage is a common plane for tumor spread.

(E) Skip metastases within the same bone are common and unrelated to prognosis.

443. A 19-year-old woman develops axillary lymphadenopathy. Biopsy reveals Hodgkin's disease, nodular sclerosing variety. Which of the following statements about staging is correct?

(A) Only one quarter of patients have advanced (stage III or IV) disease after all staging procedures.

(B) The presence of pruritus indicates stage B Hodgkin's.

(C) If B symptoms are present, chemotherapy, with or without radiation therapy, is a mandatory part of treatment.

(D) Nodular sclerosing forms of Hodgkin's disease are more commonly diagnosed at advanced stages than the lymphocyte-depleted variant.

(E) Increasing use of effective chemotherapy regimens has meant that staging laparotomy is less commonly performed.

444. The most likely presenting symptom in a young woman with Hodgkin's disease is

(A) coincidentally detected mediastinal mass

(B) fixed tender inguinal lymph node involvement

(C) mobile nontender cervical lymph nodes

(D) fixed, nontender axillary nodes

(E) mobile, tender axillary nodes

445. A 68-year-old man presents with left axillary adenopathy that on biopsy reveals a low-grade lymphocytic lymphoma. Which of the following statements is correct?

(A) Staging in this type of disorder is not relevant.

(B) If disease is widespread, early aggressive chemotherapy will result in an improved prognosis for survival.

(C) The disease is likely to be widespread at the time of diagnosis.

(D) Untreated, the prognosis is measured in months.

(E) His age is not a relevant factor in treatment.

446. Skin biopsy of a 63-year-old man reveals evidence of a lymphoma. Diagnostic evaluation does not reveal evidence of a visceral malignancy. This disease

(A) is invariably a precursor to leukemia

(B) is of T-cell origin

(C) has no specific geographic distribution

(D) has a high likelihood of cure

(E) is related to sun exposure

447. A 65-year-old man with a 45 pack/year history of smoking presents with hematuria. His hemoglobin (Hb) is 18.5 g, and his liver enzymes are twice normal. He has lost 15 pounds. Which of the following statements is correct?

   (A) His Hb level represents stress poly-cythemia.
   (B) The elevated Hb indicates a poor prognosis.
   (C) His tumor is nonresectable.
   (D) A computed tomography (CT) of the thorax is a useful test.
   (E) A palpable abdominal mass is very unlikely.

448. A 53-year-old woman presents with a 0.5-cm invasive carcinoma of the breast, detected on mammography. The appropriate local therapy for the tumor would be

   (A) simple mastectomy with axillary dissection
   (B) radiation therapy to breast and axilla
   (C) local excision plus radiation therapy
   (D) local excision and axillary dissection followed by radiation therapy
   (E) local excision and axillary sampling

449. A 68-year-old woman presents to her attending physician feeling unwell and having lost 10 pounds. Physical examination reveals left axillary lymphadenopathy. Biopsy reveals well-differentiated adenocarcinoma. Liver scan and bone scan suggest widespread metastases. Which statement concerning her further management is correct?

   (A) The response rate for metastatic adeno-carcinoma (well differentiated) of unknown primary site is so poor that no investigation or treatment is indicated.
   (B) Special stains might guide management.
   (C) Extensive work-up, including colonoscopy, abdominal CT scan, and mammography, will define subsets that benefit from treatment.

   (D) Special studies of the excised lymph node are not useful in determining the site of origin.
   (E) Metastatic breast cancer is the most common cause of adenocarcinoma of unknown primary site in women.

450. A 47-year-old woman with cancer phobia comes to the office for counseling. Which of the following statements is true?

   (A) Cancer is the most common cause of death in the United States.
   (B) Cancer is the most common cause of death in middle-aged women.
   (C) Incidence rates for cancer are generally higher in women than men.
   (D) Colon and rectum cancers have the highest mortality rate when considering both men and women.
   (E) About 25% of all cancers in the United States are due to environmental factors.

451. A 63-year-old man with chronic heartburn has an endoscopy that reveals no masses or tumors, but there is esophagitis. Biopsy of the lower esophagus reveals columnar cells. Which of the following statements is correct?

   (A) It is a major risk factor for squamous cell cancer of the esophagus.
   (B) It can be found in up to 20% of patients undergoing esophagoscopy for esophagitis.
   (C) The histologic changes include development of keratinized squamous cells.
   (D) Medical control of reflux will decrease the likelihood of malignant changes.
   (E) Only 10% of patients with Barrett's esophagus may develop malignancy.

452. A 59-year-old man develops jaundice. Endoscopic retrograde cholangiopancreatography (ERCP) suggests a cholangiocarcinoma. The most likely predisposing factor is

   (A) ulcerative colitis
   (B) gallstones
   (C) liver stones

(D) having lived most of his life in West Central Africa

(E) intestinal nematodes

DIRECTIONS (Questions 453 through 489): Each set of matching questions in this section consists of a list of lettered options followed by several numbered items. For each numbered item, select the appropriate lettered option(s). Each lettered option may be selected once, more than once, or not at all. EACH ITEM WILL STATE THE NUMBER OF OPTIONS TO SELECT. CHOOSE EXACTLY THIS NUMBER.

Questions 453 and 454

(A) Cumulative sun exposure is the only known risk factor.

(B) If clinically detectable, micrometastases are invariably present.

(C) Hormonal therapy can be beneficial.

(D) The disease is presenting at an earlier stage in the United States.

(E) Ulceration is a bad prognostic sign.

(F) A 10-year disease-free interval equals cure.

453. A 53-year-old woman has a lumpectomy for breast cancer (SELECT TWO)

454. A rapidly growing pigmented skin lesion is found on a Caucasian patient (SELECT TWO)

Questions 455 and 456

(A) untreated, survival measured in years

(B) M component level of 7 g/dL

(C) localized disease effectively treated with radiation therapy

(D) normal skeletal x-ray series

(E) when localized to stomach, surgery should be followed by chemotherapy

(F) Bence Jones protein 2 g/24 hours

(G) bone marrow plasma cells of 7%

(H) normal hemoglobin

(I) cure more likely than with an indolent lymphoma

(J) advanced age a contraindication to therapy

455. A 73-year-old man develops an aggressive lymphocytic lymphoma. Which of the statements is correct? (SELECT TWO)

456. An asymptomatic 74-year-old man has a high erythrocyte sedimentation rate (ESR) noted on routine blood work done with a yearly physical examination. A follow-up protein electrophoresis reveals a monoclonal immunoglobulin G (IgG) spike. Which of the statements would suggest a plasma cell myeloma rather than a monoclonal gammopathy of unknown significance? (SELECT TWO)

Questions 457 through 463

(A) Hispanic Americans

(B) White Americans

(C) Black Americans

(D) Native Americans

(E) Chinese Americans

(F) Japanese Americans

(G) Filipino Americans

457. Have the lowest cancer rates for both sexes (SELECT ONE)

458. Have very high rates of melanoma (SELECT ONE)

459. Have the highest rates for breast, corpus uteri, and ovarian cancer (SELECT ONE)

460. Have especially high rates for cervical cancer (SELECT ONE)

461. Have elevated rates for nasopharynx and liver cancer (SELECT ONE)

462. Have high rates for stomach cancer (SELECT ONE)

463. Have high cancer rates at least partially due to socioeconomic factors (SELECT ONE)

Questions 464 through 468

    (A) aflatoxin

    (B) alcoholic beverages

    (C) alkylating agents

    (D) anabolic steroids

    (E) arsenic

    (F) asbestos

    (G) benzene

    (H) chewing tobacco

    (I) tobacco smoke

    (J) ultraviolet radiation

    (K) Epstein–Barr virus

    (L) HBV

    (M) human papillomavirus (HPV)

    (N) vinyl chloride

464. Associated with cancer of the mouth and liver (SELECT ONE)

465. Increases risk of lung cancer twofold and cancer of peritoneum 100-fold (SELECT ONE)

466. Can cause different cancers, some secondary to intermittent severe exposure, others due to cumulative dose (SELECT ONE)

467. Is linked to cancer of the cervix, vulva, and penis (SELECT ONE)

468. Is linked to cancer even with indirect exposure (SELECT ONE)

Questions 469 through 473

    (A) cancer metastatic to the lung

    (B) squamous cell cancer of the lung

    (C) adenocarcinoma of the lung

    (D) small cell cancer of the lung

    (E) large cell cancer of the lung

469. The most common type of lung cancer in the United States (SELECT ONE)

470. Has the best prognosis of all malignant lung cancers (SELECT ONE)

471. Most likely to cause nonmetastatic hypercalcemia (SELECT ONE)

472. Associated with syndrome of inappropriate antidiuretic hormone (SIADH) (SELECT ONE)

473. Associated with myasthenic syndrome (Eaton–Lambert syndrome) (SELECT ONE)

Questions 474 through 478

    (A) methotrexate

    (B) cytarabine

    (C) 5-fluorouracil (5-FU)

    (D) bleomycin

    (E) doxorubicin

    (F) pamidronate

    (G) cisplatin

    (H) busulfan

    (I) cyclophosphamide

    (J) vincristine

474. Used for hypercalcemia (SELECT ONE)

475. Can cause hepatic fibrosis (SELECT ONE)

476. Can cause erythema, induration, thickening, and eventual peeling of the skin on the fingers, palms, and extremity joints (SELECT ONE)

477. Can cause acute cardiac failure (SELECT ONE)

478. Frequently causes hemorrhagic cystitis (SELECT ONE)

Questions 479 through 481

    (A) anaplastic thyroid cancer

    (B) follicular cancer of the thyroid

    (C) lymphoma of the thyroid

    (D) papillary cancer of the thyroid

    (E) medullary thyroid cancer

479. Has the best prognosis of all thyroid malignancies (SELECT ONE)

480. Is proportionately more common in blacks than whites (SELECT ONE)

481. Is associated with a specific marker (SELECT ONE)

Questions 482 through 485

   (A) lymphocyte-predominant Hodgkin's disease

   (B) nodular sclerosing Hodgkin's disease

   (C) mixed-cellularity Hodgkin's disease

   (D) lymphocyte-depleted Hodgkin's disease, reticular type

   (E) lymphocyte-depleted Hodgkin's disease, diffuse fibrosis type

   (F) all variants of Hodgkin's disease

482. The only form of Hodgkin's disease more common in women (SELECT ONE)

483. Reed–Sternberg cells can be difficult to locate in this variant (SELECT ONE)

484. This variant has a particularly good outcome (SELECT ONE)

485. Can be accompanied by a non-necrotizing epithelioid granulomatous reaction (SELECT ONE)

Questions 486 through 489

The following questions refer to the relief of pain in patients with metastatic cancer.

   (A) nonsteroidal anti-inflammatory drugs (NSAIDs)

   (B) opioids

   (C) amphetamines

   (D) anticonvulsants

   (E) phenothiazines

   (F) butyrophenones

   (G) steroids

486. This group of medications is particularly useful for pain from bony metastases (SELECT ONE)

487. Leukopenia and thrombocytopenia can limit the use of the most widely used drug in this category (SELECT ONE)

488. Can be particularly useful for headaches (SELECT ONE)

489. Can be useful in controlling opioid-induced sedation (SELECT ONE)

Answers and Explanations

427. **(C)** Ataxia–telangiectasia is inherited in an autosomal recessive manner. It is associated with non-Hodgkin's lymphoma, acute lymphocytic leukemia, and stomach cancer. Associated IgA (± IgE) deficiency predisposes to infection as well. All the other conditions listed are inherited in an autosomal dominant manner, and a positive family history is much more likely. (*Devita, p. 2526*)

428. **(D)** Only the chronic carrier state increases HCC risk, not previous infection. The majority, but not all, of HCC associated with HBV occurs in the setting of cirrhosis (60 to 90%). Because the latency period of HBV infection is 35 years before HCC supervenes, early life infection is strongly correlated with HCC. The chronic carrier state of HBsAg in endemic areas such as Taiwan is associated with a relative risk of over 100 for the development of HCC. Over half the chronic carriers of HBsAg in such a population will die of cirrhosis or HCC. In Taiwan, where childhood vaccination was introduced in 1984, the death rate from childhood HCC has already declined. (*Devita, pp. 158–160, 3192–3193*)

429. **(B)** Radiation-induced malignancies tend to occur at the age where that particular malignancy would normally occur. Therefore, the latency period can be 40 years or more. The latency period tends to be shortest (5 to 7 years) for leukemia. The risk for most malignancies is greatest with early-life radiation, and evidence suggests that therapeutic radiation confers excess risk as well. The amount of exposure determines the likelihood of developing malignancy, not its severity. (*Devita, pp. 197–198*)

430. **(B)** There is universal agreement on the need for regular Pap smears in young women. There is no need to screen for colon cancer (fecal occult blood) or lung tumors (CXR), particularly at this age. Mammography, if indicated for screening, would be only for older women. Many authorities recommend breast self-examination as well as physical examination by a physician. (*Devita, pp. 628–637*)

431. **(D)** An anterior mediastinal mass with ocular muscular weakness suggests the association of a thymoma with myasthenia gravis. About 5 to 10% of patients with thymoma will also have hypogammaglobulinemia. About 5% of patients with thymoma will have autoimmune pure red cell aplasia. (*Devita, pp. 1024–1025*)

432. **(D)** The history of weight loss and dysphagia suggests carcinoma of the esophagus, a disease most common in older men who drink and smoke heavily. Tylosis, a disease characterized by hyperkeratosis of the palms and soles and papillomata of the esophagus is inherited in an autosomal dominant manner. Affected individuals have a high likelihood of developing squamous cell cancer of the esophagus. (*Devita, p. 1054*)

433. **(E)** Low dietary vitamins A and C and high salt and nitrate consumption predispose to gastric cancer, as does ingestion of smoked foods. Smoking is a risk factor, but alcohol is not. (*Devita, p. 1093*)

434. **(B)** The most likely mode of action of methotrexate is by tightly binding dihydrofolate reductase (DHFR), which maintains the intracellular folate pool in its fully reduced form as tetrahydrofolates. These compounds are required in the de novo synthesis of pyrimidines and purines. *(Devita, pp. 388–389)*

435. **(D)** Adenocarcinoma comprises most of the cancers of the pancreas. The proximal pancreas is the most common site, with only 20% occurring in the body and 5 to 10% in the tail. About 95% of the tumors arise from the exocrine portion of the gland, and these are usually malignant. Most of the endocrine tumors are benign. Early development of metastases are characteristic of pancreatic adenocarcinoma. *(Devita, pp. 1126–1130)*

436. **(E)** For most patients the development of HCC is the first manifestation of their underlying liver disease. The most common presentation is with right upper quadrant (RUQ) pain, mass, and weight loss, but hepatic decompensation with jaundice and ascites is also common. About 25% of patients have hepatic bruits. *(Devita, pp. 1163–1164)*

437. **(B)** Adenocarcinoma, the most common malignancy of the small bowel is most common proximally, particularly in the duodenum. Small bowel lymphomas are most common in the ileum, but the stomach is the most common site of GI lymphoma. Carcinoids usually present with local symptoms. Carcinoid syndrome is present only with hepatic metastases. Benign tumors bleed more frequently than malignant ones. Malignant adenocarcinomas can occur in Peutz–Jeghers syndrome. *(Devita, pp. 1208–1213)*

438. **(C)** Rectal bleeding is a good prognostic sign, perhaps because surface erosion manifests early. Young age, male gender, and location in the rectum all indicate a poorer prognosis. Unlike most tumors, no correlation with tumor size and prognosis has been established for colon cancer. *(Devita, pp. 1232–1234)*

439. **(B)** Carcinoma of the cervix is common in young women. For endometrial cancer, the peak is from ages 55 to 60. Endometrial cancer is associated with nulliparity, diabetes mellitus, and obesity. Cervical cancer is associated with HPV infection. There is tremendous variation in incidence of cervical cancer based on geography, ethnicity, and sexual history. *(Devita, pp. 1526–1527, 1575–1576)*

440. **(B)** Breast cancer risk is reduced by 20% for each year that menarche is delayed. Early menopause, natural or surgical, also decreases risk. Early (age 18 or 19) full-term pregnancy and multiparity decrease the risk. Radiation exposure is a risk factor primarily in adolescence and is marginal after the age of 40. *(Devita, pp. 1652–1655)*

441. **(C)** The history of being a pipefitter suggests asbestosis. The classic associated cancer is mesothelioma. However, in 30 to 50% of cases, no history of asbestos exposure is apparent. Among the other postulated causes is therapeutic irradiation. The average age on presentation is 60, and this is typically many years after the exposure. The most common presenting symptoms are dyspnea and nonpleuritic chest pain. *(Devita, pp. 1947–1948)*

442. **(A)** Overwhelmingly, the major prognostic factor in osteosarcoma is location of the tumor. Pelvic and axial lesions do worse than those in the extremities, and survival is better in tibial tumors than femoral tumors. Lung metastases are very common. *(Devita, pp. 1910–1911)*

443. **(E)** Stage IB Hodgkin's disease is effectively treated with radiation therapy alone. Some reports suggest that stage IIB can be similarly treated. Although physical exam and CXR will initially suggest that 90% of patients with Hodgkin's disease have localized disease, by the end of staging, 60% will be stage III or IV. The purpose of staging laparotomy is to determine whether radiation alone will be used for treatment. As chemotherapy usage increases, the necessity for staging laparotomy decreases. Pruritus alone does not result in a B stage. *(Devita, pp. 2350–2362)*

444. **(C)** The most characteristic presentation of Hodgkin's disease is that of enlarged, superficial cervical or supraclavicular lymph nodes in a young person. The nodes are usually freely moveable, nontender, and not painful. Occult presentation with intrathoracic or intra-abdominal disease is unusual. *(Devita, p. 2352)*

445. **(C)** About 85% of low-grade lymphocytic lymphomas are widespread at the time of diagnosis. However, staging is still important as radiation therapy can be curative for localized (stage I, II) disease. Because the prognosis for this malignancy is measured in years, it has been difficult to demonstrate a survival benefit for aggressive chemotherapy. The poor prognosis for lymphoma in older patients might be a result of less aggressive therapy. *(Devita, p. 2277)*

446. **(B)** Cutaneous lymphomas are of T-cell origin and are more common in other parts of the world, such as Japan. Patients with adult T-cell lymphoma–leukemia (ATLL) have acute fulminant courses characterized by skin invasion and leukemic cells. This syndrome is clearly related to human T-cell lymphotropic virus-I (HTLV-I), and there is a possibility that HTLV-I or another retrovirus might be the agent for mycosis fungoides and Sézary syndrome. ATLL responds poorly to treatment, and therapy for the low-grade malignancies controls symptoms but does not result in cure. *(Devita, pp. 2316–2318)*

447. **(D)** The age, history of smoking, and polycythemia in a patient with hematuria strongly suggests a renal cell carcinoma. The elevated hemoglobin represents increased erythropoietin production and is not related to prognosis. Elevated liver enzymes and weight loss can represent nonmetastatic effects of malignancy and can reverse with resection. Almost half of patients will have a palpable abdominal mass on presentation. The CT of the thorax is a useful test because

three quarters of those with metastatic disease will have lung metastases. *(Devita, pp. 1362–1366)*

448. **(D)** Breast-conserving surgery is now recommended for small tumors. Radiation therapy will decrease local recurrence rates. For tumors less than 1 cm, adjuvant therapy is indicated only if axillary nodes are positive. Therefore, in this case, an axillary dissection will provide important therapeutic information. However, this is an area of rapidly changing knowledge and practice. *(Devita, pp. 1664–1670)*

449. **(B)** The patients with adenocarcinoma of unknown origin are typically elderly and have metastatic tumor at many sites. Generally, the prognosis is poor, but some subsets in whom effective treatment is available can be identified by clinical criteria with only moderate investigations. These include peritoneal carcinomatosis in women (responds to treatment for ovarian cancer), predominant skeletal metastases in men (can reflect prostatic cancer), and women with axillary lymphadenopathy (can reflect breast cancer). In the latter scenario, studies for estrogen and progesterone receptors are very useful in guiding therapy. *(Devita, p. 2541)*

450. **(B)** When men and women of all ages are considered, cardiovascular diseases are the most common cause of death. However, among women 35 to 74, cancer is the leading cause of death. Lung cancer is the number one cause of death from cancer when both men and women are considered. Men generally have higher incidence rates for cancer: breast, gallbladder, and thyroid cancers are the exceptions. It is felt that 75 to 80% of all cancers in the United States are due to environmental factors. The environmental contribution is estimated by comparing age-adjusted U.S. rates of specific cancers to the rates for the country with the lowest risk. *(Devita, pp. 228–250)*

451. **(B)** Barrett's esophagus, characterized by a columnar cell-lined esophageal mucosa, is a

major risk factor for adenocarcinoma of the esophagus. Although acid reflux may be a predisposing factor, there is no evidence that either medical or surgical antireflux measures alter the outcome. It is found in about 20% of patients undergoing endoscopy for esophagitis, and up to 50% may develop a malignancy. *(Devita, pp. 1055–1056)*

452. **(C)** Worldwide, the presence of liver flukes (eg, *Clonorchis sinensis*) is the most likely predisposing factor for cholangiocarcinoma. Part of this increased risk is caused by the development of hepatolithiasis. About 5 to 10% of patients with liver stones will develop cholangiocarcinoma, making this a more important risk factor than ulcerative colitis. The highest rate of cholangiocarcinoma is found in Southeast Asia. It is thought that liver flukes and a diet high in nitrosamine are the prime reasons for this. In North America, primary sclerosing cholangitis is the most common predisposing factor. *(Devita, pp. 1178–1179)*

453. **(B, C)** The size of the tumor is a prognostic factor. By the time of detection, breast cancer has gone through about 30 doublings, ample opportunity to establish distant micrometastases. Both hormonal therapy and chemotherapy can be effective as adjuvant therapy. *(Devita, pp. 1688–1696)*

454. **(D, E)** For malignant melanoma, there has been a steady increase in presentation with localized disease (81% by 1990) in the United States. As a result, thickness of the tumor is the most important prognostic factor in the majority of cases. The increasing mortality in the United States is caused by the increasing incidence of disease. Ulceration indicates a more aggressive cancer with a poorer prognosis. Although cumulative sun exposure is a major factor in melanoma (eg, more frequent near the equator), it cannot explain such things as the more common occurrence of some types in relatively young people. It is possible that brief, intense exposure to sunlight may contribute to or initiate carcinogenic events. *(Devita, pp. 2015–2018, 2023)*

455. **(E, I)** Even if disease seems to be localized, systemic chemotherapy is always required in aggressive lymphocytic lymphomas. In the GI tract, these are usually large B-cell lymphomas. Although untreated survival is dismal, the chances of a cure with current chemotherapy are about 50%, much better than in low-grade lymphomas. The poor prognosis of elderly patients might be secondary to lower doses of chemotherapy. Treatment should be based on toxicities actually experienced rather than making excessive anticipatory dose reductions for the elderly. *(Devita, pp. 2287, 2303)*

456. **(B, F)** IgG spikes greater than 3.5 g/dL or IgA greater than 2 g/dL strongly suggest myeloma rather than monoclonal gammopathies of undetermined significance (MGUS). MGUS is suggested when the spike is less than 3.5 g/dL, the marrow has fewer than 10% plasma cells, and the Bence Jones proteinuria is less than 1.0 g/24 hours. Depressed hemoglobin levels, elevated calcium levels, progressive bone lesions, and impaired renal function suggest more advanced stages of multiple myeloma. *(Devita, p. 2474)*

457. **(D)** Native Americans of both sexes have low cancer rates, but cancer rates (for women) for stomach, biliary tract, cervix, and kidney are surprisingly high. *(Devita, pp. 228–240)*

458. **(B)** Whites have high rates for melanoma, lymphoma, leukemia, and lip cancer. *(Devita, pp. 228–240)*

459. **(B)** Whites have high rates for breast, corpus uteri, testis, bladder, brain, colon, and rectum cancer. *(Devita, pp. 228–240)*

460. **(A)** Although Hispanic Americans have relatively low cancer rates (66% of that for White Americans and 54% of that for Black Americans), they do have high rates for cancer of the cervix. *(Devita, pp. 228–240)*

461. **(E)** Chinese Americans have a rate of nasopharyngeal cancer 23 times greater than

White Americans and liver cancer rates seven times greater than White Americans. *(Devita, pp. 228–240)*

462. **(F)** Japanese Americans have a threefold increase in stomach cancer rate compared to White Americans, but this is lower than rates in Japan. *(Devita, pp. 228–240)*

463. **(C)** The excess risk of cancers of the stomach, esophagus, lung, and cervix among Black Americans is diminished when socioeconomic variations are factored in. *(Devita, pp. 228–240)*

464. **(B)** Alcoholic beverages combine with tobacco smoking to increase cancer of the mouth and, by causing cirrhosis, can lead to liver cancer. *(Devita, pp. 241–250)*

465. **(F)** Asbestos exposure causes more deaths from lung cancer (twofold increase) than from mesothelioma (100-fold increase) because the latter tumor is so rare. *(Devita, pp. 241–250)*

466. **(J)** Sun exposure severe enough to cause sunburn is associated with increased risk of melanoma, whereas other skin cancers are more related to cumulative exposure. *(Devita, pp. 241–250)*

467. **(M)** Although causation is not definite, a high proportion of cervical cancers reveal HPV-16 and HPV-18 on biopsy. HPV has also been isolated from vulvar, penile, and anal cancers. *(Devita, pp. 241–250)*

468. **(I)** Tobacco smoke constituents and metabolites can be detected in the body fluids of exposed nonsmokers. Evidence suggests that nonsmoking women married to smokers have a 30% excess risk for lung cancer. *(Devita, pp. 241–250)*

469. **(C)** Adenocarcinoma is now the most common form of lung cancer, accounting for 40% of the total cases. *(Devita, p. 928)*

470. **(B)** Because of its tendency for early exfoliation and obstruction, squamous cell cancer is often detected at an earlier stage. Even correcting for this, there is some suggestion that its prognosis is still better, perhaps because of its slow growth rate. *(Devita, p. 928)*

471. **(B)** Nonmetastatic hypercalcemia occurs in up to 15% of all squamous cell cancers. *(Devita, p. 933)*

472. **(D)** SIADH occurs in up to 10% of all small cell cancers of the lung. SIADH, Cushing's syndrome, and neurologic paraneoplastic syndromes usually occur with small cell lung cancer, not non–small cell. *(Devita, p. 985)*

473. **(D)** Eaton–Lambert syndrome is unusual, but small cell lung cancer causes the majority of cases that are paraneoplastic. *(Devita, pp. 985, 2530)*

474. **(F)** Pamidronate, a bisphosphonate, is given intravenously and is associated with only minor side effects. It is poorly absorbed by mouth. There is some data to suggest it is less effective if hypercalcemia is mediated by parathyroid hormone (PTH)-related protein. Calcitonin, plicamycin (mithramycin), and steroids are also used, but less frequently. *(Devita, p. 2637)*

475. **(A)** Liver toxicity is most common when methotrexate is used on a daily basis, such as for psoriasis. Myelosuppression and GI mucositis are the most common side effects in cancer therapy. *(Devita, p. 392)*

476. **(D)** Although lung injury is the most serious complication of bleomycin, this unusual skin reaction is more frequent, occurring in almost 50% of patients. *(Devita, pp. 453–454)*

477. **(E)** Doxorubicin can cause a cumulative, dose-dependent cardiomyopathy that can result in congestive heart failure. However, an acute, non–dose-related myocarditis–pericarditis can also occur. It can cause arrhythmias, heart failure, or pericardial effusions. *(Devita, pp. 425–427)*

478. **(I)** Cyclophosphamide causes hemorrhagic cystitis in up to 10% of patients because ac-

tive metabolites are excreted. Adequate hydration and frequent urination can decrease the frequency of this complication. *(Devita, pp. 363–365)*

479. **(D)** Papillary cancer has the best prognosis of all thyroid cancers. Although it is seven times more common than follicular cancer, fewer people die from it. Even with follicular cancer, most patients will die of other diseases. In common with other thyroid cancers, age seems to be an independent risk factor for poor prognosis. *(Devita, pp. 1746–1750)*

480. **(B)** Although well-differentiated thyroid cancer is twice as common in whites than in blacks, the proportion that are follicular is more than twice as high in blacks. *(Devita, pp. 1746–1750)*

481. **(E)** Serum calcitonin elevation is specific for medullary thyroid cancer and is the most specific tumor marker now available. When combined with provocative agents (eg, calcium, pentagrastin), it is also very sensitive. In the familial syndrome, provocative tests have been superseded by genetic studies. *(Devita, p. 1757)*

482. **(B)** Nodular sclerosing Hodgkin's disease is more common in women and is particularly common in younger age groups but can occur at any age. *(Devita, p. 2347)*

483. **(A)** In lymphocyte-predominant Hodgkin's disease, multiple sections often have to be examined to find Reed–Sternberg cells. Some authorities question whether such cells are necessary for diagnosis of this form. Variants, often called L&H or popcorn cells, are often frequently found. *(Devita, p. 2345)*

484. **(A)** Most patients with lymphocyte-predominant Hodgkin's disease have clinically local-

ized disease and are asymptomatic; the prognosis is usually favorable. However, it accounts for only 4 to 5% of cases. *(Devita, p. 2346)*

485. **(F)** This is a frequent accompaniment of Hodgkin's disease and can be found in involved lymph nodes and may be extensive enough to obscure the presence of Hodgkin's disease. Rather than evidence of occult involvement, the presence of granulomas implies, stage for stage, a better prognosis than those without this reaction. *(Devita, pp. 2344–2352)*

486. **(A)** Prostaglandins play a role in bone resorption in metastatic disease, perhaps explaining the effectiveness of NSAIDs for this type of pain. Aspirin has been shown to have an antitumor effect in an animal bone tumor model. *(Devita, p. 2992)*

487. **(D)** Carbamazepine is an anticonvulsant used widely as an adjuvant analgesic for neuralgic pain caused by either tumor infiltration or surgical nerve injury. Because cancer patients commonly have compromised hematologic reserve, the leukopenia and thrombocytopenia caused by carbamazepine may limit its use. *(Devita, pp. 2993, 2999)*

488. **(G)** Steroids are useful for controlling pain in patients with leptomeningeal metastases or headache from increased intracranial pressure. *(Devita, p. 3000)*

489. **(C)** Usually, sedation can be controlled by altering opioid dosage, or switching to a drug with a shorter half-life, as well as stopping other sedating medications. If this fails, amphetamine, methylphenidate, and caffeine can be used to counteract the sedative effect. *(Devita, p. 3001)*

CHAPTER 7

Diseases of the Nervous System
Questions

DIRECTIONS (Questions 490 through 518): Each of the numbered items or incomplete statements in this section is followed by answers or by completions of the statement. Select the ONE lettered answer or completion that is BEST in each case.

490. A 69-year-old woman with worsening short-term memory impairment is tested in clinic and has poor ability to generate lists of words or copy diagrams (intersecting pentagons). She is likely to have

   (A) atrophy of the medial temporal lobes
   (B) atrophy of the entire frontal and temporal lobes
   (C) cranial nerve involvement
   (D) transient episodes of hemiplegia
   (E) atrophy of the caudate

Questions 491 through 493

491. A 38-year-old man presents with involuntary facial grimacing, shrugging of the shoulders, and jerking movements of the limb. His father was similarly affected. The progress includes

   (A) a normal life span
   (B) a 50% chance of only male children being similarly affected
   (C) mental deterioration
   (D) eventual development of rigidity
   (E) development of hemiparesis

492. At autopsy this man's brain would reveal

   (A) an intact cerebral cortex
   (B) predominant loss of cholinergic striatal interneurons
   (C) predominant loss of GABAergic striatal efferents
   (D) shrinkage, or even obliteration, of the lateral ventricles
   (E) severe involvement of the caudate nucleus with relative sparing of the putamen

493. Management options for this man include

   (A) gamma-aminobutyric acid (GABA)-mimetic agents
   (B) inhibitors of GABA metabolism
   (C) cholinergic agents
   (D) dopamine receptor blockers
   (E) centrally acting cholinesterase inhibitors

494. An 18-year-old woman has periodic episodes that begin with severely decreased vision, followed by ataxia, dysarthria, and tinnitus. The symptoms last for 30 minutes and are then followed by a throbbing occipital headache. The most likely diagnosis is

   (A) vertebral–basilar insufficiency
   (B) chronic basilar artery dissection
   (C) classic migraine
   (D) ophthalmoplegic migraine
   (E) basilar migraine

495. A 6-month-old child has recurrent seizures. Evaluation reveals a baby with impaired movement, retinal abnormalities, and x-ray evidence of brain calcification. The most likely diagnosis is

(A) Tay–Sachs disease
(B) hydrocephalus
(C) kernicterus
(D) toxoplasmosis
(E) congenital neurosyphilis

496. A 74-year-old woman develops occlusion in the right posterior cerebral artery. This is likely to cause

(A) homonymous hemianopia
(B) total blindness
(C) sudden death
(D) infarction of the right brain stem
(E) a right-sided hemiplegia

497. A 53-year-old man complains of clumsiness with both hands. Physical examination reveals fasciculations, diffuse muscle weakness, plus positive Babinski signs bilaterally. One would expect to see

(A) a long history of remissions and exacerbations
(B) sensory loss in the distribution of peripheral nerves
(C) focal seizures
(D) a progressively downhill course
(E) cogwheel rigidity

498. A 63-year-old man develops transient episodes of vertigo, slurred speech, diplopia, and paresthesias. This suggests

(A) posterior circulation transient ischemic attack (TIA)
(B) anterior communicating artery aneurysm
(C) hypertensive encephalopathy
(D) pseudobulbar palsy
(E) occlusion of the middle cerebral artery

499. A 75-year-old woman develops a right homonymous hemianopia. The lesion is located in the

(A) right optic nerve
(B) chiasm
(C) right optic radiations
(D) right occipital lobe
(E) left optic radiations

500. A 10-year-old boy with multiple tan-colored cutaneous macules present almost since birth is likely to have or develop

(A) bilateral eighth nerve tumors
(B) irregular small pupils
(C) axillary freckling
(D) cataracts
(E) hip involvement

501. A 60-year-old man with diabetes acutely develops double vision. Physical exam will reveal

(A) paralysis of the lateral gaze
(B) ptosis of the eyelid
(C) widening of the palpebral fissure
(D) inability to turn the eye downward and outward
(E) deviation of the eye inward

502. A 40-year-old man is injured in a car accident and fractures his left elbow. Neurological findings might include

(A) atrophy of the muscles of the thenar eminence
(B) wrist drop
(C) inability to oppose the thumb
(D) sensory loss of the palmar surface of the thumb, index, and middle fingers
(E) impaired adduction and abduction of the fingers

Questions 503 and 504

503. A 43-year-old man is referred from the emergency department with polyneuritis, confusion, disorientation, memory loss, and a tendency to confabulate. The most likely diagnosis is

(A) pernicious anemia

(B) alcoholism

(C) cerebrovascular disease of the carotid system

(D) Charcot–Marie–Tooth disease

(E) dermatomyositis

504. Acute treatment for this man might include

(A) prophylactic phenytoin administration

(B) prophylactic diazepam administration

(C) prophylactic carbamazepine administration

(D) calcium administration

(E) steroid administration

505. Signs and symptoms of involvement of the peripheral nerves in the form of pains, paresthesias, motor weakness, and reflex loss develop in a fairly large percentage of patients with

(A) heart disease

(B) dermatomyositis

(C) hypothyroidism

(D) diabetes mellitus

(E) adrenal insufficiency

506. A 94-year-old man develops headaches, light-headedness, drowsiness, and seizures over 6 weeks. A hyperintense clot over the left cerebral cortex is seen on computed tomography (CT) scan. This lesion

(A) is almost always of venous origin

(B) is rarely seen in infancy

(C) is due to injury to the middle meningeal artery

(D) is always chronic

(E) does not usually occur in the absence of trauma

507. A 68-year-old man has many months history of progressive hearing loss, unsteady gait, tinnitus, and facial pain. This tumor is most likely to lead to a palsy of the

(A) fourth cranial nerve

(B) sixth cranial nerve

(C) eighth cranial nerve

(D) tenth cranial nerve

(E) eleventh cranial nerve

Questions 508 through 509

508. Figure 7–1A shows a plaque of demyelination in the optic nerve as compared to a normal sample in Figure 7–1B. What is the most likely cause of this phenomenon?

(A) diabetic microvascular disease

(B) arteriosclerosis

(C) trauma

(D) multiple sclerosis

(E) Creutzfeldt–Jakob disease

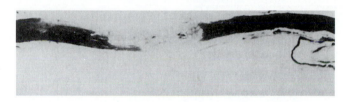

Figure 7–1A.

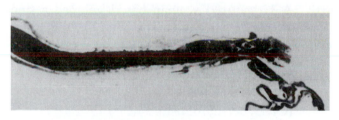

Figure 7–1B.

509. A very common presenting symptom in the disease illustrated above is

(A) limb weakness

(B) hemiplegia

(C) cervical myelopathy

(D) sphincter impairment

(E) seizures

Questions 510 and 511

510. A 25-year-old man complains of excessive sleepiness during the daytime for years despite adequate nighttime sleep. He has sought medical attention after falling asleep while driving. He is slender and otherwise healthy and on no medications. He might also complain about which of the following?

(A) excessive snoring (wife's report)
(B) automatic behavior (wife's report)
(C) restless sleep (wife's report)
(D) paresthesias
(E) morning headache

511. Treatment for this man might include

(A) a device providing continuous positive airway pressure (CPAP) at night
(B) oral surgery
(C) tracheostomy
(D) amphetamines
(E) benzodiazepines at bedtime

512. A 17-year-old woman has developed a fine tremor of her hands. The most likely diagnosis is

(A) hypopituitarism
(B) marijuana use
(C) hyperthyroidism
(D) myxedema
(E) iron overdose

513. A 19-year-old man has had progressive ataxia of gait and great difficulty in running. In the past year he has developed hand clumsiness. Physical exam reveals pes cavus, kyphoscoliosis, and both cerebellar and sensory changes in the legs. There is a positive family history. The pathologic changes would be found in

(A) spinal cord tracts
(B) basal ganglia
(C) cerebral cortex
(D) peripheral autonomic nerves
(E) peripheral motor nerves

514. An 18-year-old man presents with mild jaundice. Examination reveals rigidity and tremor. In this disease, there is usually

(A) a reduction of copper excretion in the urine
(B) an increase of the serum ceruloplasmin content
(C) no renal involvement
(D) retention of normal neurologic movements
(E) a peculiar greenish-brown pigmentation of the cornea

515. A 30-year-old woman complains of double vision. Examination reveals ptosis and impaired eye movements with normal pupillary response. The most likely diagnosis is

(A) optic atrophy
(B) ophthalmic zoster
(C) paralysis agitans
(D) Horner syndrome
(E) myasthenia gravis

516. A 47-year-old woman presents with headaches. The physical examination reveals a bitemporal hemianopsia with the upper fields more severely impaired. The most likely diagnosis is a(n)

(A) pituitary adenoma
(B) falx meningioma
(C) craniopharyngioma
(D) aneurysm of the internal carotid artery
(E) glioblastoma

517. A 45-year-old man has fasciculations in his arms and legs. The most likely diagnosis is

(A) amyotrophic lateral sclerosis (ALS)
(B) myotonic muscular dystrophy
(C) amyotonia congenita
(D) tabes dorsalis
(E) migraine

518. The most likely finding in a 79-year-old woman with Parkinson's disease is

(A) constant fine tremor
(B) muscle atrophy
(C) akinesia
(D) pupillary constriction
(E) spontaneous remission

DIRECTIONS (Questions 519 through 527): Each set of matching questions in this section consists of a list of lettered options followed by several numbered items. For each numbered item, select the appropriate lettered option(s). Each lettered option may be selected once, more than once, or not at all. EACH ITEM WILL STATE THE NUMBER OF OPTIONS TO SELECT. CHOOSE EXACTLY THIS NUMBER.

Questions 519 and 520

(A) aqueductal stenosis
(B) infectious process
(C) enlarged foramina of Luschka
(D) nutritional deficiency
(E) agenesis of the corpus callosum
(F) postvaccination
(G) acoustic neuroma

519. A 77-year-old woman with deterioration of gait has a computed tomography (CT) scan revealing enlarged ventricles (SELECT ONE)

520. Associated with central nervous system (CNS) demyelinization (SELECT THREE)

Questions 521 through 524

(A) basal ganglia hemorrhage
(B) cerebellar hemorrhage
(C) pontine hemorrhage
(D) lobar intracerebral hemorrhage
(E) cocaine-related hemorrhage
(F) subarachnoid hemorrhage
(G) arteriovenous malformation (AVM)
(H) hypertensive encephalopathy
(I) primary intraventricular hemorrhage

521. A 67-year-old man develops coma over a few minutes. He has ataxic respiration and pinpoint, reactive pupils. Oculocephalic reflexes are absent. The likely diagnosis is (SELECT ONE)

522. A 74-year-old woman develops occipital headache, vomiting, and ataxia. Over the next few hours, she develops a decline in her level of consciousness. Magnetic resonance imaging (MRI) is likely to reveal (SELECT ONE)

523. This syndrome is almost always associated with chronic hypertension (SELECT FOUR)

524. A 24-year-old man has a history of recurrent throbbing headaches. He suddenly develops mild right-sided weakness. His blood pressure in the past has been normal but is now slightly elevated (SELECT ONE)

Questions 525 through 527

(A) hyperkalemia
(B) facial nevi
(C) weakness and atrophy of the hands
(D) hypokalemia
(E) mental retardation
(F) fasciculations
(G) hypercalcemia
(H) convulsions
(I) acetazolamide useful in acute attack

525. A 20-year-old man with familial periodic paralysis (SELECT TWO)

526. An 11-year-old girl with tuberous sclerosis (SELECT THREE)

527. A 23-year-old woman with impaired pain and temperature sensation in her arms but normal light touch (SELECT TWO)

DIRECTIONS (Questions 528 through 547): Each of the numbered items or incomplete statements in this section is followed by answers or by completions of the statement. Select the ONE lettered answer or completion that is BEST in each case.

528. A 20-year-old man suffered significant head injury after a diving accident. In this situation, seizures

   (A) are inevitable
   (B) are more often generalized than focal
   (C) always indicate a brain abscess
   (D) usually occur immediately
   (E) are usually on the dominant side

529. CT scanning of the brain is superior to MRI of the brain in which circumstances?

   (A) demonstrating Chiari malformation
   (B) imaging demyelinating diseases (eg, multiple sclerosis)
   (C) imaging small lacunes
   (D) diagnosing an acute subarachnoid hemorrhage
   (E) searching for metastatic disease

530. A 77-year-old woman develops acute hoarseness and dysphagia. MRI reveals evidence of infarction in the lateral aspect of the medulla on the right side. This syndrome

   (A) is invariably caused by occlusion of the posterior–inferior cerebellar artery
   (B) causes contralateral sensory impairment
   (C) causes contralateral ataxia
   (D) causes ipsilateral paralysis of tongue
   (E) causes ipsilateral paralysis of arm and leg

531. A 27-year-old woman, a recent immigrant from the Caribbean basin, has had progressive leg weakness. Physical exam reveals increased tone of both legs with weakness, clonus, extensor plantar responses, and brisk reflexes. This disease

   (A) never shows evidence of cerebellar signs
   (B) is associated with a definite sensory level

   (C) can be spread by sexual activity
   (D) rarely involves the bladder
   (E) is characterized by rapid progression once symptoms and signs develop

Questions 532 and 533

532. A 40-year-old woman complains of episodes of severe unilateral, stabbing facial pain that is intermittent for several hours, then disappears for several days. Physical examination is entirely normal. The most likely diagnosis is

   (A) trigeminal neuralgia
   (B) herpes zoster
   (C) acoustic neuroma
   (D) Bell's palsy
   (E) diabetic neuropathy

533. The most effective therapy for this condition is

   (A) morphine
   (B) indomethacin
   (C) cimetidine
   (D) carbamazepine
   (E) lidocaine (Xylocaine) gel

534. A 63-year-old man suddenly becomes acutely ill and has a fever of 102.4°F. There is pain in the eye, and the orbits are painful to pressure. There is edema and chemosis of the conjunctivae and eyelids, and the bulbs are proptosed. Diplopia and ptosis are present, and the pupils are slow in reacting. The most likely diagnosis is

   (A) cavernous sinus thrombosis
   (B) chorioretinitis
   (C) subarachnoid hemorrhage
   (D) brain abscess
   (E) none of the above

535. A 20-year-old woman presents with a history of rapid loss of vision in one eye. Examination reveals pain on movement of the eyeball. The pupillary reactions are normal, as is the appearance of the fundi. Perimetry shows a

large central scotoma. The most likely diagnosis is

(A) optic atrophy
(B) papilledema
(C) retrobulbar neuritis
(D) amblyopia ex anopsia
(E) hysteria

536. A 67-year-old man has episodes of numbness of the left side of his body, with impaired vision in his right eye, lasting up to 5 minutes. The most likely diagnosis is

(A) posterior cerebral artery insufficiency
(B) parietal lobe neoplasm
(C) parasagittal meningioma
(D) AVM
(E) internal carotid artery insufficiency

Questions 537 and 538

537. An 18-year-old man develops fever, headache, and generalized seizures. Cerebrospinal fluid (CSF) shows mononuclear cell pleocytosis and increased protein. The electroencephalogram (EEG) shows bilateral periodic discharges from the temporal leads and slow-wave complexes at regular intervals of 2 to 3 per second. A CT scan shows bilateral, small, low-density temporal lobe lesions. The most appropriate diagnostic approach in this setting is

(A) angiography
(B) observing response to therapy
(C) cerebral biopsy
(D) acute viral titers
(E) CSF culture

538. The patient in the previous question is most likely to respond to treatment with

(A) penicillin
(B) chloramphenicol
(C) acyclovir
(D) erythromycin
(E) steroids

539. A 24-year-old woman develops bilateral foot drop, progressing over 1 week to paralysis of both legs and lower trunk. There are no constitutional symptoms or signs. The CSF protein is very high. The most likely diagnosis is

(A) diabetic neuropathy
(B) alcoholic neuropathy
(C) Guillain–Barré syndrome
(D) cyanide poisoning
(E) poliomyelitis

Questions 540 through 542

A 37-year-old woman complains of drooping eyelids at the end of the day. Further history reveals difficulty in chewing food and some weakness in climbing stairs. On examination, there is weakness of the eyelids, masticatory muscles, and thigh flexors. There is no sensory abnormality, and reflexes are normal. The chest x-ray (CXR) is shown in Figure 7–2.

540. What does the CXR show?

(A) bronchogenic carcinoma
(B) Hodgkin's disease
(C) teratoma
(D) thyroid tumor with retrosternal extension
(E) thymoma

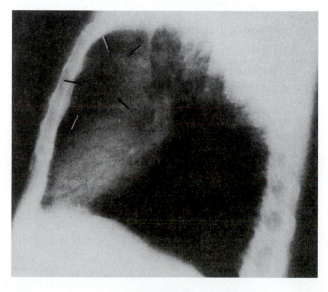

Figure 7–2.

541. The cause of the patient's symptoms is

(A) hypercalcemia
(B) myasthenia gravis
(C) multiple sclerosis
(D) thyroid storm
(E) meningeal lymphoma

542. Which of the following treatments is contraindicated in this patient?

(A) anticholinergic drugs
(B) surgery
(C) plasmapheresis
(D) cyclophosphamide
(E) high-dose prednisone

Questions 543 through 547

543. A 79-year-old woman is seen in the office for "dizziness." Which of the following findings would suggest true vertigo?

(A) The patient is taking multiple antihypertensives.
(B) The symptoms are worse on standing.
(C) She has had two falls.
(D) The room is spinning around her.
(E) A prior Holter monitor was negative during episodes of dizziness.

544. Which of the following findings suggests the vertigo is peripheral in origin?

(A) optic neuritis
(B) tinnitus
(C) bidirectional nystagmus
(D) vertical nystagmus
(E) visual fixation does not affect vertigo or nystagmus

545. Which of the following findings suggests the vertigo is central in origin?

(A) deafness
(B) mild chronic symptoms
(C) unidirectional nystagmus

(D) visual fixation inhibits vertigo and nystagmus
(E) spinning sensation is toward fast phase of nystagmus

546. Benign paroxysmal positional vertigo (BPPV) is usually caused by

(A) head trauma
(B) ischemic events
(C) benign cerebellar tumors
(D) unknown causes
(E) Ménière's disease

547. Which of the following findings on vestibular testing favors the diagnosis of BPPV over central positional vertigo?

(A) no latency period
(B) no fatigability
(C) habituation occurs
(D) mild vertigo
(E) symptoms consistently the same from one set of tests to the next

DIRECTIONS (Questions 548 through 567): Each set of matching questions in this section consists of a list of lettered options followed by several numbered items. For each numbered item, select the appropriate lettered option(s). Each lettered option may be selected once, more than once, or not at all. EACH ITEM WILL STATE THE NUMBER OF OPTIONS TO SELECT. CHOOSE EXACTLY THIS NUMBER.

Questions 548 through 552

(A) simple partial seizure
(B) complex partial seizures
(C) tonic–clonic (grand mal) seizures
(D) absence (petit mal) seizures
(E) myoclonic seizures
(F) status epilepticus

548. A 55-year-old man, recently arrived from Britain, has a long history of beef consumption. He has now developed a rapidly progressive dementia. The most likely type of seizure is (SELECT ONE)

549. A 27-year-old woman's MRI reveals temporal lobe sclerosis. The most likely form of seizure is (SELECT ONE)

550. A teenager has a long history of "daydreaming" in school. EEG reveals evidence of a generalized seizure disorder, but there has never been a history of convulsive muscular activity (SELECT ONE)

551. A 23-year-old woman has a history of repetitive involuntary movements of her right hand associated with abnormal facial movements. At times, the movements spread to involve the entire arm (SELECT ONE)

552. This form of epilepsy almost always starts in childhood (SELECT ONE)

Questions 553 through 557

(A) phenytoin
(B) carbamazepine
(C) phenobarbital
(D) primidone
(E) sodium valproate (valproic acid)
(F) ethosuximide
(G) clonazepam
(H) trimethadione

553. Used for absence attacks, it can cause ataxia, tremor, bone marrow suppression, and hepatotoxicity (SELECT ONE)

554. Is the drug of choice for myoclonic seizures (SELECT ONE)

555. Can be used for tonic–clonic (grand mal) and partial seizures and can cause gum hyperplasia and lymphadenopathy (SELECT ONE)

556. Used for tonic–clonic and partial seizures, it can increase metabolism of other drugs (SELECT ONE)

557. Useful in myoclonic seizures and absence attacks, but development of tolerance can limit its effectiveness (SELECT ONE)

Questions 558 through 562

(A) essential anisocoria
(B) Horner syndrome
(C) tonic pupils (Holmes–Adie syndrome)
(D) Argyll–Robertson pupils
(E) midbrain pupils
(F) atropinized pupils
(G) oculomotor palsy

558. A 63-year-old man with a unilateral small, round pupil with brisk response to light and near stimuli; associated with ptosis (SELECT ONE)

559. A 23-year-old woman has one large pupil and diminished reflexes (SELECT ONE)

560. A 57-year-old woman has small, irregular pupils. Accommodation is normal, but reaction to light is poor (SELECT ONE)

561. Can be caused by a parasympathetic lesion at the ciliary ganglion (SELECT ONE)

562. Commonly caused by an infection (SELECT ONE)

Questions 563 through 567

A 48-year-old man complains of muscle weakness.

(A) anterior horn cell
(B) peripheral nerve
(C) neuromuscular junction
(D) muscle

563. On examination, reflexes are decreased out of proportion to weakness (SELECT ONE)

564. He has noticed fluctuation during the day (SELECT ONE)

565. Examination reveals severe atrophy (SELECT ONE)

566. Examination reveals predominantly distal weakness and sensory abnormalities (SELECT ONE)

567. Characteristic facial features (SELECT ONE)

Answers and Explanations

490. (B) Alzheimer's disease can be quite diffuse, but there is particular involvement of the medial temporal lobes and cortical association areas. The atrophy of the hippocampus is particularly marked. Microscopic examination reveals neurofibrillary tangles and amyloid plaques. *(Victor, pp. 1110–1114)*

491. (C) This is a case of Huntington's chorea. It is an autosomal dominant gene (found on the short arm of chromosome 4), and male and female children are equally affected. Movement disorder, mental deterioration, and personality change are the hallmarks of the disease, but can be very subtle initially. The disease starts typically between ages 35 and 40 (although the variation is wide) and runs its course in about 15 years. The akinetic rigid variety (Westphal variant) of Huntington's typically has a childhood onset. *(Victor, pp. 1121–1123)*

492. (C) The caudate nucleus and putamen are both severely involved in Huntington's chorea. The degeneration of the caudate nucleus results in enlarged lateral ventricles (with a "butterfly" appearance on CT). Atrophy is very widespread in the brain and includes the cerebral cortex. A decrease in glucose metabolism as revealed on position-emission tomography (PET) scan precedes the evidence of tissue loss. *(Victor, pp. 1123–1124)*

493. (D) There are disturbances of norepinephrine, glutamic acid decarboxylase, choline acetyltransferase, GABA, acetylcholine, and somatostatin, but their significance is poorly understood. Dopamine blocking agents (eg, haloperidol) can be used to treat psychosis and ameliorate chorea but do not alter the course of disease. Presynaptic dopamine depleters such as clozapine, reserpine, or tetrabenazine can be used for chorea as well, but have significant side effects. Antidepressants are helpful for symptomatic treatment. Most patients eventually end up in an institution. *(Victor, p. 1125)*

494. (E) Basilar migraine can be very dramatic, and can resemble ischemia in the territory of the basilar posterior cerebral arteries. The visual symptoms of basilar migraine typically affect the whole of both visual fields, and can even cause temporary cortical blindness. There can also be an alarming period of coma or quadriplegia. *(Victor, pp. 183–184)*

495. (D) Toxoplasmosis is the most likely diagnosis. The infection has a predilection for the CNS and the eye and produces encephalitis in utero. Symptoms can be evident in the first few days of life. Infants born with active disease may have fever, rash, seizures, and hepatosplenomegaly at birth. *(Victor, p. 775)*

496. (A) Occlusion of the right posterior cerebral artery is most likely to cause homonymous hemianopia. This artery conveys blood to the inferior and medial portion of the posterior temporal and occipital lobes and to the optic thalamus. *(Victor, p. 839)*

497. (D) This man has amyotrophic lateral sclerosis. The disease causes neuronal loss in the anterior horns of the spinal cord and motor nuclei of the lower brain stem. The disease is one of constant progression rather than remissions and exacerbations, and death usually occurs within 5 years. There is no sensory loss and no seizure diathesis, because only the motor system is involved. There can be signs of hyperreflexia and spasticity, depending on the balance of upper and lower motor neuron damage, but not cogwheel rigidity. *(Victor, pp. 1152–1157)*

498. **(A)** Posterior circulation TIA is suggested by the transient episodes. The basilar artery is formed by the two vertebral arteries and supplies the pons, the midbrain, and the cerebellum. With vertebrobasilar TIAs, tinnitus, vertigo, diplopia, ataxia, hemiparesis, and bilateral visual impairment are common findings. *(Victor, pp. 838–841)*

499. **(E)** The hemianopia is due to a lesion of the left optic radiations. The posterior cerebral artery arises from the basilar artery but is sometimes a branch of the internal carotid. With posterior cerebral artery lesions affecting the occipital cortex, it is possible for the hemianopia to be an isolated finding. *(Victor, p. 831)*

500. **(C)** The two common forms of neurofibromatosis (NF-1 and NF-2) are genetically distinct. NF-1 is the type with multiple café au lait spots and is associated with axillary or inguinal freckling, iris hamartomas (Lisch nodules), peripheral neurofibromas, and bony abnormalities (including kyphoscoliosis). NF-2 is associated with CNS tumors, particularly bilateral eighth nerve tumors. Skin lesions are spare or absent, and early lens opacities can occur. *(Victor, pp. 1074–1076)*

501. **(B)** Third nerve palsy can result in ptosis of the eyelid. There is also loss of the ability to open the eye, and the eyeball is deviated outward and slightly downward. With complete lesions, the pupil is dilated, does not react to light, and loses the power of accommodation. In diabetes, the pupil is often spared. The sixth cranial nerve can also be affected by diabetes, but this is much less common. *(Victor, pp. 282, 1396)*

502. **(E)** Injury to the ulnar nerve results in impaired adduction and abduction of the fingers. The fibers arise from the eighth cervical and the first thoracic segments. The ulnar is a mixed nerve with sensory supply to the medial hand. *(Victor, p. 1434)*

503. **(B)** The combination of symptoms is typical of chronic alcohol abuse. The mental symptoms are suggestive of Korsakoff syndrome. A distal limb sensory–motor neuropathy is also typical of alcoholism. The confusion and disorientation are typical for acute alcohol intoxication. *(Victor, pp. 1237–1249)*

504. **(B)** Prophylactic administration of diazepam in a withdrawing alcoholic can prevent or reduce severe syndromes such as delirium tremens (DTs). Prophylactic phenytoin, however, is not helpful. A calm, quiet environment with close observation and frequent reassurance is very important. Vitamin administration (especially thiamine) is important, but frequently, severe magnesium depletion slows improvement. *(Victor, p. 1244)*

505. **(D)** These signs and symptoms develop in a fairly large percentage of patients with diabetes mellitus. Loss of proprioceptive sensation together with absent reflexes superficially resembles tabes dorsalis. If sensory loss is severe, Charcot joints can develop. *(Victor, p. 1398)*

506. **(A)** A subdural hematoma is almost always of venous origin and secondary to a minor or severe injury to the head, but may occur in blood dyscrasias or cachexia in the absence of trauma. Acute subdural hematomas commonly present with a fluctuating level of consciousness and significant cerebral damage. Chronic subdurals may also present with seizures or papilledema. *(Victor, pp. 938–940)*

507. **(C)** An acoustic neuroma is most likely to lead to a palsy of the eighth cranial nerve. Deafness, headache, ataxia, tinnitus, and diplopia are seen, as well as facial paresthesias. Acoustic neuromas represent 5 to 10% of all intracranial tumors. They develop from

Schwann cells and generally grow very slowly. They may be very large before symptoms develop. *(Victor, pp. 709–712)*

508. **(D)** Visual loss in multiple sclerosis varies from slight blurring to no light perception. Other eye symptoms include diplopia and pain. The classic syndrome of optic or retrobulbar neuritis occurs commonly at some point in the disease, and it is the presenting symptom in 25% of cases. *(Victor, pp. 961–965)*

509. **(A)** Weakness or numbness in one or more limbs is the initial manifestation of disease in about half the patients. Other common initial presentations include optic neuritis (25%) and acute myelitis. Hemiplegia, seizures, and cervical myelopathy (in older patients) occur occasionally as the initial manifestation. Sphincter impairment usually occurs later in the disease. *(Felig, p. 963)*

510. **(B)** The early age of onset and otherwise good health suggest a diagnosis of narcolepsy, which is usually accompanied by other symptomatology. Hypnagogic hallucinations are almost always visual. They occur most frequently at the onset of sleep, either during the day or at night. They are generally very vivid. Cataplexy is a brief loss of muscle power without loss of consciousness. The patient is fully aware of what is going on. The paralysis may be complete or partial. Automatic behavior with amnesia is a common manifestation of the narcolepsy–cataplexy syndromes, occurring in 50% of cases. Automatic behavior can be confused with complex partial seizures. Paresthesias are not part of the narcolepsy syndrome. Snoring, restless sleep, and morning headache suggest sleep apnea. *(Victor, pp. 422–424)*

511. **(D)** This man does not have risk factors for sleep apnea (older age, snoring, obesity) and likely has narcolepsy. Adrenergic stimulant drugs such as methylphenidate or amphetamines help the sleepiness, and tricyclic compounds can help the cataplexy. Strategically planned naps can also be helpful. *(Victor, p. 424)*

512. **(C)** In hyperthyroidism, neurologic symptoms include tremors of the hands, exophthalmos, lid lag, stare, and muscle weakness. The muscle weakness of hyperthyroidism affects the pelvic girdle and, to a lesser extent, the shoulder girdle. Reflexes are normal or increased, and sensation is normal. It must be differentiated from myasthenia gravis, which may also accompany thyrotoxicosis. *(Victor, pp. 100–101, 1519–1520)*

513. **(A)** This young man has Friedreich's ataxia, associated with a gene defect on chromosome 9. The pathologic changes are found in the spinal cord tracts. Degeneration is seen in the posterior columns, the lateral corticospinal tract, and the spinocerebellar tracts. Ataxia, sensory loss, nystagmus, reflex changes, clubfeet, and kyphoscoliosis are the characteristic findings. The heart is frequently involved, and cardiac disease is a common cause of death. *(Victor, pp. 1145–1147)*

514. **(E)** In Wilson's disease, there is usually a reduction of the serum ceruloplasmin content. Signs and symptoms of injury to the basal ganglia are accompanied by cirrhosis of the liver. Renal involvement is characterized by persistent aminoaciduria. The most common neurologic finding is tremor. The corneal pigmentation (Kayser–Fleischer ring) is the most important diagnostic finding on physical examination. If it is absent, any neurologic findings cannot be ascribed to Wilson's disease. *(Victor, pp. 1026–1029)*

515. **(E)** In myasthenia gravis, weakness of the facial and levator palpebrae muscles produces a characteristic expressionless face, with drooping of the eyelids. Weakness of the ocular muscles may cause paralysis or weakness of individual muscles, paralysis of conjugate gaze, ophthalmoplegia, or a pattern similar to internuclear ophthalmoplegia. The presence of normal pupillary responses to light and accommodation with weakness of extraocular muscles, levators, and orbicularis oculi is almost completely diagnostic of myasthenia. *(Victor, pp. 1536–1537)*

516. (A) Adenomas of the pituitary gland constitute approximately 7% of intracranial tumors, with the chromophobic type being the most common. With macroadenomas, some degree of pituitary insufficiency is common, and half the patients have headaches. With microadenomas, the other pituitary functions may be completely normal. *(Victor, pp. 713–717)*

517. (A) The most common initial symptom of ALS is weakness and wasting of the extremities. The fasciculations can be a very prominent part of the disease. This is rare in other neurologic disorders. *(Victor, p. 1153)*

518. (C) The characteristic triad in Parkinson's disease (tremor, rigidity, akinesia) has been expanded to include postural instability. This forms the mnemonic TRAP. Autonomic instability is also common. Findings on exam also include masklike facies, dysarthria, stooped posture, and abnormal gait. *(Victor, pp. 1128–1137)*

519. (A) Adults may develop hydrocephalus as a result of occlusion of CSF pathways by tumors in the third ventricle, brain stem, or posterior fossa. In adults, the symptoms of obstructive hydrocephalus include headache, lethargy, malaise, incoordination, and weakness. Seizures do not usually occur. Dementia, altered consciousness, ocular nerve palsies, papilledema, ataxia, or corticospinal tract signs may be present. *(Victor, pp. 660–665)*

520. (B, D, F) Myelin is a complex protein lipid carbohydrate structure, which forms part of the cell membrane of the oligodendroglia. Vascular lesions cause demyelination because of ischemia. Papovaviruses can cause progressive multifocal leukoencephalopathy in patients with human immunodeficiency virus (HIV) infection, or less commonly, malignancy. Acute disseminated encephalomyelitis has been described after smallpox or rabies vaccination. Nutritional deficiencies can also cause demyelination (eg, pernicious anemia with vitamin B_{12} deficiency). *(Victor, pp. 954, 1205–1229)*

521. (C) Pontine hemorrhage is associated with impaired oculocephalic reflexes and small, reactive pupils. It generally evolves over a few minutes, usually with coma and quadriplegia. The prognosis is poor, and death often occurs within hours. *(Braunwald, p. 2386)*

522. (B) Cerebellar hemorrhage, when mild, may present with only headache, vomiting, and ataxia of gait. Patients may complain of dizziness or vertigo. The eyes may be deviated to the side opposite the hemorrhage. Nystagmus is not common, but an ipsilateral sixth nerve palsy can occur. This is the only type of intracerebral hemorrhage that commonly benefits from surgical intervention. *(Braunwald, p. 2386)*

523. (A, B, C, H) Intracerebral hemorrhage into the cerebellum, pons, and thalamus are usually due to spontaneous rupture of small, penetrating arteries and are usually associated with hypertension, although hemorrhagic disorders and neoplasms are possible causes. Hypertensive encephalopathy is an unusual complication of chronic hypertension and nowadays is almost never the initial presentation of hypertension. Cocaine-related hemorrhage is caused by acute hypertension. Subarachnoid hemorrhage is more likely caused by an aneurysm and lobar intracerebral hemorrhage is frequently caused by nonhypertensive factors such as amyloid angiopathy, AVMs, and aneurysms. *(Braunwald, pp. 2386–2387)*

524. (G) AVMs are more frequently seen in men and, although present from birth, do not usually become symptomatic until later in life. The peak incidence of symptoms is between ages 10 and 30. The headaches can be similar to migraine, or it can be more diffuse. It can also present with seizure or rupture. Hemorrhage can be massive or minimal when rupture does occur. *(Braunwald, pp. 2390–2391)*

525. (A, I) The most common familial periodic paralysis syndrome is usually associated with low potassium, but there are less common forms characterized by high or normal potassium. It is characterized by recurrent attacks of weakness or paralysis of the somatic musculature, with loss of the deep tendon reflexes. Preventive therapy includes potassium supplementation and possibly a low carbohydrate, low salt, high potassium diet. Imipramine and acetazolamide are said to be useful in acute attacks. *(Victor, pp. 1560–1562)*

526. **(B, E, H)** Tuberous sclerosis is an autosomal dominant disease with a wide variety of clinical phenotypes. Lesions occur in the nervous system, skin, bones, retina, kidney, and elsewhere. The skin lesions include facial nevi (fibroma molluscum) and patches of skin fibrosis. Hard nodules are found throughout the brain. Seizures and mental retardation can occur. *(Victor, pp. 1069–1072)*

527. **(C, F)** Syringomyelia is characterized by a dissociated sensory loss. Atrophy of the muscles can result in a clawhand deformity. Fasciculations are commonly found. *(Victor, pp. 1337–1338, 1476)*

528. **(B)** In the majority of cases, seizures do not develop until several months after the injury, 6 to 18 months being the most common interval. The more severe the injury, the greater the likelihood of seizures. For severe injuries, some authorities recommend prophylactic anticonvulsants for 1 to 2 years. There is no firm evidence for this, however. *(Victor, pp. 943–944)*

529. **(D)** CT scan is still superior to MRI in certain circumstances, particularly in the emergency setting, for diagnosing acute subarachnoid hemorrhage and fractures of the face, temporal bone, and base of the skull. CT is useful in evaluating patients with osseous spinal stenosis and spondylosis, but MRI is preferred if there are neurological defects. *(Braunwald, pp. 2337–2338)*

530. **(B)** The lateral medullary syndrome causes ipsilateral numbness but also contralateral involvement of pain and thermal sense by affecting the spinothalamic tract. It can be caused by occlusion of the vertebral arteries; posterior–inferior cerebellar arteries; and superior, middle, or inferior medullary arteries. Ipsilateral ataxia and falling to the side of the lesion are common. Ipsilateral paralysis of the tongue is characteristic of medial medullary syndrome, which also causes contralateral paralysis of arm and leg. Paralysis of the body is not characteristic of lateral medullary syndrome, but ipsilateral paralysis of palate and vocal cord does occur. Ipsilateral Horner syndrome, nystagmus, diplopia, vertigo, nausea, and vomiting are characteristic. *(Braunwald, p. 2376)*

531. **(C)** Tropical spastic paraparesis (TSP) is frequently associated with a retroviral (human T-lymphotropic virus-I) infection that can be spread through blood transfusion, sexual contact, intravenous drug use, and vertical transmission from mother to child. It is slowly progressive, and bladder involvement is characteristic. Sensory symptoms are usually mild, and a true sensory level is almost never found. On occasion, cranial nerve findings, frontal release signs, and cerebellar signs (tremor, dysmetria) are present. *(Braunwald, pp. 1133–1134, 2431)*

532. **(A)** The cause of trigeminal neuralgia (tic douloureux) is unknown, although some cases may be caused by compression of the trigeminal nerve by arteries or veins of the posterior fossa. The pain occurs in paroxysms and is strictly limited to one or more branches of the fifth cranial nerve. Paroxysms may be brief or last up to 15 minutes. There is no objective sensory loss, but the patient may complain of hyperesthesia of the face. Watering of the eye on the involved side may occur during an attack. *(Victor, pp. 196–198)*

533. **(D)** This anticonvulsant drug is given in doses varying from 600 to 1200 mg/day. Phenytoin has also been used. The two drugs can also be used in combination. Operative procedures include alcohol injection of the nerve or ganglion, partial section of the nerve in the middle or posterior fossa, decompres-

sion of the root, and medullary tractotomy. Radiofrequency surgery can destroy pain fibers but spare motor fibers. *(Victor, p. 198)*

534. **(A)** Cavernous sinus thrombosis is usually secondary to traumatic, neoplastic, or suppurative processes in the orbit, the nasal sinuses, or the upper half of the face. The optic discs are swollen, and there may be numerous surrounding small or large hemorrhages if the orbital veins are occluded. Visual acuity is normal or moderately impaired. *(Victor, pp. 288, 1462)*

535. **(C)** In the vast majority of cases, retrobulbar neuritis occurs as an episode in a demyelinating disease such as multiple sclerosis. It is the first manifestation of multiple sclerosis in 15% of cases and occurs at some point in 50% of all patients with the disease. The course of the retrobulbar neuritis is that of gradual spontaneous improvement. *(Victor, pp. 261–262, 962–963)*

536. **(E)** Internal carotid artery insufficiency is the most likely diagnosis. Abnormalities are found in the extracranial arteries in more than one half of the patients with symptomatic cerebral infarction. Current treatment is carotid endarterectomy for severe stenosis and aspirin therapy for lesser degrees of stenosis. *(Victor, pp. 859–860)*

537. **(B)** The patient's findings strongly suggest herpes simplex encephalitis. This is generally caused by herpes simplex virus type 1 (HSV-I). When the disease is suspected, appropriate antiviral therapy (acyclovir) should be started immediately. CT scan is not helpful in diagnosis because it becomes positive only late in the disease, but MRI scans may be helpful. Brain biopsy, once the diagnostic test of choice, is the most definitive test but is rarely performed. *(Victor, pp. 793–794)*

538. **(C)** Acyclovir selectively inhibits viral deoxyribonucleic acid (DNA) polymerase. Acyclovir is currently the treatment of choice because of better efficacy and less toxicity than previous drugs. Because it is so nontoxic,

therapy can be started even if the diagnosis is only presumptive. *(Victor, pp. 794–795)*

539. **(C)** Guillain–Barré syndrome often appears days to weeks after a viral upper respiratory or gastrointestinal (GI) infection. The initial symptoms are due to symmetric limb weakness. Paresthesias may be present. Unlike most other neuropathies, proximal muscles may be affected more than distal muscles early in the disease. Tendon reflexes are usually lost within a few days. Protein content of the CSF is usually high within a few days of onset. *(Victor, pp. 1381–1384)*

540. **(E)** The thymus tissue is often abnormal, with encapsulated tumors occurring in about 15% of cases. Almost all thymomas occur in patients over age 30. Even without thymoma, thymectomy can result in remission in patients with generalized myasthenia. Its benefit is delayed for months or more, so it is not an emergency treatment for myasthenia. *(Victor, pp. 1537–1546)*

541. **(B)** The most common presenting symptoms relate to weakness of eye muscles, causing ptosis or diplopia. Difficulty in chewing, dysarthria, and dysphagia are also common. The differential diagnosis includes all diseases that cause weakness of oropharyngeal or limb muscles. These include the muscular dystrophies, ALS, and progressive bulbar palsies, among others. Most other conditions do not improve after injection of edrophonium or neostigmine. *(Victor, pp. 1537–1546)*

542. **(A)** Anticholinergic drugs exacerbate the underlying defects. Cholinergic drugs are largely inhibitors of cholinesterase. Prednisone may improve as many as 80% of patients. Thymectomy helps patients with no thymoma, but thymoma patients do not do as well. Plasmapheresis benefits most patients but needs to be repeated at intervals. *(Victor, pp. 1546–1547)*

543. **(D)** Vertigo is defined as an illusory or hallucinatory feeling of movement of the body or environment, usually spinning. Dizziness can

be caused by multiple factors in the elderly, including orthostatic hypotension, hypoglycemia, and depression. *(Braunwald, p. 116)*

544. **(B)** Tinnitus and deafness may be found in peripheral vertigo, but not central. The nystagmus is usually unidirectional and is never vertical. Visual fixation inhibits vertigo and nystagmus during testing in peripheral vertigo. *(Braunwald, p. 117)*

545. **(B)** In central vertigo, the vertigo can be mild and chronic. In peripheral disease, the symptoms are generally more severe, but finite (although often recurrent). *(Braunwald, p. 117)*

546. **(D)** Although BPPV can occur after head trauma, there is usually no obvious precipitating factor. It generally abates spontaneously and can be treated with vestibular rehabilitation. *(Braunwald, pp. 117–118)*

547. **(C)** Patients with BPPV, in contrast to those with central positional vertigo, have a latent period from the time of onset of the offending position to development of symptoms. With maintenance of the position, patients with BPPV become less symptomatic (fatigability) and repeated positioning also lessens the symptoms (habituation). As well, in BPPV, although the symptoms are usually severe, they can be quite variable from one testing period to the next. *(Braunwald, p. 117)*

548. **(E)** Myoclonic seizures are sudden, brief, single, or repetitive muscle contractions involving one body part or the entire body. Loss of consciousness does not occur unless other types of seizures coexist. These seizures can be idiopathic or associated with Creutzfeldt–Jakob disease, uremia, hepatic failure, subacute leukoencephalopathies, and some hereditary disorders. Recent evidence has linked a variant form of Creutzfeldt–Jakob disease with bovine spongiform encephalopathy (BSE), a prior disease of cattle. This variant form usually presents with ataxia and behavior changes prior to myoclonus and dementia. *(Braunwald, pp. 2489–2490)*

549. **(B)** Complex partial seizures were once classified as temporal lobe epilepsy. Although the temporal lobe (especially the hippocampus or amygdala) is the most common site of origin, some seizures have been shown to originate from mesial parasagittal or orbital frontal regions. *(Braunwald, pp. 2355–2357)*

550. **(D)** Pure absence seizures consist of the sudden cessation of ongoing conscious activity without convulsive muscular activity or loss of postural control. They can be so brief as to be inapparent but can last several minutes. There is usually no period of postictal confusion. *(Braunwald, pp. 2355–2356)*

551. **(A)** Simple partial seizures can occur with motor, sensory, autonomic, or psychic symptoms. When a partial motor seizure spreads to adjacent neurons, a "Jacksonian march" can occur (eg, right thumb to right hand and right arm to right side of face). Face and hand movements are frequently linked because their cortical controlling regions are adjacent. *(Braunwald, p. 2355)*

552. **(D)** Absence seizures almost always begin in young children (age 6 to 14). They may first present as learning difficulties in school. The EEG is diagnostic, revealing brief 3-Hz spike and wave discharges occurring synchronously throughout all the leads. *(Braunwald, pp. 2355–2356)*

553. **(E)** Valproic acid can be used for typical and atypical seizures, myoclonic seizures, and tonic–clonic seizures. It causes little sedation and does not impair cognition. However, the blood count and liver tests must be monitored for a time after initiation of therapy to ensure the safety of the patient. *(Braunwald, pp. 2363–2365)*

554. **(E)** Valproic acid is the drug of choice for atypical absence seizures and myoclonic seizures. *(Braunwald, pp. 2363–2365)*

555. **(A)** Phenytoin can cause gum hyperplasia and hirsutism, which are particularly unpleasant side effects in young women. Lym-

phadenopathy, ataxia, incoordination, confusion, and cerebellar toxicity can also occur. *(Braunwald, pp. 2363–2365)*

556. **(C)** Phenobarbital is effective for tonic–clonic and partial seizures. It has few, if any, systemic side effects but can cause sedation and dulling of intellect. It induces liver enzymes, which can enhance the metabolism of other drugs. *(Braunwald, pp. 2363–2365)*

557. **(G)** Clonazepam is used in the treatment of typical and atypical absence seizures as well as myoclonic seizures. It causes drowsiness and irritability but few systemic symptoms. Unfortunately, the development of tolerance can limit its effectiveness. *(Braunwald, pp. 2363–2365)*

558. **(B)** Horner syndrome results in a small, round pupil on one side. Light and near reaction is brisk, and response to mydriatics and miotics is normal. The affected pupil will not dilate in the dark, so darkness accentuates the anisocoria. The syndrome is often idiopathic but can be caused by neoplasm, brain stem stroke, or carotid dissection. *(Braunwald, pp. 165–166)*

559. **(D)** The tonic pupil can be associated with Shy–Drager syndrome, amyloidosis, or diabetes. However, it is most commonly seen in otherwise healthy young women. *(Braunwald, pp. 165–166)*

560. **(D)** Argyll–Robertson pupils are small, irregular, and often bilateral. The response to light is impaired, but the response to near vision is preserved. *(Braunwald, pp. 165–166)*

561. **(C)** The tonic pupil (Holmes–Adie syndrome) is caused by a parasympathetic lesion at or distal to the ciliary ganglion. The pupil is large and usually unilateral, with absent response to light. A bright room, by causing constriction of the normal pupil, accentuates the anisocoria. *(Braunwald, pp. 165–166)*

562. **(D)** Argyll–Robertson pupils can be a manifestation of syphilis, a treponemal infection. It can also be associated with lesions of the dorsal midbrain (obstructive hydrocephalus, pineal region tumors) and after aberrant regeneration. *(Braunwald, pp. 165–166)*

563. **(B)** Peripheral nerve lesions result in reflex loss greater than the degree of weakness. Reflex loss is variable in anterior horn cell disease and decreased proportionately in muscle disease. In neuromuscular junction disorders, reflexes are characteristically normal. *(Braunwald, pp. 119–121, 2516)*

564. **(C)** Diurnal fluctuations and pathologic fatigue are common in disorders of neuromuscular transmission (eg, myasthenia gravis). *(Braunwald, pp. 2516–2517)*

565. **(A)** In diseases of the anterior horn cell, atrophy is marked and early. Muscle disease can result in marked atrophy, but much later in the course of the disease. Atrophy is generally moderate in peripheral nerve disease and absent in disorders of the neuromuscular junction. *(Braunwald, pp. 119–121)*

566. **(B)** Peripheral nerve disease is the most likely to cause distal weakness and is the only one of the four to also cause sensory symptoms. *(Braunwald, pp. 2498–2506)*

567. **(D)** Certain muscle diseases such as myotonic dystrophy and facioscapulohumeral dystrophy have virtually pathognomonic facial features. Most will present earlier in life. *(Braunwald, pp. 2530–2534)*

CHAPTER 8

Kidneys
Questions

DIRECTIONS (Questions 568 through 605): Each of the numbered items or incomplete statements in this section is followed by answers or by completions of the statement. Select the ONE lettered answer or completion that is BEST in each case.

568. Which substance is filtered through the glomerulus but unaffected by tubular secretion?

   (A) potassium
   (B) hydrogen ion
   (C) penicillin
   (D) urea
   (E) creatinine

569. Ten days after a kidney transplant, a 32-year-old man develops allograft enlargement, fever, oliguria, and hypertension. The most likely cause is

   (A) steroid hyperglycemia
   (B) erythrocytosis
   (C) hyperacute rejection
   (D) acute rejection
   (E) renal artery stenosis

570. A 19-year-old man develops acute glomerulonephritis. The most characteristic urinary finding is

   (A) proteinuria
   (B) microhematuria
   (C) granular casts
   (D) erythrocyte casts
   (E) hyaline casts

571. A 24-year-old woman has a renal biopsy. If this is poststreptococcal, the electron microscopy will reveal

   (A) diffuse mesangial deposits
   (B) no deposits
   (C) electron-dense endothelial deposits
   (D) closed capillary lumen
   (E) subepithelial humps

572. A 74-year-old man has a catheter inserted to relieve urinary obstruction. In the following diuresis, the urine is likely

   (A) high in sodium
   (B) low in potassium
   (C) concentrated
   (D) acidic
   (E) to have an osmolality of 500 or greater

573. A 68-year-old woman has used large amounts of analgesic for years to relieve severe headaches and arthritis. The most prominent renal effect is

   (A) glomerulosclerosis
   (B) papillary necrosis
   (C) cortical necrosis
   (D) tubular necrosis
   (E) nephrolithiasis

574. A 64-year-old woman has an elevated bicarbonate level with normal P_{CO_2} on blood gas elevation. This is most likely caused by

(A) extracellular fluid (ECF) volume expansion
(B) hyperkalemia
(C) mineralocorticoid excess
(D) decreased distal salt delivery
(E) bicarbonate deprivation

575. Evaluation of kidney function in a 32-year-old man with sickle-cell anemia is likely to reveal

(A) an inability to acidify the urine
(B) a decrease in glomerular filtration
(C) an inability to concentrate the urine
(D) pyuria
(E) a salt-losing state

576. A 63-year-old man with an 8-year history of recurrent severe arthritis in his large toes has an elevated creatinine level. Evaluation of renal impairment is likely to reveal

(A) glomerulonephritis
(B) rapid progression
(C) sodium urate stones
(D) distal tubular atrophy
(E) nonspecific changes

577. Intravenous pyelography (IVP) must be performed with special caution in patients with

(A) hyperparathyroidism
(B) pyelonephritis
(C) nephrolithiasis
(D) hypernephroma
(E) multiple myeloma

578. A 64-year-old man has amyloid detected on renal biopsy. Which statement concerning his renal evaluation is correct?

(A) It is caused by primary amyloidosis.
(B) Hypertension is present.
(C) Nephrotic syndrome is likely.
(D) There is impaired tubular function.
(E) Hematuria is present.

579. A 74-year-old man with anemia and an immunoglobulin G (IgG) paraprotein is likely to develop renal involvement resulting in

(A) nitrogen retention
(B) hypertension
(C) retinitis
(D) edema
(E) hematuria

580. A 77-year-old man with a mass in the lung develops hyponatremia, increased effective circulating volume, and high urine osmolality. He most likely has

(A) nephrotic syndrome
(B) syndrome of inappropriate antidiuretic hormone (SIADH) production
(C) renal metastases from lung cancer
(D) lung metastases from hypernephroma
(E) renal tubular acidosis

581. A 69-year-old man has lost a friend to prostate cancer and would like to be evaluated for the disease. The highest positive predictive value for detection of cancer is

(A) ultrasound
(B) digital rectal exam (DRE)
(C) IVP
(D) prostate specific antigen (PSA)
(E) none of the above

582. A 63-year-old woman has type 2 diabetes mellitus. Which of the following will directly attenuate the course of renal disease?

(A) calcium channel blockers
(B) angiotensin-converting enzyme (ACE) inhibitors
(C) hepatic hydroxymethylglutaryl-coenzyme A (HMG-CoA) inhibitors
(D) dietary carbohydrate restriction
(E) weight reduction

583. A 68-year-old man is found to have a low magnesium level. The most likely cause is

(A) cerebellar hemangioma
(B) pernicious anemia
(C) chronic alcoholism

(D) inadequate diet

(E) poorly controlled diabetes mellitus

584. A 32-year-old man had trace proteinuria on dipstick. A 24-hour urine collection revealed 280 mg of urine. Which of the following statements concerning this degree of protein-uria is correct?

(A) It rarely requires any investigation.

(B) In systemic diseases, it has no prognostic values.

(C) It can be caused by fever.

(D) It is rarely reversible.

(E) It is usually caused by tubular defects.

585. A 69-year-old woman presents with left flank pain and hematuria. Physical examination suggests a left-sided abdominal mass. Labo-ratory investigation might reveal

(A) polycythemia

(B) thrombocytopenia

(C) hypocalcemia

(D) leukocytosis

(E) high-renin hypertension

586. A 60-year-old woman with heart failure and normal renal function is started on fur-osemide (Lasix) 80 mg/day. A subsequent nephropathy might be characterized by

(A) tubular damage

(B) glomerular damage

(C) erythrocyte casts

(D) granular casts

(E) renal potassium wasting

587. A 57-year-old man, otherwise fine, is found to have a low serum sodium on routine lab testing. His serum osmolality is low, but his urine osmolality is > 150 mOsm/kg. Evalua-tion is like to reveal

(A) massive edema

(B) hyperkalemia

(C) dehydration

(D) elevated urea nitrogen

(E) an intrathoracic lesion

588. In a normal kidney, the largest volume of wa-ter is reabsorbed at the

(A) collecting ducts

(B) proximal tubule

(C) distal tubule

(D) ascending loop of Henle

(E) descending loop of Henle

589. Figure 8–1 is a selective renal arteriogram done on a 64-year-old man who was admit-ted for hematuria after slipping on icy pave-ment. What is the most likely diagnosis?

(A) renal cell carcinoma

(B) kidney contusion and laceration

(C) transitional cell carcinoma

(D) renal hamartoma

(E) renal hemangioma

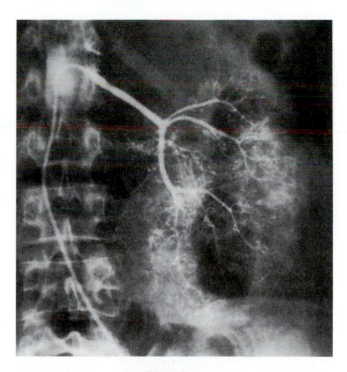

Figure 8–1.

590. A 68-year-old woman develops acute dysuria. Urinalysis reveals numerous white cells. The most likely coexisting condition is

(A) anemia
(B) exercise
(C) diabetes mellitus
(D) influenza
(E) analgesic drug use

591. A 28-year-old woman develops acute glomerulonephritis. Chest x-ray (CXR) is abnormal, and serology reveals positive antineutrophil cytoplasmic antibodies. The most likely diagnosis is

(A) Wegener's granulomatosis
(B) bacterial endocarditis
(C) Goodpasture syndrome
(D) lupus erythematosus
(E) poststreptococcal disease

592. A 42-year-old man develops gross edema including periorbital edema. The most likely diagnosis is

(A) sickle-cell disease
(B) medullary sponge kidney
(C) radiation nephritis
(D) staphylococcal infection
(E) amyloid disease

593. A 74-year-old woman develops acute renal failure requiring dialysis. Peritoneal dialysis might be selected if there is coexistent

(A) cerebral trauma
(B) hypercatabolic states
(C) severe lung disease
(D) atrial premature beats
(E) drug overdose

594. A pregnant woman develops hypertension, proteinuria, and hyperuricemia at 34 weeks' gestation. The most likely diagnosis is

(A) first pregnancy
(B) diabetes mellitus
(C) twin pregnancy

(D) extreme of reproductive age
(E) sickle-cell anemia

595. A 30-year-old man with hematuria has renal cysts on ultrasound. His father had a similar condition. In this syndrome

(A) frequently only one kidney is affected
(B) pregnancy aggravates the disease
(C) episodic oliguria is common
(D) other organs do not contain cysts
(E) renal transplantation is often indicated

596. A 15-year-old boy develops renal colic. The stone is not recovered, but urinalysis reveals hexagonal crystals, and a cyanide–nitroprusside test on the urine is positive. The most likely diagnosis is

(A) cystinuria
(B) thalassemia
(C) hereditary glycinuria
(D) primary hyperoxaluria
(E) sarcoidosis

597. A 29-year-old man is stable 1 year post–kidney transplant. He is most likely to die as a consequence of

(A) atherosclerotic disease
(B) opportunistic infection
(C) metabolic bone disease
(D) lung cancer
(E) lymphoma

598. A 37-year-old immunosuppressed patient with renal failure develops sepsis. Which of the following antibiotics, if used, would require a major reduction in dosage?

(A) erythromycin
(B) doxycycline
(C) tobramycin
(D) isoniazid (INH)
(E) amphotericin B

599. A 63-year-old diabetic woman develops a sudden deterioration in renal function. The most likely diagnosis is

(A) papillary necrosis
(B) progressive proteinuria
(C) chronic pyelonephritis
(D) renal calculi
(E) polyposis of the bladder

600. A 24-year-old woman is dipstick positive for blood in her urine. This is repeated twice between menstrual periods and remains positive. Microscopic evaluation reveals red blood cells, some of which are deformed. The most likely cause of the hematuria is

(A) urinary tract stones
(B) immunoglobulin A (IgA) nephropathy
(C) trauma
(D) malignant renal tumor
(E) benign renal tumor

Questions 601 through 605

601. A 63-year-old man becomes oliguric 2 days following an open cholecystectomy. Which of the following findings would suggest that prerenal acute renal failure (ARF) is a major factor in etiology?

(A) postural hypotension
(B) fractional excretion of sodium is 2%
(C) specific gravity is 1.012
(D) the urine sodium concentration is 30 mmol/L
(E) heme granular casts on urine microscopy

602. Which of the following results concerning the levels of blood urea nitrogen (BUN) and creatinine are true for prerenal azotemia?

(A) markedly elevated BUN, unchanged creatinine
(B) unchanged BUN, elevated creatinine
(C) little change in either creatinine or BUN for several days after oliguria develops

(D) BUN/creatinine ratio is 10
(E) BUN/creatinine ratio is 25

603. The next day, complete oliguria develops in this patient. The most important test would be

(A) abdominal ultrasound
(B) blood cultures
(C) urine cultures
(D) inferior vena cavagram with selective renal venogram
(E) BUN/creatinine ratio

604. Which of the following tests would suggest that renal vein thrombosis is a contributor to the renal failure?

(A) white cell casts on urinalysis
(B) heme granular casts
(C) heavy proteinuria
(D) urine supernatant pink and tests positive for heme
(E) specific gravity > 1.020

605. Which of the following medications should be held during the recovery phase from this man's ARF?

(A) acetaminophen
(B) digoxin
(C) lorazepam
(D) celecoxib
(E) simvastatin

DIRECTIONS (Questions 606 through 647): Each set of matching questions in this section consists of a list of lettered options followed by several numbered items. For each numbered item, select the appropriate lettered option(s). Each lettered option may be selected once, more than once, or not at all. EACH ITEM WILL STATE THE NUMBER OF OPTIONS TO SELECT. CHOOSE EXACTLY THIS NUMBER.

Questions 606 through 609

   (A) hypothalamic diabetes insipidus
   (B) nephrogenic diabetes insipidus
   (C) primary polydipsia
   (D) osmotic diuresis
   (E) hypercalcemia

606. A 21-year-old woman develops polydipsia and polyuria during pregnancy (SELECT TWO)

607. A 19-year-old man develops polyuria and polydipsia after a head injury (SELECT TWO)

608. A 19-year-old man and one of his two brothers have had polyuria and polydipsia since birth. Neither his sisters nor his parents are affected (SELECT ONE)

609. A 27-year-old woman with well-controlled bipolar affective disorder treated with lithium develops polyuria and polydipsia (SELECT ONE)

Questions 610 through 614

   (A) metabolic acidosis
   (B) metabolic alkalosis
   (C) respiratory acidosis
   (D) respiratory alkalosis

610. A 19-year-old girl develops diarrhea. The anion gap is normal (SELECT ONE)

611. A 75-year-old man with severe chronic lung disease is given codeine after a tooth extraction and develops somnolence and confusion (SELECT ONE)

612. A 74-year-old woman is treated with furosemide 80 mg/day for heart failure (SELECT ONE)

613. A 53-year-old woman is being treated for tuberculosis (SELECT ONE)

614. A 69-year-old woman is taking large amounts of aspirin for osteoarthritis (SELECT ONE)

Questions 615 through 620

   (A) nephrogenic diabetes insipidus
   (B) central diabetes insipidus
   (C) primary polydipsia
   (D) solute diuresis
   (E) natriuretic syndrome

615. May occur during course of acute tubular necrosis (SELECT ONE)

616. Causes the greatest amount of medullary washout (SELECT ONE)

617. Can be caused by hypokalemia (SELECT ONE)

618. Can be caused by major tranquilizers (SELECT ONE)

619. Little or no response to vasopressin after fluid deprivation test (SELECT ONE)

620. Can be caused by high-protein tube feeds (SELECT ONE)

Questions 621 through 626

A 75-year-old man is referred from a local nursing home with a serum sodium of 120. For each of the following clinical findings, match the correct diagnosis.

   (A) congestive heart failure (CHF)
   (B) extrarenal fluid losses
   (C) SIADH
   (D) polydipsia
   (E) essential hyponatremia
   (F) renal failure
   (G) endocrine cause of hyponatremia

(H) renal fluid losses

(I) artifactual

(J) osmotic

(K) impaired diuresis

621. Blood pressure 100/50, neck veins not visible, urine sodium 30 mmol/L (SELECT ONE)

622. Left hemiplegia (SELECT ONE)

623. Depression being treated with amitriptyline (SELECT ONE)

624. Postural drop in blood pressure, urine sodium 5 mmol/L (SELECT ONE)

625. Pitting edema (SELECT ONE)

626. Uric acid low, urinary sodium 40 mmol/L (SELECT ONE)

Questions 627 through 631

A 30-year-old woman is found to have a low potassium level. For each of the following clinical findings, match the correct diagnosis.

(A) lower gastrointestinal (GI) losses

(B) prior use of diuretics

(C) renal tubular acidosis (RTA)

(D) current use of diuretics

(E) malignant hypertension

(F) primary hyperaldosteronism

(G) glucocorticoid excess

627. Normal blood pressure, urine potassium 15 mmol/L, bicarbonate above normal (SELECT ONE)

628. Hypertension, low plasma renin, low plasma aldosterone (SELECT ONE)

629. Normal blood pressure, urine potassium 40 mmol/L, low serum bicarbonate (SELECT ONE)

630. Hypertension, low plasma renin, high plasma aldosterone (SELECT ONE)

631. Normal blood pressure, urine potassium 15 mmol/L, bicarbonate low (SELECT ONE)

Questions 632 through 636

(A) metabolic acidosis and respiratory acidosis

(B) metabolic acidosis and respiratory alkalosis

(C) metabolic alkalosis and respiratory acidosis

(D) metabolic alkalosis and respiratory alkalosis

(E) metabolic alkalosis and metabolic acidosis

632. Salicylate overdose (SELECT ONE)

633. Sepsis (SELECT ONE)

634. Chronic pulmonary disease on steroids (SELECT ONE)

635. Renal failure with vomiting (SELECT ONE)

636. Hepatic cirrhosis complicated by acute renal failure (SELECT ONE)

Questions 637 through 641

(A) diffuse proliferative glomerulonephritis (GN)

(B) crescentic GN

(C) focal proliferative GN

(D) membranoproliferative GN

(E) minimal change GN

(F) focal segmental GN

(G) membranous GN

(H) deposition diseases

(I) nonimmune basement membrane abnormalities

637. A 14-year-old girl develops purpuric skin lesions and abdominal pain. Her stools test positive for blood, and urinalysis reveals red blood cells (RBCs) and RBC casts. Her renal function deteriorates rapidly over several days. Renal biopsy will likely show (SELECT ONE)

638. A 28-year-old woman has a 2-year history of facial rash, hair loss, arthralgias, and thrombocytopenia. She then develops an elevated serum creatinine. Renal biopsy might reveal (SELECT FOUR)

639. A 47-year-old woman with rheumatoid arthritis (RA) is being treated with nonsteroidal anti-inflammatory drugs (NSAIDs) and gold. She develops acute shortness of breath with hypoxemia and is admitted to the hospital. Admission urinalysis reveals 4$^+$ proteinuria but no active sediment. Renal biopsy will show (SELECT ONE)

640. A 19-year-old man, who is otherwise healthy, is found to have RBCs in his urine. There is no proteinuria. Evaluation of his family reveals that his mother also has hematuria. She has minimal renal impairment and, other than being hard-of-hearing, is in good health. Renal biopsy will show (SELECT ONE)

641. A 33-year-old man from Southeast Asia, without human immunodeficiency virus (HIV) infection, is diagnosed as having pulmonary tuberculosis. He is started on multiple medications, including INH and rifampin. Three months later, he has developed edema. Liver tests are normal, and serum creatinine is increased by 30% over baseline. Urinalysis reveals 4$^+$ proteinuria. The most likely diagnosis is (SELECT ONE)

Questions 642 through 645

   (A) polycystic kidney disease
   (B) medullary sponge kidney
   (C) medullary cystic disease
   (D) Liddle syndrome
   (E) Bartter syndrome
   (F) congenital nephrogenic diabetes insipidus
   (G) renal tubular acidosis type I
   (H) renal tubular acidosis type II
   (I) X-linked hypophosphatemia
   (J) cystinuria
   (K) Fanconi syndrome

642. A 14-year-old boy is short in height and has had several fractures with minimal trauma. Physical exam reveals prominent costochondral junctions and bowed legs. This syndrome could be secondary to (SELECT FOUR)

643. A 43-year-old man had a subarachnoid hemorrhage from an intracranial aneurysm 8 years ago. He has also had progressive renal impairment associated with hematuria. The most likely diagnosis is (SELECT ONE)

644. An 18-year-old man is found to have metabolic alkalosis and hypokalemia. This could be secondary to (SELECT TWO)

645. A 28-year-old man presents with a kidney stone. He is married to his first cousin, and 6 months earlier his 8-year-old son had a kidney stone as well. The most likely diagnosis is (SELECT ONE)

Questions 646 and 647

   (A) urinary osmolality > 500
   (B) urinary sodium > 40
   (C) urinary sodium < 20
   (D) fractional sodium excretion > 1
   (E) RBCs in urine
   (F) granular casts in urine

646. A 21-year-old woman develops hypovolemia and prerenal azotemia. Evaluation will reveal (SELECT TWO)

647. A 63-year-old woman develops acute tubular necrosis (ATN) in the setting of sepsis. Evaluation will reveal (SELECT FOUR)

Answers and Explanations

568. **(D)** Urea is filtered at the glomerulus, and thereafter any movement in or out of tubules is a passive process depending on gradients, not secretion. Reabsorption of urea in the distal tubule and collecting duct when urine flow is reduced results in the disproportionate elevation of urea nitrogen over creatinine in prerenal azotemia. *(Goldman, p. 568)*

569. **(D)** Renal scans initially show a reduction in excretion with cortical retention. This is the most common type of rejection. Most acute rejections will respond to immunosuppressive agents if diagnosed early. In contrast, immediate nonfunction of a graft can be caused by damage to the kidney during procurement and storage. Such problems are becoming less frequent. Obstruction, vascular compression, and ureteral compression are other causes of primary nonfunction of a renal graft. *(Goldman, pp. 584–585)*

570. **(D)** Both granular and erythrocyte casts are present, but the latter indicate bleeding from the glomerulus and are most characteristically seen. Red cells reach the urine probably via capillary wall "gaps" and form casts as they become embedded in concentrated tubular fluid with a high protein content. Proteinuria is invariably present but is not as specific. *(Goldman, p. 591)*

571. **(E)** These humps are discrete, electron-dense nodules that persist for about 8 weeks and are highly characteristic of the disease. Light microscopy reveals diffuse proliferation, and immunofluorescence reveals granular IgG and C3. Most patients will recover spontaneously. *(Goldman, p. 590)*

572. **(A)** The urine contains large amounts of potassium, magnesium, and sodium. The large volume is often appropriate to pre-existing volume expansion, but careful attention to fluid and electrolytes is important to prevent hypokalemia, hypomagnesemia, hyponatremia or hypernatremia, and volume depletion. *(Goldman, p. 607)*

573. **(B)** Chronic analgesic ingestion may lead to papillary necrosis. Complete understanding of the pathogenesis is lacking, and may vary with different analgesics. Depletion of reducing equivalents such as glutathione may also play a role. *(Goldman, p. 597)*

574. **(C)** Mineralocorticoid excess leads to metabolic alkalosis, primarily because of renal bicarbonate generation. Other major mechanisms for metabolic alkalosis include ECF volume contraction, potassium depletion, and increased distal salt delivery. Less common causes are Liddle syndrome, bicarbonate loading (posthypercapneic alkalosis), and delayed conversion of administered organic acids. *(Goldman, pp. 564–567)*

575. **(C)** In sickle-cell anemia, the kidney is characterized by an inability to concentrate the urine. Papillary necrosis may also occur in patients with homozygous sickle-cell disease or sickle-cell trait. *(Goldman, p. 899)*

576. **(E)** The typical renal lesions in gout are urate crystals in the medulla or pyramids, with surrounding mononuclear and giant cell reaction. The degree of renal impairment, however, does not correlate with the hyperuricemia and the decline in renal function correlates with aging, hypertension, renal calculi, or unrelated nephropathy. (*Goldman, p. 1545*)

577. **(E)** Danger of acute renal failure after IVP has led to caution, especially in patients with multiple myeloma. The patient should not be dehydrated if the IVP is necessary. The risk is also increased in patients with diabetes mellitus or chronic renal failure. (*Goldman, pp. 530, 982*)

578. **(C)** Renal amyloidosis can occur in primary or secondary amyloidosis. The hallmark finding, nephrotic syndrome, is present in 25% of patients at presentation and probably develops ultimately in over 50%. (*Goldman, pp. 588, 986*)

579. **(A)** Nitrogen retention is characteristic of renal involvement in multiple myeloma. Hypercalcemia may produce transient or irreversible renal damage as do amyloid and myeloma cell infiltrates. (*Goldman, pp. 981–982*)

580. **(B)** The urine osmolality in patients with SIADH need not be hypertonic to plasma, but only inappropriately high compared with serum. The major characteristics of SIADH include hyponatremia, volume expansion without edema, natriuresis, hypouricemia, and normal or reduced serum creatinine level, with normal thyroid and adrenal function. (*Goldman, pp. 548–551*)

581. **(D)** Although an elevated PSA (> 4) has the best positive predictive value, combining it with DRE is probably the most effective screening process. (*Goldman, p. 636*)

582. **(B)** It is very likely that control of hypertension and excellent glucose control will slow the development and course of renal disease in type 2 diabetes mellitus. ACE inhibitors seem to decrease proteinuria and slow progression of renal disease. As renal function deteriorates, limiting dietary protein intake can also be beneficial. Calcium channel

blockers have no extra effect beyond their antihypertensive effect. (*Goldman, pp. 610–612*)

583. **(C)** Magnesium deficiency is usually accompanied by hypocalcemia. Symptoms include lethargy, weakness, and irritability. Tetany, with positive Chvostek's and Trousseau's sign, may result from the accompanying hypocalcemia. (*Goldman, pp. 1137–1138*)

584. **(C)** Persistent proteinuria should always be investigated and, if no cause can be found, yearly follow-up instituted. Mild proteinuria has significant prognostic value in diabetes. Mild proteinuria can be caused by glomerular or tubular causes. Functional causes of proteinuria such as fever, orthostasis, exercise, and heart failure are usually reversible. (*Goldman, p. 528*)

585. **(A)** This patient likely has a hypernephroma. Polycythemia is caused by the production of erythroprotein-like factors. There is no relationship to hypertension. The tumor frequently presents as metastatic disease. (*Goldman, pp. 631–632*)

586. **(A)** Hypokalemia can result in tubular damage to the kidney, paralytic ileus, rhabdomyolysis, weakness, and cardiac repolarization abnormalities. (*Goldman, p. 555*)

587. **(E)** Intrathoracic lesions may be benign or malignant, and the latter may secrete a substance similar to lysine vasopressin. Bronchogenic carcinoma is the most common intrathoracic lesion causing SIADH. (*Goldman, pp. 548–550*)

588. **(B)** The largest volume of water is reabsorbed in the nephron at the proximal convolution. Maximally concentrated urine depends on ADH, which allows distal convoluted tubes and collecting ducts to become permeable to water. (*Goldman, pp. 535–538*)

589. **(A)** The diagnosis is renal cell carcinoma. There is marked hypervascularity of the left kidney. The arteries are irregular and tortuous, following a random distribution. There

are small vessels within the renal vein that indicate the blood supply of the neoplastic thrombosis involving the renal vein. The kidney is enlarged and abnormally bulbous in the lower pole. Computed tomography (CT) scans have dramatically decreased the need for arteriography in evaluating renal lesions. (*Goldman, p. 632*)

590. **(C)** Urinary tract infections (UTIs) are increased in diabetes mellitus as well as pregnancy, sickle cell disease, polycystic disease, and structural abnormalities of the urinary tract. (*Goldman, p. 614*)

591. **(A)** Numerous diseases are associated with renal and pulmonary manifestations, including lupus, Goodpasture syndrome, and Wegener's granulomatosis. Wegener's is typically associated with antineutrophil cytoplasmic antibodies. (*Braunwald, pp. 590, 1529–1532*)

592. **(E)** In addition to amyloid disease, other conditions associated with the nephrotic syndrome are secondary syphilis, malaria, and treatment with gold salts. Minimal change nephrotic syndrome, focal glomerular sclerosis, membranous nephropathy, and membranoproliferative glomerulonephritis are the primary renal diseases that present as nephrotic syndrome. (*Goldman, p. 587*)

593. **(A)** Peritoneal dialysis is preferred with cerebral trauma as well as severe heart failure because of risk of hemorrhage or hypotension with hemodialysis. In particular, peritoneal dialysis does not require any anticoagulation and is safer if head trauma has occurred. (*Goldman, p. 571*)

594. **(B)** Diabetes mellitus, chronic hypertension, multifetal gestation, and prior preeclampsia are associated with preeclampsia. When toxemia occurs in the first trimester, however, hydatidiform mole must be considered. The clinical manifestations of severe preeclampsia include headache, epigastric pain, visual disturbances, and hypertension. (*Goldman, pp. 1351–1352*)

595. **(E)** Renal transplantation is utilized in end-stage renal failure. The transplanted kidney

cannot be affected by the disease. Hepatic and pancreatic cysts are also common in autosomal dominant polycystic kidney disease. Intracranial aneurysms are also more frequent. (*Goldman, pp. 627–629*)

596. **(A)** Cystinuria is a congenital disorder associated with decreased tubular resorption of cystine, arginine, ornithine, and lysine. Only cystine is insoluble and is the cause of renal calculi. The typical hexagonal crystals are most likely to be seen on an acid early-morning urine specimen. A positive cyanidenitroprusside screening test should be confirmed by chromatography. (*Goldman, p. 607*)

597. **(A)** Increase in neoplasms in renal transplant recipients include cervical carcinoma, lymphoma, and cutaneous malignancies. Osteoporosis and persistent hyperparathyroidism are other bony complications. Risk of infection is related to degree of immunosuppression. Nevertheless, the most common causes of death are cardiovascular and tend to occur earlier than in the general population. (*Goldman, pp. 585–586*)

598. **(C)** Amikacin and vancomycin are other antibiotics that require dose reduction in renal failure. Newer antibiotics are often used instead of aminoglycosides to reduce the risk of renal damage. (*Goldman, p. 97*)

599. **(A)** Severe infection of the renal pyramids in association with vascular disease or obstruction leads to papillary necrosis. Diabetes also predisposes to emphysematous pyelonephritis. (*Goldman, p. 615*)

600. **(B)** Isolated hematuria is usually of urologic cause (eg, tumor, trauma, or stone) but can also be glomerular in origin. The finding of red cell casts or dysmorphic red cells (best appreciated by phase microscopy) confirms the glomerular source of bleeding. (*Goldman, p. 528*)

601. **(A)** Although evidence of volume contraction cannot confirm prerenal ARF, as this can progress into intrinsic renal failure, it suggests that prerenal factors are contributing. In prerenal ARF the specific gravity is usually above 1.020 and the sodium concentration is < 10 mmol/L. The fractional excretion of sodium relates sodium clearance to creatinine clearance and is more sensitive than direct measurements of sodium excretion. In prerenal azotemia, sodium is avidly resorbed from glomerular filtrate, but not in intrinsic renal azotemia because of tubular epithelial cell injury. Creatinine is resorbed less efficiently in both conditions. Therefore, the fractional excretion of sodium is less than 1% in prerenal azotemia (often much less) whereas it is greater than 1% in intrinsic renal azotemia.

Fractional excretion of sodium % = $\dfrac{U_{Na}\,P_{Cr}}{P_{Na}\,U_{Cr}} \times 100$

(Braunwald, pp. 1546–1547)

602. **(E)** The ratio of BUN/creatinine is usually < 10 to 15 in intrinsic renal disease and > 20 in prerenal azotemia. *(Braunwald, p. 1546)*

603. **(A)** Oliguria suggests that obstruction is a possible explanation for the renal failure. Imaging is very sensitive for obstruction, but if bladder obstruction secondary to a large prostate is suspected, bladder catheterization would be the first step. *(Braunwald, p. 1547)*

604. **(C)** Renal vein thrombosis is associated with heavy proteinuria and hematuria. Flank pain and pulmonary embolism can also occur. *(Braunwald, p. 1546)*

605. **(D)** Although all drugs should be reassessed at this time, and if appropriate the dosage adjusted, drugs with known nephrotoxicity, such as ACE inhibitors and NSAIDs, should be stopped. *(Braunwald, p. 1549)*

606. **(A, D)** Gestational diabetes can result in hyperglycemia and polyuria with subsequent polydipsia. Vasopressin is catabolized by a placental enzyme, and hypothalamic diabetes insipidus may result. *(Goldman, pp. 1227–1231)*

607. **(A, C)** Head injury can result in hypothalamic diabetes insipidus. This can develop abruptly or gradually. Head injuries can result in primary polydipsia. *(Goldman, pp. 1227–1231)*

608. **(B)** Nephrogenic diabetes insipidus can be inherited on the X chromosome. Its X-linked recessive nature means that males are predominantly affected. Only women who are homozygous are affected. *(Goldman, p. 1228)*

609. **(B)** Lithium is one of the drugs that causes nephrogenic diabetes insipidus. Hypercalcemia and hypocalcemia can also cause the syndrome. *(Goldman, p. 1228)*

610. **(A)** The anion gap is calculated as the sodium concentration minus the chloride plus the bicarbonate concentration. Other causes of bicarbonate loss with normal anion gap include proximal renal tubular acidosis and primary hyperparathyroidism. *(Goldman, p. 562)*

611. **(C)** Causes of acute respiratory acidosis include narcotic overdose, myasthenia gravis, airway obstruction, and trauma to the chest. Acute increases in Pa_{CO_2} result in carbon dioxide narcosis. This starts with somnolence and confusion and can lead to coma. Asterixis may be present. Cerebral vasodilation may result in frank papilledema. *(Goldman, p. 566)*

612. **(B)** The disorder can occur in volume-expanded patients in which the alkalosis is unresponsive to sodium chloride loading, as in primary hyperaldosteronism or volume contraction with secondary hyperaldosteronism, as in this case. *(Goldman, pp. 564–565)*

613. **(A)** INH can result in impaired oxygen utilization, leading to lactic acidosis, accumulation of lactate, and increased anion gap. *(Goldman, p. 562)*

614. **(D)** During acute hyperventilation, plasma bicarbonate concentrations fall by approximately 3 mEq/L when the arterial pressure of CO_2 falls to about 25 mm Hg. Acute respi-

ratory alkalosis can be caused by anxiety, central nervous system (CNS) disorders, drugs, or fever. Chronic respiratory alkalosis occurs in pregnancy and liver disease as well. *(Goldman, p. 566)*

615. **(E)** The diuretic phase of acute tubular necrosis is characterized by large losses of sodium and water. *(Braunwald, pp. 267–268)*

616. **(C)** Primary polydipsia can cause greater medullary washout than either nephrogenic or central diabetes insipidus because primary polydipsia tends to cause expansion of the ECF volume. This tends to increase total delivery of sodium chloride and water to the inner medulla. It also increases renal blood flow, and increased flow through the vasa recta reduces ability to trap solutes in the medulla. *(Braunwald, pp. 267–268)*

617. **(A)** Nephrogenic diabetes insipidus can be caused by hypokalemia as well as hypercalcemia. *(Braunwald, pp. 267–268)*

618. **(C)** Both thioridazine and chlorpromazine have been associated with primary polydipsia. *(Braunwald, pp. 267–268)*

619. **(C)** There is little or no response to vasopressin after fluid deprivation in primary polydipsia because of medullary wash-out, not vasopressin deficiency. Complete nephrogenic diabetes insipidus also will not respond; however, incomplete nephrogenic diabetes insipidus will show some response. *(Braunwald, pp. 267–268)*

620. **(D)** High protein tube feeds may cause a solute diuresis because of excessive excretion of urea. Other causes of solute diuresis include glucosuria, mannitol, radiographic contrast media, and chronic renal failure. *(Braunwald, pp. 267–268)*

621. **(H)** The combination of ECF volume contraction with a high urinary sodium (20 mmol/L) suggests renal fluid loss. This is commonly caused by diuretics or glucosuria. *(Braunwald, pp. 274–276)*

622. **(C)** SIADH is associated with many CNS diseases including meningitis, encephalitis, tumors, trauma, stroke, and acute porphyria. It is assumed that ADH in these patients is secreted in response to direct stimulation of the hypothalamic osmoreceptors. *(Braunwald, pp. 274–276)*

623. **(C)** Amitriptyline is one of the psychoactive drugs that cause SIADH. Others include phenothiazines, serotonin reuptake inhibitors, and monoamine oxidase inhibitors (MAOIs). Antineoplastic drugs such as vincristine and cyclophosphamide also cause SIADH, as does the hypoglycemic agent chlorpropamide. *(Braunwald, p. 2058)*

624. **(B)** The combination of ECF volume contraction and a low urinary sodium (< 10 mmol/L) suggests extrarenal sodium loss. Common causes are vomiting, diarrhea, or excessive sweating. *(Braunwald, pp. 274–276)*

625. **(A)** The hyponatremia associated with nephrotic syndrome, cirrhosis, or CHF is characterized by edema. It is believed that the hyponatremia is caused by a decrease in "effective" circulating volume secondary to decreased cardiac output or sequestration of fluid. *(Braunwald, pp. 274–276)*

626. **(C)** SIADH is characterized by a low uric acid and a urine sodium greater than 20 mmol/L. *(Braunwald, pp. 274–276)*

627. **(B)** In patients who have prior diuretic use resulting in hypokalemia at the time of evaluation, the bicarbonate tends to be elevated and the urine potassium low (< 25 mmol/L). *(Braunwald, pp. 279–281)*

628. **(G)** Glucocorticoid and licorice ingestion can result in hypertension with low plasma renin and aldosterone levels. *(Braunwald, pp. 279–281)*

629. **(C)** RTA types I and II cause hypokalemia with high potassium excretion (> 25 mmol/L) and a low bicarbonate in the absence of hypertension. Diabetic ketoacidosis can also result in this constellation of findings. *(Braunwald, pp. 279–281)*

630. **(F)** Primary hyperaldosteronism is characterized by hypertension with high plasma aldosterone and low plasma renin. *(Braunwald, pp. 279–281)*

631. **(A)** In lower GI loss (diarrhea), the blood pressure is normal, the urine potassium is low (< 25 mmol/L), and the bicarbonate is either normal or low. *(Braunwald, pp. 279–281)*

632. **(B)** Metabolic acidosis and respiratory alkalosis are seen in salicylate overdose. *(Braunwald, p. 284)*

633. **(B)** Sepsis can cause cardiovascular insufficiency with lactic acidosis, whereas the fever and endotoxemia stimulate the respiratory center, causing respiratory alkalosis. *(Braunwald, pp. 286, 290)*

634. **(C)** Chronic pulmonary disease often causes respiratory acidosis, whereas the steroids frequently used in therapy may cause a metabolic alkalosis. *(Braunwald, pp. 288–289)*

635. **(E)** Renal failure causes metabolic acidosis, whereas the loss of H^+ ions in vomiting cause a metabolic alkalosis. *(Braunwald, p. 284)*

636. **(B)** Hepatic cirrhosis frequently results in chronic respiratory alkalosis. Acute renal failure with metabolic acidosis is common in patients with cirrhosis. *(Braunwald, p. 284)*

637. **(A)** This is a case of Henoch–Schönlein purpura (HSP). Diffuse proliferative GN is characterized by the acute nephritic syndrome: acute renal failure over days to weeks, with hypertension, edema, oliguria, and active urine sediment. Less severe clinical presentation correlates with a more benign biopsy. The pattern of glomerular involvement is similar to IgA nephropathy. *(Braunwald, pp. 1592, 1965)*

638. **(A, C, D, G)** Systemic lupus erythematosus (SLE) can cause a wide variety of renal disorders, and can progress to end-stage renal failure (ESRF). It is difficult to diagnose the type of glomerular involvement in SLE without a biopsy. *(Braunwald, p. 1593)*

639. **(G)** Gold is one of the drugs causing nephrotic syndrome secondary to membranous GN. Captopril and penicillamine have also been implicated. Signs and symptoms of nephrotic syndrome (low albumin, edema, hyperlipidemia) are common, and membranous GN is also associated with a thrombotic diathesis. *(Braunwald, p. 1595)*

640. **(I)** This presentation is typical for an inherited disorder of basement membranes such as Alport syndrome. It is inherited as an X-linked dominant disorder. It is relatively benign in women but frequently progresses to ESRF in men. It is often associated with sensorineural hearing loss. *(Braunwald, pp. 1595–1596)*

641. **(E)** Rifampin can cause minimal change disease as well as more severe renal damage. The described case is typical for minimal change GN with nephrotic syndrome. Drug-induced minimal change GN frequently has an associated interstitial nephritis. INH is not usually associated with renal disease. *(Braunwald, p. 1595)*

642. **(G, H, I, K)** Rickets and osteomalacia can be secondary to a variety of renal tubular defects. There are also two variants of vitamin D–dependent rickets caused by renal tubular defects. In one variant, there is impaired production of $1,25(OH)_2 D_3$, and in the other, there is renal resistance to the action of the hormone. *(Braunwald, pp. 1602–1605)*

643. **(A)** The autosomal dominant form of polycystic kidney disease is often associated with hepatic cysts, intracranial aneurysms, and colonic diverticuli. The occurrence of renal failure is usually in the third decade or later. Complications include infection, obstruction by stone or clot, and gross hematuria. *(Braunwald, pp. 1598–1600)*

644. **(D, E)** Bartter syndrome and Liddle syndrome can be inherited in an autosomal dominant fashion. Patients with Liddle syndrome have hypertension, whereas those with Bartter syndrome do not. In both syndromes, hypokalemia is prominent. *(Braunwald, p. 1563)*

645. **(J)** Many of the listed disorders can cause nephrolithiasis, but cystinuria is the most common cause of stones in childhood. It is a common inborn error of amino acid transport and is inherited as an autosomal recessive trait. The disorder affects transport of all dibasic amino acids (lysine, arginine, ornithine, and cystine) in the kidney and the gut, but symptoms arise from the overexcretion of cystine because it is the least soluble. *(Braunwald, p. 1619)*

646. **(A, C)** In prerenal acute renal failure (ie, no histologic damage), the urinalysis reveals only hyaline casts. The urinary osmolality is high (> 500), and the urine sodium is low (< 20). The fractional excretion of sodium is less than one. *(Goldman, pp. 567–570)*

647. **(B, D, E, F)** In acute renal failure, the urinalysis can reveal red cells, white cells, granular casts, and tubular cells. The fractional excretion of sodium is greater than one, and the urinary sodium is generally greater than 40. *(Goldman, pp. 567–570)*

CHAPTER 9

Muscles and Joints
Questions

DIRECTIONS (Questions 648 through 711): Each of the numbered items or incomplete statements in this section is followed by answers or by completions of the statement. Select the ONE lettered answer or completion that is BEST in each case.

648. A 42-year-old man of eastern European Jewish descent develops aseptic necrosis of the femoral head. The other femur shows evidence of osteopenia, and there is diffuse osteopenia of the spine with some collapse. Review of medical records reveals he has had splenomegaly and mild pancytopenia for years. The most likely cause is

(A) insulin deficiency
(B) abnormal elastic tissue
(C) excess iron in tissue
(D) homocystinuria
(E) abnormal lysosomal enzymes

649. An 18-year-old man has had fever for several weeks. The fever occurs on an almost daily basis and is associated with an evanescent salmon-colored truncal rash. He has diffuse arthralgias, and an extensive investigation for infections and malignancy is negative. The diagnosis is likely to be established by

(A) high-titer rheumatoid factor
(B) postive antinuclear antibody (ANA)
(C) response to steroid therapy
(D) response to nonsteroidal anti-inflammatory drug (NSAID) therapy
(E) lymph node biopsy

650. A 32-year-old man develops symptoms secondary to a dry mouth and dry eyes. He has enlarged salivary glands. Studies for autoantibodies to Ro/SS-A are negative. A salivary gland biopsy reveals lymphocytic infiltration. The most likely diagnosis is

(A) sarcoidosis
(B) primary Sjögren syndrome
(C) human immunodeficiency virus (HIV) infection
(D) lymphoma
(E) amyloidosis

651. A young woman presents with a facial rash, arthralgias, and thrombocytopenia. The most diagnostically helpful eye finding would be

(A) cytoid bodies
(B) microaneurysm
(C) Argyll–Robertson pupil
(D) macular degeneration
(E) nystagmus

652. The most common portion of the gastrointestinal (GI) tract to become involved in scleroderma is the

(A) esophagus
(B) stomach
(C) duodenum
(D) ileum
(E) colon

653. A 22-year-old woman develops a syndrome associated with color change in her fingers with cold exposure. The fingers turn white, then blue, and finally red. This phenomenon

(A) may lead to gangrene of the fingers
(B) is almost always due to scleroderma
(C) occurs when scleroderma is already well established
(D) causes fingers to turn red in cold water
(E) affects the sexes equally

654. A 63-year-old man develops pain and swelling in his knee. Pseudogout can be distinguished from gout by means of

(A) positive birefringent crystals
(B) acute onset
(C) involvement of single joints
(D) involvement of large joints
(E) association with diabetes

655. A 10-year-old child with recurrent signs and symptoms of palpable purpura on the buttocks, arthralgias, colicky abdominal pain, diarrhea, and microscopic hematuria is most likely to have

(A) influenza
(B) immune complex vasculitis
(C) juvenile rheumatoid arthritis (RA)
(D) systemic lupus erythematosus (SLE)
(E) Wegener's granulomatosis

Questions 656 and 657

656. A 75-year-old woman has abrupt onset of soreness and severe stiffness of the shoulders and upper thighs with low-grade fever. Physical examination is entirely normal, but the erythrocyte sedimentation rate (ESR) is over 100 mm/hr. The most likely diagnosis is

(A) dermatomyositis
(B) osteoarthritis
(C) polymyalgia rheumatica
(D) midline granuloma
(E) sarcoidosis

657. This woman is most likely to require treatment with

(A) intravenous high-dose steroids
(B) acetylsalicylic acid
(C) indomethacin
(D) low-dose steroids by mouth
(E) topical steroid creams

658. A 63-year-old man has a 60 pack/year history of smoking. He develops hemoptysis, and chest x-ray (CXR) reveals a lung mass with mediastinal widening. The most likely musculoskeletal manifestation of this disease would be

(A) SLE
(B) scleroderma
(C) dermatomyositis (DM)
(D) polyarteritis
(E) Weber–Christian disease

659. A 24-year-old woman develops pain in her left arm. The radial pulse is not palpable, and there are numerous vascular bruits. This syndrome is characterized by

(A) high pressure in the legs and low pressure in the arms
(B) low pressure in the legs and high pressure in the arms
(C) high-pitched diastolic murmur
(D) a relentless course to death
(E) hypertension

660. Figure 9–1 is an x-ray of a 40-year-old caucasian man with symptoms of sinusitis and an incidental finding in the skull. The most likely diagnosis would be

(A) normal variant
(B) osteomyelitis
(C) Paget's disease
(D) hemangioma
(E) metastatic disease

Questions 661 and 662

661. A mucin clot test is shown in Figure 9–2 with the normal control on the left and the patient's fluid on the right. The patient's most likely diagnosis is

(A) degenerative joint disease
(B) traumatic arthritis
(C) SLE
(D) scleroderma
(E) gout

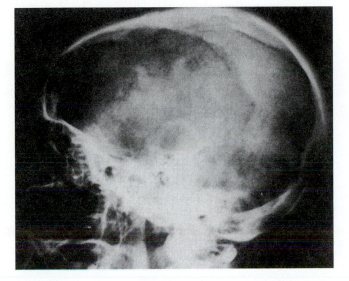

Figure 9–1.

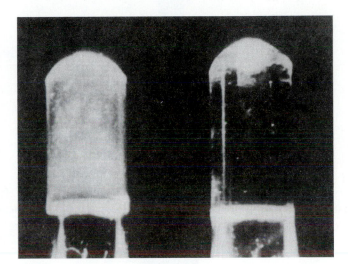

Figure 9–2.

662. It is also helpful to analyze the fluid for

(A) autoantibodies
(B) lactic dehydrogenase (LDH)
(C) glucose
(D) protein
(E) leukocytes

663. The usual cause of death in the condition pictured in Figure 9–3 is

(A) ruptured esophageal varices
(B) berry aneurysm
(C) aortic aneurysm
(D) respiratory failure
(E) sepsis

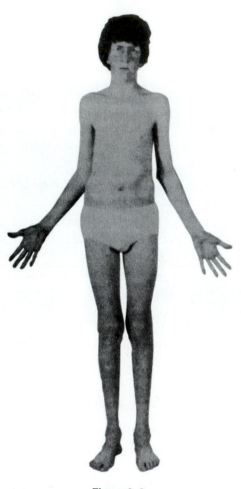

Figure 9–3.

664. Leukopenia is a common finding in

(A) periarteritis nodosa
(B) SLE
(C) scleroderma
(D) dermatomyositis
(E) osteoarthritis

665. A 69-year-old man develops clubbing of his fingers. This syndrome is associated with

(A) rheumatoid factor
(B) aortic stenosis
(C) periosteal inflammation
(D) crystal-induced arthritis
(E) diffuse osteoarthritis

666. A 67-year-old man has a long history of symmetrical small joint arthritis with deformities. There are no respiratory symptoms. The pulmonary pathology most likely to be detected at autopsy is

(A) pleuritis
(B) cavitating lesions
(C) intrapulmonary nodules
(D) interstitial fibrosis
(E) diffuse pneumonitis

667. A 32-year-old woman has a long history of bloody diarrhea. The best description of the accompanying arthritis is

(A) symmetric migratory polyarthritis involving the large joints of the legs
(B) usually associated with disease flares
(C) a progressive, crippling course
(D) symmetrical small joint involvement
(E) seropositive

668. A 19-year-old man has a chronic papulosquamous skin disorder. Arthritis is most likely to occur in the setting of

(A) eye findings
(B) GI disease
(C) nail lesions
(D) major involvement of the knees
(E) elevated uric acid

669. The rheumatoid factor (RF)

   (A) is positive in 10 to 20% of people over age 65
   (B) is positive in almost 100% of "classical" RA
   (C) is seen only in RA
   (D) has a molecular weight of about 160,000
   (E) is frequently present in osteoarthritis

670. A 45-year-old man has had intermittent swelling and pain in the superior part of his auricles for several years. Mild arthritis usually accompanies these episodes. Last year he also had redness, pain, and swelling over the bridge of his nose. This syndrome is characterized by

   (A) a rapidly fatal course
   (B) an increase in hemoglobin
   (C) lymphocytosis
   (D) inflammatory subcutaneous nodules
   (E) infectious etiology

671. Ehlers–Danlos syndrome is characterized by

   (A) thickening of the skin
   (B) mental retardation
   (C) an increased incidence of skin carcinoma
   (D) thrombocytopenia
   (E) habitual dislocation of joints

672. A 19-year-old man injures his right knee in a car accident. Examination of synovial fluid is likely to reveal

   (A) clear fluid
   (B) xanthochromic fluid
   (C) normal viscosity
   (D) 5000 to 50,000 white blood cells (WBCs)/mm^2
   (E) no cells

673. A 24-year-old man develops a lilac-colored rash on his eyelids and knuckles. He is having difficulty getting out of a chair. The course of the disease is best monitored by repeated

   (A) testing of muscle strength
   (B) sedimentation rates
   (C) urine transaminase enzymes
   (D) electromyography
   (E) alkaline phosphatase

674. Which of the following statements concerning renal disease in SLE is correct?

   (A) Evidence of any pathological change on renal biopsy indicates a poor prognosis.
   (B) Rapidly deteriorating renal function and an active urine sediment require prompt renal biopsy.
   (C) About 50% of patients with SLE have immunoglobulins in glomeruli.
   (D) Presence of anti–deoxyribonucleic acid (DNA) antibodies is associated with active nephritis.
   (E) Mesangial involvement suggests a poor prognosis.

675. Which of the following statements concerning the articular manifestations of RA is correct?

   (A) Wrists are rarely involved.
   (B) Involvement of hands is characteristically asymmetric.
   (C) Fever up to 104°F is common with joint involvement.
   (D) Ulnar deviation at the wrist is common.
   (E) Absence of morning stiffness makes RA an unlikely cause of articular symptoms.

Questions 676 through 679

A 22-year-old man has a history of low back pain and stiffness. After several months of mild symptoms, he notes more severe stiffness at night and hip pain. On physical examination, there is paravertebral muscle tenderness and limited flexion of the lumbar spine. A diastolic murmur is heard. Figure 9–4 shows an x-ray of the lumbar spine.

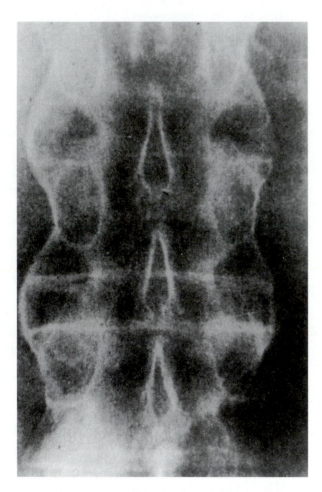

Figure 9–4.

676. The most likely diagnosis is

(A) Reiter syndrome
(B) Marfan syndrome
(C) ankylosing spondylitis (AS)
(D) RA
(E) pseudogout

677. The diastolic murmur is likely to be

(A) mitral stenosis
(B) tricuspid stenosis
(C) aortic insufficiency
(D) pulmonic insufficiency
(E) tetralogy of Fallot

678. The most likely extra-articular manifestation of this disease is

(A) colitis
(B) acute anterior uveitis
(C) psoriasis
(D) urethritis
(E) cardiac conduction disturbances

679. The standard drug used in treatment is

(A) indomethacin
(B) phenylbutazone
(C) azathioprine
(D) acetaminophen
(E) prednisone

Questions 680 and 681

A very tall, slender, 16-year-old boy is referred for evaluation. Physical examination reveals long fingers, pectus excavation, and a high arched palate.

680. Chest x-ray (CXR) is most likely to reveal

(A) dextrocardia
(B) aortic dilatation
(C) pneumothorax
(D) apical interstitial fibrosis
(E) rib notching

681. Musculoskeletal morbidity can be prevented by

(A) a vigorous exercise program
(B) bisphosphate therapy
(C) mechanical back bracing
(D) a prophylactic surgical procedure
(E) appropriate footwear

Questions 682 through 688

A 29-year-old woman develops painful swelling of both hands. She is also very stiff in the morning. Physical examination reveals involvement of the proximal interphalangeal joints and the metacarpophalangeal joints.

682. The most likely cause of the inflammation in her joints is

(A) activated T cells
(B) activated B cells
(C) microvascular injury
(D) interleukin-4 (IL-4)
(E) precipitated rheumatoid factor

683. She is most likely to develop extra-articular features if

(A) her knees are involved early
(B) there is a poor articular response to disease-suppressing medication
(C) humoral immunity is suppressed
(D) cellular immunity is suppressed
(E) she develops an antibody to her own immunoglobulin

684. The most likely place for her to develop vasculitis is

(A) kidneys
(B) heart
(C) lungs
(D) bowel
(E) skin

685. A CXR done 2 years after diagnosis reveals a pleural effusion. If this is secondary to her primary disease, it will reveal

(A) low glucose and low complement levels
(B) high glucose and high complement levels
(C) high glucose and low complement levels
(D) low glucose and high complement levels
(E) low protein and high complement levels

686. Three years later, at a time when her joints are quiescent, she develops neutropenia. This is most likely associated with

(A) cytotoxic therapy
(B) rheumatoid nodules disrupting bone marrow architecture
(C) splenomegaly
(D) her African-American heritage
(E) pancytopenia

687. The most likely drug to relieve the signs and symptoms of disease is

(A) D-penicillamine
(B) an antimalarial
(C) methotrexate
(D) aspirin
(E) gold

688. The most frequently used drug to prevent the progression of disease is

(A) D-penicillamine
(B) an antimalarial
(C) methotrexate
(D) aspirin
(E) gold

Questions 689 through 694

A 22-year-old woman develops a red rash over her cheeks and pain and swelling in both knees, as well as several small joints in her hand. Medical evaluation reveals oral ulceration and 3+ proteinuria.

689. The most sensitive test for diagnosis is

(A) lupus erythematosus (LE) cells
(B) ANAs
(C) anti-Sm
(D) anti-Ro
(E) antiphospholipid

690. The most specific test for diagnosis is

(A) LE cells
(B) ANAs
(C) anti-Sm
(D) anti-Ro
(E) antiphospholipids

691. The most likely cardiac manifestation is

(A) pericarditis
(B) myocarditis
(C) aortic regurgitation
(D) nonbacterial endocarditis
(E) myocardial vasculitis with infarction

692. The most likely drug to mimic this syndrome is

(A) hydralazine
(B) procainamide
(C) isoniazid (INH)
(D) chlorpromazine
(E) methyldopa

693. Renal damage is generally secondary to

(A) vasculitis
(B) microemboli
(C) anti–basement membrane antibodies
(D) deposition of circulating immune complexes
(E) primary tubular atrophy

694. In the course of this disease, the most common symptoms are related to

(A) renal pathology
(B) cardiopulmonary pathology
(C) musculoskeletal pathology
(D) thrombotic events
(E) GI pathology

Questions 695 through 698

A 39-year-old man has had several weeks of fever, weight loss, and lack of energy. Three days prior to assessment, he developed a left foot drop. Physical exam confirms left peroneal nerve damage and a bilateral sensory peripheral neuropathy in both legs. Lab evaluation reveals an ESR of 105, a neutrophilia of 14,000, and a positive serologic test for antineutrophil cytoplasmic antibody (ANCA). Eosinophil count is normal.

695. A reasonable method of establishing a diagnosis would be

(A) testicular biopsy
(B) skin biopsy
(C) spiral computed tomography (CT) of chest
(D) further serologic testing
(E) abdominal angiography

696. Renal involvement in this syndrome is characterized by

(A) nephrotic syndrome
(B) diffuse glomerulonephritis
(C) granuloma formation
(D) necrotizing vasculitis of vessels
(E) exclusively small vessel involvement

697. Evidence for viral involvement in the pathogenesis of this disease includes

(A) high cytomegalovirus (CMV) titers
(B) herpesvirus material in circulating immune complexes
(C) hepatitis B material in circulating immune complexes
(D) epidemiologic relationship to coxsackie B virus
(E) triggering of symptoms following viral gastroenteritis secondary to rotavirus infection

698. Initial treatment will include

(A) plasmapheresis
(B) steroid therapy alone
(C) combination therapy with steroids and cyclophosphamide
(D) cyclophosphamide therapy alone
(E) combination therapy with steroids and methotrexate

Questions 699 through 701

A 32-year-old woman has had a year of intermittent pain and swelling in both knees. The symptoms last weeks at a time and then improve. She has always been healthy. Her only past medical history is that of a round, pruritic skin lesion in her left groin 2 years earlier, which appeared shortly after a camping trip.

699. The pathogenesis of this syndrome

(A) autoimmune
(B) viral infection
(C) spirochetal infection
(D) circulating immune complexes
(E) metabolic (abnormal crystal metabolism)

700. Diagnosis of active disease is confirmed by

(A) positive antibody studies
(B) synovial fluid analysis
(C) skin biopsy
(D) clinical symptoms
(E) synovial biopsy

701. The treatment of choice for this syndrome will include

(A) high-dose glucocorticoids
(B) low-dose glucocorticoids
(C) high-dose NSAID therapy
(D) long-term penicillin
(E) long-term doxycycline

Questions 702 through 706

702. A 74-year-old man comes to the office with a history of headaches for 3 months. Which of the following signs or symptoms is most helpful in the diagnosis?

(A) throat pain on swallowing
(B) pain in the jaw when chewing
(C) malaise
(D) fatigue
(E) sweating

703. This disorder is often seen with another syndrome. The common presentation of this syndrome includes

(A) heliotrope rash
(B) proximal muscle weakness
(C) painful peripheral neuropathies

(D) stiffness and pain of proximal muscles
(E) hematuria

704. The most useful laboratory investigation to start the diagnostic process would be

(A) immunoelectrophoresis
(B) c-ANCA levels
(C) ESR
(D) creatine phosphokinase (CPK)
(E) hemoglobin and red cell indices

705. The definitive diagnostic test in this man would reveal

(A) immune complex deposition
(B) arteritis with giant cells
(C) lymphocytic infiltration
(D) type II muscle fiber atrophy
(E) polyphasic potentials on electromyography (EMG)

706. The most feared complication in this man would be

(A) blindness
(B) cortical stroke
(C) limb claudication
(D) renal infarction
(E) aortic aneurysm

Questions 707 through 711

707. Which of the following is a risk factor for osteoarthritis?

(A) being Chinese
(B) being Native American
(C) being male
(D) being underweight
(E) hyperthyroidism

708. Osteoarthritis would be best described as a disease of

(A) the synovial membrane
(B) articular cartilage
(C) the entire joint
(D) subchondral bone
(E) ligaments

709. The first change in the pathogenesis of osteoarthritis is likely

(A) abnormal chondrocyte function

(B) a defect in the extracellular matrix of cartilage

(C) inflammatory changes in subchondral bone

(D) ligament inflammation

(E) synovial inflammation

710. Which of the following statements about joint pain in osteoarthritis is correct

(A) synovial inflammation is not the cause

(B) ligament inflammation is a common cause

(C) clinically visible (via plain x-ray) fractures are a common cause of pain

(D) osteophytes can cause pain

(E) muscles are not involved

711. Which is the most common location for osteoarthritis?

(A) hip

(B) base of thumb

(C) knee

(D) spine

(E) distal interphalangeal joints of hand

DIRECTIONS (Questions 712 through 721): Each set of matching questions in this section consists of a list of lettered options followed by several numbered items. For each numbered item, select the appropriate lettered option(s). Each lettered option may be selected once, more than once, or not at all. EACH ITEM WILL STATE THE NUMBER OF OPTIONS TO SELECT. CHOOSE EXACTLY THIS NUMBER.

Questions 712 through 716

(A) associated with hemolysis

(B) seen in mixed connective tissue disease

(C) most sensitive test for SLE

(D) most sensitive test for drug-induced LE

(E) causes false-positive VDRL (Venereal Disease Research Laboratory)

(F) relatively disease specific

712. ANAs (SELECT ONE)

713. Anti-double-stranded (ds) DNA (SELECT ONE)

714. Antiphospholipid (SELECT ONE)

715. Antihistone (SELECT ONE)

716. Anti-RNP (ribosomal nuclear protein) (SELECT ONE)

Questions 717 through 721

(A) Felty syndrome

(B) rheumatoid vasculitis

(C) episcleritis

(D) Sjögren syndrome

(E) rheumatoid nodules

(F) rheumatoid pleural involvement

(G) Caplan syndrome

(H) pericardial disease

717. May present as small brown spots in the nail folds (SELECT ONE)

718. Most common form of eye involvement (SELECT ONE)

719. Associated with increased frequency of infections (SELECT ONE)

720. Found in association with occupational lung disease (SELECT ONE)

721. Commonly involves Achilles tendon (SELECT ONE)

DIRECTIONS (Questions 722 through 730): Each of the numbered items or incomplete statements in this section is followed by answers or by completions of the statement. Select the ONE lettered answer or completion that is BEST in each case.

722. Rickets and osteomalacia differ because

(A) the mineralization defect is less severe in osteomalacia

(B) osteomalacia is only produced by vitamin D deficiency, unlike rickets

(C) the skeleton is at a different stage when affected

(D) parathyroid hormone levels are only routinely elevated in rickets

(E) rickets always is characterized by hypocalcemia

723. Resistance to the effects of vitamin D can be caused by

(A) excess parathyroid hormone secretion

(B) insufficient parathyroid hormone secretion

(C) defective receptors for 25 (OH) vitamin D

(D) defective receptors for 1,25 (OH)$_2$ vitamin D

(E) mineralocorticoid excess

724. The primary defect in vitamin D metabolism that causes osteopenia associated with aging is

(A) impaired intestinal absorption of vitamin D

(B) impaired liver hydroxylation of vitamin D

(C) impaired renal hydroxylation of 1 (OH) vitamin D

(D) low parathyroid hormone levels

(E) low phosphate levels

725. Which of the following clinical findings is characteristic of both osteomalacia and rickets?

(A) frontal bossing in the skull

(B) muscle weakness

(C) prominent costochondral junctions

(D) defects in tooth enamel

(E) knock knees

Questions 726 and 727

726. An 84-year-old man, previously well except for chronic osteoarthritis, develops a hot, red, painful knee. Physical exam reveals an exquisitely tender, swollen knee. The most likely finding on investigation of synovial fluid would be

(A) staphylococcal infection

(B) gonococcal infection

(C) calcium hydroxyapatite crystals

(D) calcium pyrophosphate crystal deposition

(E) calcium oxalate

727. If this man gets frequent attacks, the most effective prophylaxis would be

(A) allopurinol

(B) continuous NSAIDs

(C) low dose glucocorticoids

(D) continuous antibiotic therapy

(E) colchicine

728. A 79-year-old woman on chronic hemodialysis presents with an acute, swollen knee. The most characteristic finding from joint aspiration in this situation would be

(A) uric acid crystals

(B) calcium pyrophosphate crystals (CPPD disease)

(C) calcium hydroxyapatite crystals

(D) calcium oxalate crystals

(E) crystallized urea

729. An 81-year-old woman develops progressive pain and immobility of her right shoulder. A series of x-rays over 8 months reveals destruction of the shoulder joint and an aspiration reveals blood in the effusion. Her only other articular manifestations are mild episodes of pain in her knees. What is the likely cause?

(A) a chronic bacterial infection

(B) uric acid deposition

(C) CPPD disease

(D) calcium oxalate deposition

(E) calcium hydroxyapatite deposition

730. A 59-year-old woman with rheumatoid arthritis under reasonable control with methotrexate develops acutely, a hot, swollen, red knee. Joint aspiration reveals a white count of 100,000/μL, predominantly neutrophils. This likely represents

(A) uric acid deposition

(B) CPPD deposition

(C) staphylococcal infection

(D) reactivation of rheumatoid arthritis

(E) calcium hydroxyapatite deposition

DIRECTIONS (Questions 731 through 735): Each set of matching questions in this section consists of a list of lettered options followed by several numbered items. For each numbered item, select the appropriate lettered option(s). Each lettered option may be selected once, more than once, or not at all. EACH ITEM WILL STATE THE NUMBER OF OPTIONS TO SELECT. CHOOSE EXACTLY THIS NUMBER.

(A) polyarteritis nodosa (PAN)

(B) Churg–Strauss disease

(C) Henoch–Schönlein purpura

(D) vasculitis associated with infectious diseases

(E) vasculitis associated with connective tissue diseases

(F) Wegener's granulomatosis

(G) giant cell arteritis

(H) Kawasaki disease

(I) Behçet syndrome

731. Pulmonary involvement and peripheral eosinophilia are common (SELECT ONE)

732. Aneurysms and renal involvement are characteristic (SELECT ONE)

733. Associated with a specific serum test when the disease is active (SELECT ONE)

734. Most common in children and often remits spontaneously after several episodes (SELECT ONE)

735. Characterized by oral and genital ulceration (SELECT ONE)

Answers and Explanations

648. (E) Each syndrome in the lysosomal storage diseases is caused by a mutation-produced deficiency in the activity of a lysosomal enzyme. For example, Tay–Sachs disease is caused by a deficiency of hexosaminidase A, resulting in accumulation of GM2 ganglioside. Gaucher's disease is caused by a deficiency of b-glucocerebrosidase, resulting in an accumulation of glucosylceramide. It has several forms and, as in this case, is most common in Ashkenazi (Eastern European) Jews. Type I Gaucher disease as described in this case is the most common type. Severe bone disease and hepatosplenomegaly is characteristic. Lipid-laden macrophages (Gaucher cells) are found in the bone marrow. *(Braunwald, p. 2280)*

649. (D) Still's disease (juvenile RA) in an adult may present as fever of unknown origin. Unfortunately, rheumatoid factor is often negative, and a response to NSAIDs along with exclusion of other diseases confirms the diagnosis. *(Braunwald, pp. 804–808)*

650. (C) The sicca syndrome is a recognized complication of HIV infection. Primary Sjögren syndrome is most common in middle-aged women, whereas HIV infection is more common in young men. Sjögren syndrome is more likely to have positive serology. Both have lymphocytic infiltration; in HIV, it is predominantly by CD8+ lymphocytes, whereas in Sjögren syndrome, the infiltration is by CD4+ lymphocytes. In sarcoidosis, biopsy reveals granulomas. *(Braunwald, p. 1948)*

651. (A) Cytoid bodies are a diagnostically helpful ophthalmic finding in SLE. Cytoid bod-ies are white exudates in the retina. Because they indicate a retinal vasculitis that can lead to blindness, aggressive immunosuppression should be instituted. *(Braunwald, p. 1925)*

652. (A) Esophageal symptoms are present in more than 50% of patients. They are due to the reduced tone of the gastroesophageal sphincter and dilation of the distal esophagus. Gastric and small intestinal motility problems can also occur. Vascular ectasia in the GI tract can result in bleeding. *(Braunwald, pp. 1941–1942)*

653. (A) Raynaud's phenomenon may lead to gangrene of the fingers. It can be primary (Raynaud's disease) or secondary to other disease, especially scleroderma, in which it can be the presenting symptom. In women, the primary form is common (over 50%), and the phenomenon is generally much more frequent in women. Digital infarction is much more common in relationship to scleroderma than it is in primary Raynaud's disease. *(Braunwald, pp. 1438–1439)*

654. (A) Pseudogout is distinguishable from gout by positive birefringent crystals. Calcium pyrophosphate crystals are short, blunt rhomboids, and urate crystals are needle-shaped with negative birefringence. *(Braunwald, pp. 1995–1996)*

655. (B) The child most likely has Henoch–Schönlein purpura, an immune complex vasculitis affecting the skin, GI tract, and renal glomeruli. Inciting antigens include upper respiratory tract infections, drugs, foods, and insect bites. *(Braunwald, p. 1965)*

656. **(C)** Difficulty in getting out of bed or rising from a chair may suggest polymyositis, but the muscles are normal. In general, polymyalgia rheumatica causes painful muscles, not weak muscles. However, pain may lead to profound disuse atrophy and apparent muscle weakness. In these cases, the normal creatine kinase (CK) and nonspecific muscle biopsy still allow accurate differentiation from polymyositis. *(Braunwald, p. 123)*

657. **(D)** The response of pain and stiffness to 20 mg of prednisone is dramatic. Long-term treatment with 5 mg of prednisone prevents symptoms. Mild cases may respond to NSAIDs. *(Braunwald, pp. 123, 2521)*

658. **(C)** The most common tumors associated with DM have been bronchogenic carcinomas, ovarian cancers, breast cancers, and melanoma but many others have occurred. The malignancy may antedate or postdate the myositis. Older age makes malignancy more likely. The extent of the work-up for malignancy if DM is the presentation depends on clinical circumstances, but history and physical exam, not x-rays, are the cornerstones of evaluation. *(Braunwald, p. 2525)*

659. **(A)** High pressure in the legs and low pressure in the arms characterize Takayasu syndrome. Clinical manifestations include easy fatigability of the arms and atrophy of the soft tissues of the face. The course is variable, and spontaneous remissions can occur. The disease predominantly affects young women. *(Braunwald, p. 1964)*

660. **(C)** There is a rarefied area involving the frontal and parietal bones. This is an early stage of Paget's disease in which calvarial thickening and foci or radiopacity are not present within the radiolucent area. At this stage of the disease, a cross-section through the margin of the lesion reveals a compact inner and outer table in the normal portion, whereas the diploë widens and extends to

the outer and inner surfaces of the calvarium without a change in the calvarial thickness in the lesion. *(Braunwald, p. 2238)*

661. **(E)** When acetic acid is added, a good, ropy clot forms in normal joint fluid, but a poor clot forms in severe inflammatory arthritis, including gout and RA. *(Braunwald, p. 1982)*

662. **(E)** Testing for autoantibodies, LDH, glucose, or protein in synovial fluid is rarely helpful. A white blood count over 50,000 suggests infection and may be associated with turbidity of the fluid. *(Braunwald, p. 1982)*

663. **(C)** The patient has Marfan syndrome. Aortic involvement occurs in about 80%, with degenerative changes predominating. *(Braunwald, p. 2299)*

664. **(B)** Leukopenia occurs in almost two thirds of the SLE patients, and the differential count is usually normal. Lymphocytes and platelets can also be reduced. *(Braunwald, p. 1924)*

665. **(C)** Mononuclear cell infiltration and edema develop in the periosteum, synovial membrane, and joint capsule. Secondary hypertrophic osteoarthropathy (HOA) (eg, lung cancer) is more common than primary HOA. *(Braunwald, pp. 2008–2010)*

666. **(A)** Pleural involvement is very common at autopsy but infrequently causes symptoms. If present, pleural fluid is low in glucose and complement levels. *(Braunwald, p. 1932)*

667. **(A)** In inflammatory bowel disease there are two common types of arthritis involvement. The first is a symmetric, migratory polyarthritis that affects the large joints of the lower extremities and is closely related to the activity of the bowel disease. Spondylitis is also common (though not always symptomatic) and is not always related to activity of bowel disease. *(Braunwald, p. 2004)*

668. **(C)** Most patients with psoriatic arthritis also have nail involvement. Only about a quarter actually develop a progressive, destructive dis-

ease. Uric acid may be elevated because of high tissue turnover but is not part of the pathogenesis of joint disease. *(Braunwald, p. 2003)*

669. **(A)** The presence of RF has little predictive power in determining the diagnosis of rheumatoid arthritis. However, it is useful in determining prognosis, as high titers of RF is associated with more severe and progressive disease, as well as extra-articular manifestations. *(Braunwald, p. 1933)*

670. **(D)** The disease is relapsing polychondritis and is characterized by frequent remissions and exacerbations of lesions and is rarely fatal. Auricular chondritis and nasal chondritis are the most common manifestations. It can also be secondary to SLE, rheumatoid arthritis, Sjögren's syndrome, and vasculitis. *(Braunwald, pp. 2005–2007)*

671. **(E)** In Ehlers–Danlos syndrome, skin hyperextensibility, fragility, and bruisability are marked, and this condition may create difficulties at operation. Habitual dislocation of joints is also a characteristic of this syndrome. *(Braunwald, pp. 2295–2296)*

672. **(C)** In traumatic arthritis, swellings, ecchymoses, muscular spasms, and tenderness tend to be present, but fractures must be excluded. Synovial fluid is bloody, but the fluid is of normal viscosity, so a "string" test is usually positive. *(Braunwald, p. 1982)*

673. **(A)** The course of muscle necrosis in dermatomyositis can be best followed by repeated CK determinations. Repeated muscle biopsies are rarely required. However, the goal of therapy is to increase muscle strength and function, so following muscle strength is the key issue. *(Braunwald, p. 2528)*

674. **(D)** Presence of high titer of anti-ds DNA, persistently abnormal urinalysis, and low complement increase the risk of severe nephritis. Although most patients have immunoglobulin deposition in the glomeruli, only half develop clinical nephritis. Some patterns of involvement, mesangial or mild

focal proliferative nephritis, have a good prognosis. Rapidly deteriorating renal function with an abnormal urine sediment mandates urgent treatment, but not necessarily urgent biopsy. *(Braunwald, pp. 1922–1924)*

675. **(E)** As in most inflammatory arthritides, the patient with RA generally has morning stiffness for more than 1 hour. Wrist involvement is nearly universal and is associated with radial deviation (unlike the ulnar deviation of the digits) and carpal tunnel syndrome. Hand involvement characteristically involves the proximal interphalangeal and metacarpophalangeal joints in a symmetric involvement. High fever (> 100.4°F), even with active synovitis, should suggest an intercurrent problem such as infection. *(Braunwald, pp. 1931–1933)*

676. **(C)** AS occurs in 1 to 6% of adults inheriting HLA-B27. However, the prevalence in B27-positive relatives of patients with AS is up to 30%. Men are three times more likely to be affected. *(Braunwald, p. 1949)*

677. **(C)** The frequency of aortic insufficiency has been about 4%. Other cardiac valve anomalies are not increased in incidence. Rarely, congestive heart failure or third-degree heart block can occur as well. *(Braunwald, p. 1950)*

678. **(B)** Acute anterior uveitis is the most common extra-articular manifestation. Pain, photophobia, and increased lacrimation are the usual symptoms. Attacks are unilateral and tend to recur, often in the other eye. Cataracts and secondary glaucoma are not uncommon sequelae. *(Braunwald, p. 1950)*

679. **(A)** Indomethacin and phenylbutazone are equally effective, but indomethacin is safer. Exercise and maintaining proper posture are very important. The iritis is usually managed with local glucocorticoid administration in association with a mydriatic agent. *(Braunwald, p. 1952)*

680. **(B)** In Marfan syndrome, inheritance is autosomal dominant, and the aortic lesion is a

cystic medial necrosis with loss of elastic tissue, resulting in aneurysm formation. Pneumothorax can occur but is not as characteristic. Mitral valve prolapse can also be part of the syndrome. Dislocation of the lens is the most apparent eye abnormality. Severe chest deformities and long limbs are characteristic. High, arched palate; high pedal arches; and pes planus are common. (Braunwald, p. 2299)

681. **(C)** The major musculoskeletal issue is progressive scoliosis, which is usually treated with physiotherapy and mechanical bracing. Only severe scoliosis is treated with surgery. Vigorous exercise and pregnancy are felt by some experts to increase the rate of aortic root dilatation. (Braunwald, p. 2299)

682. **(A)** Numerous mediators of inflammation are found in the synovium of patients with RA. The evidence favoring activated T cells as the initiators of the inflammation include the predominance of CD4$^+$ T cells in the synovium, the increase in soluble interleukin-2 (IL-2) receptors (a product of T-cell activation), and amelioration of symptoms by T-cell removal. (Braunwald, pp. 1841, 1929–1930)

683. **(E)** Extra-articular manifestations of RA generally develop in patients with high titers of autoantibody to the Fc component of immunoglobulin G (also known as rheumatoid factor). (Braunwald, p. 1933)

684. **(E)** Although widespread vasculitis resembling PAN can occur, most often the skin is involved. This presents as crops of small brown spots in the nailbeds, nail folds, and digital pulp. Mononeuropathy is another relatively common presentation of rheumatoid vasculitis. (Braunwald, p. 1932)

685. **(A)** Pleuritis is common at autopsy in patients with RA but is not usually symptomatic. Typically, the pleural fluid shows low glucose and low complement levels. Pleuropulmonary manifestations are more common in men with RA. (Braunwald, p. 1932)

686. **(C)** The triad of chronic rheumatoid arthritis, splenomegaly, and neutropenia is called Felty syndrome. It is associated with high titers of RF and extra-articular disease. The increased susceptibility to infections is secondary to both decreased neutrophil number and function. Felty syndrome is rare in African Americans. (Braunwald, pp. 1932–1933)

687. **(D)** Aspirin or other nonsteroidal agents are effective medications for relieving the signs and symptoms of disease. They do little to modify the course of the disease, however. The new generation of NSAIDs that are more specific inhibitors of cyclo-oxygenase 2 cause less gastrointestinal toxicity. Glucocorticoids are very powerful at suppressing signs and symptoms of disease and may alter disease progression. (Braunwald, p. 1934)

688. **(C)** Methotrexate, 7.5 to 20 mg once weekly, is the most commonly recommended disease-modifying drug, because its effect is more rapid and patients are able to tolerate it for longer periods of time. Maximum improvement with methotrexate occurs after 6 months of therapy. Toxicity includes GI upset, oral ulceration, and liver function abnormalities. The GI upset in particular may be ameliorated by concurrent folic acid administration. Pneumonitis has also been reported. (Braunwald, p. 1935)

689. **(B)** ANAs are present in 98% of patients with SLE. Repeatedly negative tests make the diagnosis of SLE very unlikely. Unfortunately, the test is not specific and may be positive in normal people (especially in older individuals), or secondary to infections, drugs, or other autoimmune disorders. (Braunwald, pp. 1923, 1925)

690. **(C)** Anti-Sm detects a protein complexed to six species of small nuclear ribonucleic acid (RNA). It is believed to be very specific for SLE. However, only 30% of patients have a positive test. In the case presented, there are enough clinical criteria (four) to confirm the diagnosis of SLE with 98% specificity and 97% sensitivity. (Braunwald, pp. 1923, 1925)

691. (A) Pericarditis, sometimes leading to tamponade, is the most common manifestation of cardiac disease. Myocarditis does occur and can cause arrhythmias, sudden death, or heart failure. Libman–Sachs endocarditis is associated with thrombotic events or, less commonly, valvular regurgitation. Myocardial infarction is more commonly a result of atherosclerotic disease than vasculitis. *(Braunwald, p. 1924)*

692. (B) All the drugs listed can cause lupus, but only procainamide and hydralazine do so with any frequency. About 50 to 75% of patients treated chronically with procainamide will develop ANA positivity (compared with 25 to 30% for hydralazine). About 10 to 20% of patients with ANA positivity will develop systemic symptoms compatible with lupus, particularly arthralgias. Genetic variation in drug acetylation rates might be a predisposing factor. *(Braunwald, p. 1926)*

693. (D) Renal disease is usually secondary to deposition of circulating immune complex. Although most patients with SLE have such deposits, only half have clinical nephritis as defined by proteinuria. Renal biopsy can provide both prognostic and therapeutic information. *(Braunwald, p. 1923)*

694. (C) About 95% of patients will develop musculoskeletal symptoms during the course of SLE. Arthralgias and myalgias predominate, but arthritis, hand deformities, myopathy, and avascular necrosis of bone also occur. About 85% of patients will have hematologic disease, and 80% will have skin manifestations. *(Braunwald, p. 1924)*

695. (E) This patient likely has PAN. The positive test for p-ANCA is nonspecific and does not indicate a diagnosis of Wegener's granulomatosis the way a positive test for c-ANCA would. The optimal diagnostic strategy is biopsy of an affected organ. However, abnormal angiography to look for aneurysms of small and medium-sized arteries is generally higher yield than blind biopsy of unaffected organs. The lungs are not a character-

istic site of involvement. *(Braunwald, pp. 1958–1960)*

696. (D) In classic PAN, unlike microscopic polyangitis, both small and medium vessels are involved. The renal lesions are ischemic secondary to fibrinoid necrosis of the vessels. In microscopic polyangitis, a diffuse glomerulonephritis is frequently present. The most common organ systems involved are the kidneys, musculoskeletal system, and peripheral nervous system. *(Braunwald, pp. 1958–1960)*

697. (C) About 20 to 30% of patients with PAN have hepatitis B antigenemia. Circulating immune complexes containing hepatitis B antigen and immunoglobulin have been detected, and immunofluorescence of blood vessel walls have also demonstrated hepatitis B antigen. Antiviral therapy has been used in these cases. *(Braunwald, p. 1959)*

698. (C) Current treatment for PAN mimics that of Wegener's granulomatosis in the initial treatment with combination steroid and cyclophosphamide therapy. This will result in up to a 90% long-term remission rate even after discontinuation of therapy. In cases associated with hepatitis B infection, plasmapheresis is sometimes used as initial therapy. *(Braunwald, p. 1960)*

699. (C) This story is typical of Lyme disease. The spirochete involved *(Borrelia burgdorferi)* is transmitted by ixodic ticks and is most common in the northeastern and midwestern parts of the United States. The host animal varies depending on the exact type of tick. *(Braunwald, pp. 1061–1062)*

700. (D) Because antibody studies cannot differentiate between active and inactive disease, the appropriate constellation of symptoms is also required for diagnosis. *(Braunwald, p. 1063)*

701. (E) Treatment is briefer and more effective earlier in the course of the disease. Presuming that this woman is not pregnant, the treatment of choice is doxycycline 100 mg bid for 1 to 2 months. Amoxicillin is a second-choice drug. *(Braunwald, p. 1064)*

702. **(B)** Although malaise, fatigue, and sweating are common in temporal arteritis, they are too nonspecific to help in making the diagnosis. Claudication of the jaw and tongue, while not very sensitive for temporal arteritis, are more specific than the constitutional symptoms. Odynophagia is not a characteristic of this disease. *(Braunwald, p. 1963)*

703. **(D)** Temporal arteritis is frequently associated with polymyalgia rheumatica. This disorder is characterized by stiffness, aching, and pain in proximal muscle groups in the neck, shoulders, back, hips, and thighs. It is considerably more common than temporal arteritis. Both diseases are almost exclusively seen in the over 50 age group. *(Braunwald, p. 1963)*

704. **(C)** Almost all patients with temporal arteritis will have an elevated ESR. Although a high ESR cannot make the diagnosis, a normal ESR helps in excluding the diagnosis. C-ANCA is a diagnostic tool for Wegener's granulomatosis. Elevated CPK is not seen in temporal arteritis, even with associated polymyalgia rheumatica. The normochromic, or slightly hypochromic, anemia often seen in temporal arteritis is too nonspecific to be of much diagnostic help. *(Braunwald, p. 1963)*

705. **(B)** Temporal artery biopsy is required for definitive diagnosis because of the relatively nonspecific nature of the presenting symptoms, signs, and routine laboratory tests. The arteritis can be segmental, however, and great care must be taken in the pathological assessment. *(Braunwald, p. 1964)*

706. **(A)** Although all these complications have been reported, the only one with a significant likelihood is blindness secondary to ischemic optic neuropathy. Thus, if the disease is suspected, urgent diagnosis and treatment is required. *(Braunwald, p. 1963)*

707. **(B)** There are numerous diseases and risk factors associated with the development of osteoarthritis. People of Chinese and African heritage have a lower risk than Caucasians, while Native Americans have a higher risk. Women are more affected than men, and obesity is a significant risk factor. Hyperthyroidism is not one of the many metabolic/endocrine disorders associated with osteoarthritis.

708. **(C)** Although the hallmark of osteoarthritis is the progressive loss of articular cartilage, it is best considered as a disease of the entire organ, the synovial joint, rather than of any of its component tissues. In fact, all areas of the joint, bone, cartilage, synovium, meniscus, and ligaments are involved. *(Braunwald, p. 1988)*

709. **(B)** It is most likely that the primary change in osteoarthritis occurs in the cartilage. It is possible that there is a disruption of the collagen network of the cartilage, specifically a disruption of the "glue" holding together adjacent fibers. *(Braunwald, p. 1989)*

710. **(D)** Osteophytes can cause pain by stretching periosteal nerve endings. Synovial inflammation is frequently seen in osteoarthritis, but not ligament inflammation. Microfractures, but not macrofractures, commonly cause pain. Muscle spasm can be an important factor in the joint pain. *(Braunwald, p. 1989)*

711. **(E)** Heberden's nodes, bony enlargement of the distal interphalangeal joints of the hand, are the most common type of osteoarthritis. Although they can present acutely with pain and inflammation, they are frequently slow in developing, and relatively asymptomatic. *(Braunwald, p. 1990)*

712. **(C)** Although not specific, ANA is positive in 95% of patients with SLE. A repeatedly negative test makes SLE unlikely. *(Braunwald, p. 1923)*

713. **(F)** Anti-ds DNA is relatively disease specific and associated with nephritis and clinical activity. Anti–single-stranded (ss) DNA is not very specific. *(Braunwald, p. 1923)*

714. **(E)** The presence of anticardiolipin antibodies is associated with false-positive VDRL, vascular thrombosis, and spontaneous abortion. *(Braunwald, p. 1923)*

715. **(D)** Antihistone antibodies are seen in 95% of patients with drug-induced LE and in 70% of those with SLE. *(Braunwald, p. 1923)*

716. **(B)** Anti-RNP is found in high titer in syndromes with features of polymyositis, scleroderma, lupus, and mixed connective tissue disease. *(Braunwald, p. 1923)*

717. **(B)** Although widespread vasculitis is rare, limited forms of vasculitis are not, particularly in white patients with high titers of rheumatoid factor. Cutaneous vasculitis usually presents as crops of small brown spots in the nailbeds, nail folds, and digital pulp. *(Braunwald, p. 1932)*

718. **(D)** Direct eye involvement with the rheumatoid process (episcleritis or scleritis) occurs in less than 1% of patients. However, 15 to 20% may develop Sjögren syndrome with attendant keratoconjunctivitis sicca. *(Braunwald, p. 1932)*

719. **(A)** Felty syndrome consists of chronic RA, splenomegaly, and neutropenia. The increased frequency of infections is due to both decreased number and function of neutrophils. *(Braunwald, pp. 1932–1933)*

720. **(G)** Caplan syndrome is a diffuse, nodular fibrotic process that may result when rheumatoid nodules occur in the lungs of patients with pneumoconiosis. *(Braunwald, p. 1932)*

721. **(E)** Rheumatoid nodules occur in 20 to 30% of patients with RA. Common locations include the olecranon bursa, the proximal ulna, the Achilles tendon, and the occiput. *(Braunwald, p. 1932)*

722. **(C)** Both rickets and osteomalacia are disorders in which mineralization of the organic matrix of the skeleton is defective. Rickets is the name when this disorder occurs in a growing skeleton, whereas osteomalacia occurs after the epiphyseal plates are closed. *(Braunwald, p. 2201)*

723. **(D)** Deficient or defective 1,25 $(OH)_2$ vitamin D receptors will result in vitamin D resistance. Parathyroid hormone levels increase secondary to decreased vitamin D effect. The 1 (OH) vitamin D is an intermediate metabolite. *(Braunwald, p. 2202)*

724. **(C)** Aging decreases the responsiveness of the renal 25 (OH) D-1-hydroxylase to PTH, thus decreasing circulatory levels of the active metabolite 1,25 $(OH)_2$ vitamin D. This results in decreased calcium absorption from the gut. There is not a close relationship of 1 (OH) vitamin D levels and osteopenia. *(Braunwald, p. 2202)*

725. **(B)** Muscle weakness is common in both rickets and osteomalacia, and proximal leg muscles are particularly involved. The combination of leg deformity and muscle weakness in rickets can result in inability to walk. The presentation of osteomalacia is more insidious in the elderly, but the proximal myopathy may be severe enough to cause a waddling gait and mimic a primary muscle disorder. The other clinical findings listed are found only in rickets. *(Braunwald, p. 2203)*

726. **(D)** The term *pseudogout* refers to crystal deposition disease not due to uric acid (gout). By far the most common cause of pseudogout is calcium pyrophosphate deposition (CPPD). The major predisposing factors are advanced age and pre-existing joint disease. The knee is the most common joint involved, and presentation can mimic acute gout. However, in the majority of cases, the deposition of calcium pyrophosphate seems to be asymptomatic. *(Braunwald, p. 1996)*

727. **(E)** Unfortunately, there is no medical means to remove the deposits of CPPD. Colchicine does seem to decrease the rate of recurrence. NSAIDs, steroids (systemic or intra-articular), and colchicine are all helpful in acute attacks. *(Braunwald, p. 1996)*

728. **(C)** Although gout and CPPD disease are found in chronic renal failure, hydroxyapatite deposition is characteristic of end-stage renal failure. The crystals are very small, nonbirefringent, and only seen on election microscopy. Treatment is symptomatic, and similar to the treatment of gout or CPPD disease. *(Braunwald, p. 1997)*

729. **(E)** "Milwaukee shoulder" represents an unusual manifestation of calcium hydroxyapatite deposition disease. Once destruction changes start occurring, medical management is relatively unsuccessful. The exact reason why destructive arthritis occurs is not understood. The knee is the other joint affected in this manner. *(Braunwald, p. 1997)*

730. **(C)** The high white cell count suggests infection. In rheumatoid arthritis and crystal-induced arthritis the white cell count is usually less than 50,000/μL. *Staphylococcus aureus* infection is the most common type in rheumatoid arthritis. *(Braunwald, pp. 1998–1999)*

731. **(B)** Churg–Strauss is a granulomatous vasculitis. Pulmonary involvement often dominates the clinical presentation with severe asthma attacks and pulmonary infiltrates. Peripheral eosinophilia is present in virtually all cases. *(Braunwald, p. 1960)*

732. **(A)** PAN is a multisystem, necrotizing vasculitis of small and medium-sized muscular arteries. Aneurysmal dilations of the arteries are characteristic. Nonspecific signs and symptoms are the usual method of presentation. Renal involvement is clinically present in 60% of cases and is the most common cause of death in untreated cases. *(Braunwald, p. 1959)*

733. **(F)** A high percentage of patients with Wegener's develop ANCAs. In particular, cytoplasmic or c-ANCAs are both sensitive and specific for Wegener's. However, tissue diagnosis is still required. *(Braunwald, p. 1962)*

734. **(C)** Henoch–Schönlein purpura, characterized by palpable purpura, arthralgias, GI symptoms, and glomerulonephritis, can be seen in any age group but is most common in children. It can resolve and recur several times over a period of weeks or months and can resolve spontaneously. *(Braunwald, p. 1965)*

735. **(I)** Behçet syndrome is a leukocytoclastic venulitis characterized by episodes of oral ulcers, genital ulcers, iritis, and cutaneous lesions. Eye involvement can rapidly progress to blindness. *(Braunwald, pp. 1956, 1967)*

CHAPTER 10

Infection
Questions

DIRECTIONS (Questions 736 through 767): Each of the numbered items or incomplete statements in this section is followed by answers or by completions of the statement. Select the ONE lettered answer or completion that is BEST in each case.

736. A 22-year-old recent immigrant to the United States has never been vaccinated for tetanus. He sustains a minor, but soil-contaminated, injury. Which of the following statements is correct?

   (A) Tetanus usually develops within 2 weeks following exposure.
   (B) Tetanus always develops within 4 hours following exposure in patients who have not been previously immunized.
   (C) Tetanus may develop many months or years following exposure in susceptible individuals.
   (D) The usual incubation period for tetanus is 48 hours.
   (E) Tetanus may be prevented with penicillin.

737. A 19-year-old man has donated blood for the first time. Despite having no risk factors for human immunodeficiency virus (HIV) infection, his blood tests positive for HIV by enzyme immunoassay (EIA). Which of the following statements is correct?

   (A) EIA is currently the most specific test for HIV.
   (B) He might have a false-positive secondary to an unsuspected collagen-vascular disease.
   (C) He has a 75% chance of truly being infected with HIV.

   (D) EIA is an excellent screening test.
   (E) A Western Blot test would be more sensitive.

738. A 23-year-old woman develops vesicular lesions on an erythematous base on her vulvar area. She has tender lymphadenopathy and dysuria as well. The causative organism is likely

   (A) cytomegalovirus (CMV)
   (B) gonococcus
   (C) herpes simplex virus type 2 (HSV-2)
   (D) *Treponema pallidum*
   (E) varicella zoster

739. A 32-year-old man, previously well, develops a fever and dry cough. Chest x-ray (CXR) reveals a diffuse interstitial infiltrate. The most likely organism is a

   (A) bacterium
   (B) mycoplasma
   (C) fungus
   (D) rickettsia
   (E) spirochete

740. A 25-year-old man is admitted with fever and rust-colored sputum. The CXR is shown in Figure 10–1. The most likely diagnosis is

(A) right middle lobe pneumonia
(B) loculated pleural effusion
(C) aspergilloma
(D) aspiration pneumonia
(E) right lower lobe pneumonia

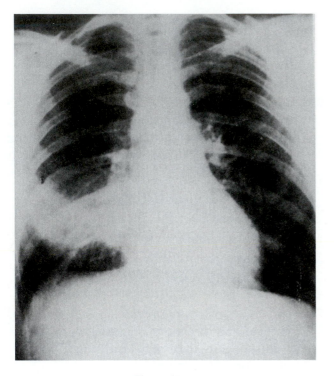

Figure 10–1.

741. A 30-year-old man develops pustular lesions at the site of a cat scratch, followed by malaise, fever, and lymphadenopathy. These are likely to be caused by a

(A) gram-negative bacillus
(B) coccobacillus
(C) acid-fast bacillus
(D) rickettsia
(E) fungus

742. A 7-year-old child, unvaccinated because of his parents' religious beliefs, develops malaise, cough, coryza, and conjunctivitis with a high fever. Examination of his mouth reveals blue-white spots on a red base beside his second molars. The next day he develops an erythematous, nonpruritic, maculopapular rash at his hairline and behind his ears, which spreads over his body. The most likely complication causing death would be

(A) pneumonia
(B) mastoiditis
(C) meningitis
(D) dehydration
(E) pancreatitis

743. A 60-year-old man presents with fever and malaise 6 weeks after mitral valve replacement. Examination reveals a loud mitral regurgitant murmur. The causative organism is likely

(A) *Staphylococcus aureus*
(B) a fungus
(C) *Staphylococcus saprophytricus*
(D) pneumococcus
(E) *Staphylococcus epidermidis*

744. A 63-year-old man develops headache, fever, cough, sore throat, malaise, and severe myalgia during a community outbreak affecting numerous individuals. He suddenly becomes hypoxic, and CXR reveals a new infiltrate. The most likely cause is

(A) primary viral pneumonia
(B) an autoimmune reaction
(C) a gram-negative bacterium
(D) *Staphylococcus*
(E) *Neisseria catarrhalis*

745. Infection of an 8-year-old boy with an enterovirus is most likely to cause

(A) fever
(B) aseptic meningitis
(C) myalgia
(D) exanthems
(E) diarrhea

746. An 18-year-old woman has eaten homemade preserves. Eighteen hours later, she develops diplopia, dysarthria, and dysphagia. This is most likely due to

(A) *Clostridium botulinum* toxin
(B) staphylococcal toxin
(C) salmonellosis
(D) brucellosis
(E) shigellosis

747. A previously healthy 19-year-old female university student develops myalgia, headache, fever, and malaise. Blood tests reveal lymphocytosis, with 20% of the lymphocytes being atypical. She remains tired and unwell for 6 weeks, but repeated tests for heterophil and antibody are negative. She most likely has

(A) Epstein–Barr virus (EBV) infection
(B) primary HIV infection
(C) human herpes virus type 7 (HHV-7)
(D) CMV infection
(E) toxoplasmosis

748. A 43-year-old man developed a cough shortly after returning from California. CXR reveals a thin-walled cavity, and sputum reveals fungal elements. The most likely cause is

(A) ringworm
(B) *Cryptococcus neoformans*
(C) *Candida albicans*
(D) mycobacteria
(E) coccidioidomycosis

Questions 749 and 750

749. An 8-year-old boy from an impoverished inner-city area has never been vaccinated appropriately. He develops fever, cough, and coryza. The next day, blue-white spots develop on the buccal mucosa. On the third day, an erythematous, nonpruritic maculopapular rash develops on the face and spreads over the entire body. The most likely complication is

(A) pneumonia
(B) encephalitis

(C) otitis media
(D) bronchitis
(E) mastoiditis

750. Prior to mass vaccination for this disease, delayed neurologic effects could result in

(A) meningitis
(B) pure motor paralysis
(C) autonomic neuropathy
(D) dementia
(E) stocking-glove peripheral neuropathy

751. Live rubella vaccine should be given to

(A) children between 1 year old and puberty
(B) infants less than 1 year old
(C) all adults
(D) pregnant women
(E) all exposed patients

752. A 23-year-old woman, recently arrived to study in the United States from southern India, presents with a chronic vulvar ulcer. The lesion began as a papule and then ulcerated. She has had the lesion for several months. Currently, physical exam reveals a painless elevated area of beefy-red, friable granulation tissue. She has been sexually active for several years. This disease is most likely caused by a(n)

(A) spirochete
(B) gram-positive coccus
(C) intracellular gram-negative bacteria
(D) chronic viral infection
(E) fungus

753. A renal transplant patient develops severe cough and dyspnea. Bronchial brushings show clusters of cysts that stain with methenamine silver. The best treatment is

(A) amphotericin B
(B) cephalosporins
(C) trimethoprim–sulfamethoxazole
(D) aminoglycosides
(E) penicillins

754. Three hours after a church social, eight people develop severe diarrhea. Food served included chicken salad and cream-filled pastries. This is most likely caused by

(A) staphylococcal enterotoxin
(B) *C. botulinum*
(C) *Clostridium perfringens*
(D) *Salmonella* species
(E) ptomaine poisoning

755. A young woman complains of hair loss, loss of hair luster, and intense scalp irritation. A Wood's light examination is positive. The most likely cause is

(A) seborrhoeic dermatitis
(B) *Aspergillus*
(C) *Trichophyton*
(D) neurosis
(E) excess androgen levels

756. Coxsackie A virus infection may result in

(A) roseola
(B) diarrhea
(C) aseptic meningitis
(D) basophilia
(E) acute hepatitis

757. A young man has recently come into contact with a wild bat. The most serious infection that might be transmitted

(A) may be further transmitted from human to human through exchange of body fluids
(B) comes from infected blood of the bat
(C) is treated only if symptoms develop
(D) has symptoms that uniformly include hyperexcitability
(E) may include finding Negri bodies in nerve cells as confirmation of the diagnosis

758. The most likely malignancy to contain EBV deoxyribonucleic acid (DNA) in a non-HIV patient in the United States is

(A) gastric cancer
(B) well-differentiated thyroid cancer

(C) anaplastic nasopharyngeal carcinoma
(D) Burkitt's lymphoma
(E) Hodgkin's disease

759. A 40-year-old man develops erythema nodosum, conjunctivitis, and a pleural effusion. Over several weeks, pulmonary lesions lead to cavitation and a large, thin-walled cavity. The most likely cause is

(A) *Streptococcus*
(B) coccidioidomycosis
(C) candidiasis
(D) *Staphylococcus*
(E) *Pneumocystis carinii*

760. A patient undergoing emergency surgery for trauma receives 20 blood transfusions during the operation. Four weeks later, she develops a syndrome resembling infectious mononucleosis. The most likely cause is

(A) EBV
(B) hepatitis C virus
(C) delayed hemolysis
(D) CMV
(E) serum sickness

761. A 32-year-old woman acutely develops high fever, hypotension, and rash. In the hospital, evidence of multiorgan failure develops. This syndrome is most likely associated with

(A) menstruation
(B) streptococcal infection
(C) clostridial infection
(D) high-level bacteremia
(E) recent sexual activity

762. Initial management for the neutropenic cancer patient with high fever should include

(A) an aminoglycoside and a cephalosporin
(B) tetracycline
(C) acetaminophen alone until culture results are available
(D) an anthracycline and a folate inhibitor
(E) serial, empiric addition of one drug at a time

763. An elderly, bedridden patient in the hospital develops a cough and right lower lobe infiltrate. This syndrome is likely to be associated with

    (A) aerobic and anaerobic organisms

    (B) an afebrile course

    (C) multilobar involvement

    (D) *Haemophilus influenzae* infection

    (E) sterile pneumonitis

764. Which of the following are characteristic of pneumonia caused by *Legionella pneumophila?*

    (A) usually very mild disease

    (B) heavy sputum production

    (C) transmitted by blood transfusion

    (D) high fever is common

    (E) indigenous to northeastern United States

765. The dental condition illustrated in Figure 10–2 is usually associated with

    (A) osteoporosis

    (B) high forehead

    (C) Paget's disease of bone

    (D) absent radius

    (E) anterior bowing of tibiae

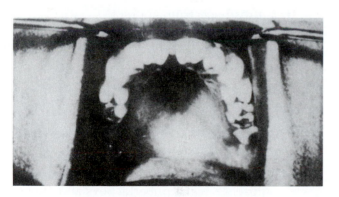

Figure 10–2.

766. A 53-year-old man with stable alcoholic cirrhosis has no ascites. Which statement concerning spontaneous bacterial peritonitis (SBP) is correct?

    (A) Pre-existing ascites is present in only 50% of the cases.

    (B) Most cases present with fever.

    (C) The microbiology reveals a polymicrobial infection.

    (D) A white blood count (WBC) of less than 1000 polymorphonuclear neutrophils (PMNs) per microliter virtually excludes the diagnosis.

    (E) Over 70% of cirrhotic patients will develop SBP over the course of their illness.

767. Which of the following statements concerning Lyme disease is correct?

    (A) The incubation period is 3 months.

    (B) After an initial brisk immune response, immunity wanes with continuous infection.

    (C) The disease is caused by a spirochete.

    (D) The disease is caused by a tick.

    (E) The characteristic skin lesion of erythema migrans is found in over 95% of cases.

DIRECTIONS (Questions 768 through 795): This section consists of clinical situations, each followed by a series of questions. Study each situation, and select the ONE best answer to each question following it.

Questions 768 through 772

An 18-year-old woman visits her physician because of 3 weeks of malaise, 2 weeks of fever, and a sore throat. Physical examination shows pharyngeal infection with enlarged tonsils and a patchy, white exudate; enlarged, palpable anterior and posterior cervical, axillary, and inguinal lymph nodes; tenderness in the right upper quadrant; and minimal splenomegaly. Laboratory data show: hemoglobin, 14% g; hematocrit, 42%; platelets, 380,000; WBC, 8500, with 35% segmented neutrophils, 1% eosinophils, and 64% lymphocytes, of which 36 were atypical.

768. The most likely diagnosis is

    (A) infectious hepatitis

    (B) lymphocytic leukemia

    (C) infectious mononucleosis

    (D) Hodgkin's disease

    (E) cat scratch fever

769. The diagnosis is most likely to be proved by

(A) lymph node biopsy

(B) bone marrow

(C) erythrocyte sedimentation rate (ESR)

(D) Paul–Bunnell heterophil antibody (sheep cell agglutination) test

(E) hepatic biopsy

770. The treatment of choice for this disease is

(A) gamma globulin

(B) adequate rest

(C) chlorambucil

(D) chloramphenicol

(E) radiation therapy

771. Which of the following rare complications can be associated with this disease?

(A) retinitis

(B) esophagitis

(C) splenic rupture

(D) Kaposi's sarcoma

(E) hemorrhage

772. The most common virus that can mimic this virus is

(A) herpes simplex

(B) echovirus

(C) CMV

(D) coxsackie virus

(E) reovirus

Questions 773 through 777

A 20-year-old woman visits your office because of headache, anorexia, chilly sensations, pain and drawing sensations in both sides of her jaw, and pain in both lower abdominal quadrants. Physical examination reveals bilateral, enlarged parotid glands that are doughy, elastic, and slightly tender; reddened orifice of Stensen's duct; bilateral lower quadrant abdominal tenderness; a temperature of 102°F; and a pulse rate of 92/min. Laboratory data show hemoglobin, 13% g; hematocrit, 40%; WBC, 9000, with 35% segmented neutrophils, 7% monocytes, and 58% lymphocytes.

773. The most likely diagnosis is

(A) cervical lymphadenitis

(B) Mikulicz syndrome

(C) parotid gland tumor

(D) uveoparotid fever

(E) mumps

774. The patient's abdominal pain and tenderness is most likely due to

(A) mesenteric lymphadenitis

(B) oophoritis

(C) gonorrhea

(D) peritoneal metastases

(E) intestinal hyperperistalsis

775. Which of the following laboratory tests help confirm the diagnosis of epidemic parotitis?

(A) single blood sample for a specific immunoglobulin G (IgG)

(B) blood cell count

(C) blood culture

(D) single blood test for a specific IgM

(E) serum amylase

776. The best treatment for this disease is

(A) symptomatic

(B) convalescent serum

(C) broad-spectrum antibiotics

(D) sulfonamides

(E) steroids

777. Which of the following statements concerning this disease is true?

(A) The disease is caused by a herpesvirus.

(B) The incubation period is 3 to 5 days.

(C) The most common complication of this disease in postpubertal boys and men is orchitis.

(D) Recurrent infections may occur.

(E) An increased serum amylase is proof of the existence of pancreatitis as a complication.

Questions 778 through 780

A 19-year-old woman was traveling in a rural area of South America. She returned 1 month ago and, over the past few days, has gradually developed lower abdominal pain and diarrhea. She is afebrile, and her stool is mostly comprised of blood and mucus.

778. She most likely has

    (A) *Escherichia coli* infection
    (B) *Salmonella* infection
    (C) *Shigella* infection
    (D) *Vibrio parahemolyticus* infection
    (E) *Entamoeba histolytica* infection

779. Diagnosis is confirmed by

    (A) stool culture
    (B) stool toxin assay
    (C) examination of a dried stool specimen
    (D) immunofluorescence of stool specimen
    (E) examination of a wet stool specimen

780. The most likely site of extraintestinal involvement would be

    (A) genitals
    (B) pleura
    (C) pericardium
    (D) liver
    (E) cerebral cortex

Questions 781 through 785

An 18-year-old man develops fever, neck stiffness, and delirium. There are no reported similar cases in the community.

781. The most organism causing this syndrome is

    (A) *Neisseria meningitidis*
    (B) *Streptococcus pneumoniae*
    (C) *H. influenzae*
    (D) *Staphylococcus*
    (E) *Listeria* species

782. The source of infection was most likely

    (A) bacteremia from an infected heart valve
    (B) middle ear

    (C) skin
    (D) oral ingestion
    (E) pharynx

783. If he had been 2 years old rather than 18, the most likely organism would be

    (A) *N. meningitidis*
    (B) *S. pneumoniae*
    (C) *H. influenzae*
    (D) *Staphylococcus*
    (E) *Listeria* species

784. Had he been the second case in a six-story university dormitory, the most likely organism would be

    (A) *N. meningitidis*
    (B) *S. pneumoniae*
    (C) *H. influenzae*
    (D) *Staphylococcus*
    (E) *Listeria* species

785. In the case of a student's developing meningococcal meningitis in the dormitory, chemoprophylaxis should be provided to

    (A) everybody in the dormitory, with oral amoxicillin
    (B) close contacts only, with oral amoxicillin
    (C) everybody in the dormitory, with oral rifampin
    (D) close contacts only, with oral rifampin
    (E) everybody in the dormitory, with meningococcal vaccine

Questions 786 through 788

A 43-year-old businesswoman is developing a new enterprise in Mexico. On her most recent trip, she developed diffuse watery diarrhea with severe cramps.

786. The most likely causative organism is

    (A) *Campylobacter*
    (B) *E. coli*
    (C) *Salmonella*
    (D) *Shigella*
    (E) rotavirus

787. She has no fever and no blood in her stools. Appropriate treatment would include

    (A) amoxicillin
    (B) symptomatic therapy with loperamide
    (C) doxycycline
    (D) oral rehydration only
    (E) specific antitoxin

788. To prevent future episodes during business trips, as well as being more careful in eating, she should take prophylactic

    (A) loperamide
    (B) trimethoprim–sulfamethoxazole
    (C) ciprofloxacin
    (D) doxycycline
    (E) bismuth subsalicylate

Questions 789 through 791

A 22-year-old man is an avid spelunker (cave explorer) and has recently been exploring several caves. A routine CXR taken for a new job reveals hilar adenopathy and two patches of pneumonitis. Careful questioning reveals he has just gotten over a "cold" with mild fever, cough, and malaise.

789. The most likely diagnosis is

    (A) tuberculosis
    (B) sarcoidosis
    (C) candidiasis
    (D) histoplasmosis
    (E) coccidioidomycosis

790. Dissemination of the disease

    (A) requires no specific therapy
    (B) can result in Addison's disease
    (C) causes splenic infarction
    (D) requires long-term therapy with a fluoroquinolone
    (E) is seen only in immunocompromised individuals

791. Eight years later, he presents with a red face and grossly distended neck veins. This complication is a result of

    (A) lymphomatous transformation
    (B) a late secondary spread of infection
    (C) a secondary autoimmune phenomenon
    (D) infectious emboli
    (E) progressive fibrosis

Questions 792 through 795

A previously well 28-year-old female has developed gradual onset of fever and malaise over 2 to 3 weeks. She also complains of arthralgias and myalgias. Repeated measurement of her temperature reveals a low-grade fever between 101.3 and 102.2°F. Physical examination reveals an oval retinal hemorrhage with a clear, pale center; a pansystolic cardiac murmur heard best at the apex; and small, tender nodules on her fingertips.

792. The most likely organism in this woman is

    (A) *S. aureus*
    (B) *S. epidermidis*
    (C) *Streptococcus*
    (D) enterococcus
    (E) *Candida*

793. Had she been an intravenous drug abuser, the most likely organism would be

    (A) *S. aureus*
    (B) *S. epidermidis*
    (C) *Streptococcus viridans*
    (D) enterococci
    (E) *Candida*

794. Pending identification of the causative organism in this woman, treatment should be directed against

    (A) *S. aureus*
    (B) *S. epidermidis*
    (C) *Streptococcus viridans*
    (D) enterococci
    (E) *Candida*

795. Impairment of renal function with proteinuria and red cell casts suggests

    (A) septic emboli
    (B) cardiac failure with prerenal azotemia

(C) a high level of circulating immune complexes

(D) fungal disease

(E) inevitable progression to renal failure

DIRECTIONS (Questions 796 through 805): Each set of matching questions in this section consists of a list of lettered options followed by several numbered items. For each numbered item, select the appropriate lettered option(s). Each lettered option may be selected once, more than once, or not at all. EACH ITEM WILL STATE THE NUMBER OF OPTIONS TO SELECT. CHOOSE EXACTLY THIS NUMBER.

Questions 796 through 800

(A) *S. aureus*

(B) *Candida*

(C) *P. carinii*

(D) *Giardia lamblia*

(E) gram-negative enteric bacilli

(F) *H. influenzae*

(G) *Neisseria* species

(H) *Nocardia* species

(I) *Salmonella*

(J) rubella virus

796. Cytotoxic chemotherapy (SELECT ONE)

797. Selective IgA deficiency (SELECT ONE)

798. Defect in alternate pathology of complement (SELECT ONE)

799. T-lymphocyte deficiency/dysfunction (SELECT ONE)

800. Microbicidal defect (SELECT ONE)

Questions 801 through 805

(A) *S. aureus*

(B) *C. perfringens*

(C) *Vibrio cholerae*

(D) enterotoxigenic *E. coli*

(E) *Salmonella*

(F) *Shigella*

(G) *V. parahaemolyticus*

(H) *Bacillus cereus*

801. Occurs 3 hours after a meal of a ham sandwich and potato salad (SELECT ONE)

802. Most common cause of travelers' diarrhea (SELECT ONE)

803. Causes bloody diarrhea 24 hours after a salad (SELECT ONE)

804. Causes watery diarrhea 24 hours after raw oyster ingestion (SELECT ONE)

805. Can cause both early-onset vomiting and later-onset diarrhea (SELECT ONE)

DIRECTIONS (Questions 806 through 822): This section consists of clinical situations, each followed by a series of questions. Study each situation, and select the ONE best answer to each question following it.

Questions 806 through 810

A 19-year-old man is seen in the office 9 days after a hiking trip in Colorado. He has a fever, headache, myalgia, and nausea. He reports that he had numerous insect bites during his hike.

806. This disease is likely caused by a

(A) gram-positive bacterium

(B) gram-negative bacterium

(C) virus

(D) type of rickettsia

(E) type of chlamydia

807. The patient is started on a broad-spectrum cephalosporin, and 2 days later develops macules around his wrists and ankles. The likely diagnosis at this point is

(A) circulating immune complex disease

(B) a drug reaction

(C) infective endocarditis

(D) Rocky Mountain spotted fever

(E) *S. aureus* sepsis

808. The most frequently affected part of the body is the

(A) microcirculation
(B) liver
(C) heart
(D) brain
(E) kidney

809. The most common type of central nervous system presentation is

(A) hemiplegia
(B) cranial nerve abnormalities
(C) paraplegia
(D) encephalitis
(E) ataxia

810. The treatment of choice for severe disease is

(A) plasmapheresis plus glucocorticoids
(B) ampicillin
(C) vancomycin
(D) erythromycin
(E) doxycycline

811. A 22-year-old sexually active man presents with painful urination. The diagnosis of urethritis can be confirmed by

(A) history alone
(B) milking of the urethra
(C) routine urinalysis
(D) gram stain of a midstream urine specimen
(E) urine culture

812. The most likely organism causing this man's symptoms would be

(A) *Neisseria gonorrhoeae*
(B) *Chlamydia trachomatis*
(C) herpes simplex virus (HSV)
(D) *Ureaplasma ureolyticum*
(E) mycoplasma genitalium

813. Microscopic examination of the appropriate specimen reveals only numerous neutrophils, without evidence of gram-negative intracel-

lular diplococci. The correct management would be

(A) await culture results for *N. gonorrhoeae*
(B) treat for chlamydia infection with azithromycin
(C) treat for *N. gonorrhoeae* infection with cefixime
(D) treat for *N. gonorrhoeae* infection with penicillin
(E) treat with azithromycin and cefixime

814. A 22-year-old woman has been sexually active only with her husband. She complains of vulvar itching and burning and pain when urine is passed. Physical examination reveals some vulvar ulceration but no vaginal discharge. The likely diagnosis is:

(A) HSV infection
(B) *Trichomonas vaginalis* infection
(C) *N. gonorrhoeae* infection
(D) *C. trachomatis* infection
(E) mycoplasma genitalium infection

815. *Candida albicans* infection is discovered in a young woman with vulvovaginal itching. Appropriate management for her asymptomatic male sexual partner would be

(A) azole cream to the penis
(B) oral fluconazole
(C) standard urethritis investigation
(D) no investigation or treatment
(E) azithromycin plus cefixime

816. Which of the following statements concerning the epidemiology of *S. pneumoniae* is correct?

(A) Most children are nasopharyngeal carriers.
(B) In the adult, the presence of the bacterium is almost always associated with disease.
(C) Bacteremia is most common in people over 55.

(D) In adults, bacteremia is most common in midwinter.

(E) The likelihood of invasive disease depends solely on the serotype of the organism.

817. The most specific immunological defense against pneumococcal infection is

(A) an IgG antibody directed against *S. pneumoniae* nuclear antigens

(B) a complement fixing IgM antibody

(C) an IgG antibody directed against capsular antigens

(D) alveolar macrophages

(E) specific classes of killer T cells

818. Otitis media caused by *S. pneumoniae* is the result of

(A) hematogenous spread

(B) direct extension from the nasopharynx

(C) direct inoculation on the ear

(D) spread through lymphatic tissue

(E) associated dental disease

819. In an outbreak of pneumococcal pneumonia in a military barracks, the most common predisposing cause for symptomatic pneumonia is likely

(A) immotile cilia syndrome

(B) previous viral infection

(C) asthma

(D) cigarette-induced chronic lung disease

(E) allergies

820. The most common complication of pneumococcal pneumonia is

(A) peritonitis

(B) empyema

(C) pericarditis

(D) endocarditis

(E) osteomyelitis

821. The most common presenting symptoms of *Mycoplasma pneumoniae* infection are cough and

(A) sputum

(B) shortness of breath

(C) headache

(D) shaking chills

(E) pleuritic chest pain

822. The most common skin manifestation of *M. pneumoniae* is

(A) erythema nodosum

(B) erythema multiforme

(C) maculopapular rash

(D) vesicular rash

(E) urticaria

DIRECTIONS (Questions 823 through 842): Each set of matching questions in this section consists of a list of lettered options followed by several numbered items. For each numbered item, select the appropriate lettered option(s). Each lettered option may be selected once, more than once, or not at all. EACH ITEM WILL STATE THE NUMBER OF OPTIONS TO SELECT. CHOOSE EXACTLY THIS NUMBER.

Questions 823 through 827

(A) beta-lactams (penicillins and cephalosporins)

(B) vancomycin

(C) erythromycin

(D) sulfonamides and trimethoprim

(E) ciprofloxacin

823. Major cellular target is interference with cell metabolism (SELECT ONE)

824. Work by inhibiting DNA synthesis (SELECT ONE)

825. Resistance can be caused by drug inactivation (SELECT ONE)

826. Work by inhibiting protein synthesis (SELECT ONE)

827. Decreased intracellular accumulation can result in resistance (SELECT ONE)

Questions 828 through 832

    (A) erythromycin

    (B) ciprofloxacin

    (C) tetracycline

    (D) sulfonamides

    (E) metronidazole

    (F) rifampin

828. Can cause unwanted pregnancy (SELECT ONE)

829. Can contribute to hypoglycemia in non–insulin-dependent diabetes mellitus (NIDDM) (SELECT ONE)

830. Can cause severe reaction to alcohol (SELECT ONE)

831. Drug interaction can result in rejection for transplant recipients (SELECT ONE)

832. Can result in phenytoin toxicity (SELECT ONE)

Questions 833 through 837

    (A) brucellosis

    (B) coccidioidomycosis

    (C) histoplasmosis

    (D) leprosy

    (E) leptospirosis

    (F) infectious mononucleosis

    (G) tuberculosis

    (H) tularemia

833. Oropharyngeal ulcerations (SELECT ONE)

834. Thin-wall pulmonary cavitation (SELECT ONE)

835. Positive Mantoux test (SELECT ONE)

836. Iowa hog farmers (SELECT ONE)

837. Infected rabbits (SELECT ONE)

Questions 838 through 842

    (A) toxoplasmosis

    (B) tetanus

    (C) syphilis

    (D) *Streptococcus*

    (E) *Staphylococcus*

    (F) smallpox

    (G) salmonellosis

838. Darkfield examination (SELECT ONE)

839. Congenital hydrocephalus (SELECT ONE)

840. Abdominal pain and diarrhea (SELECT ONE)

841. Preventive measures not used any longer (SELECT ONE)

842. Treated with muscle relaxants (SELECT ONE)

Answers and Explanations

736. (A) In tetanus, an acute onset is usual. The median onset is 7 days, and 90% present within 14 days of injury. The organism is an anaerobic, motile gram-positive rod. It has the ability to survive for years in the form of spores, which are resistant to disinfectants and heat. Tetanus can occur in nonimmunized individuals, or those who have neglected their booster shots. Penicillin or metronidazole are used in treatment, but their efficacy is not clear. (*Braunwald, pp. 918–920*)

737. (D) The EIA is an excellent screening test for HIV infection as it is positive in over 99.5% of cases. However, it lacks specificity, and in low risk populations only about 10% of EIA positive results are true positives. Recent influenza vaccination, acute viral infections, and liver disease are common causes for false positives. The Western Blot test is more specific and is the usual confirmatory test, although even more specific tests are now available. (*Braunwald, p. 1876*)

738. (C) HSV-2 genital infections may be associated with fever, malaise, and anorexia. Vesicular lesions usually ulcerate rapidly and become covered with exudate. There is a 90% chance of recurrent symptoms in the first year following a primary infection. HSV-1 genital infections are similar, but the chance of recurrence is less. (*Braunwald, p. 1102*)

739. (B) Mycoplasmas have no cell walls and have filtration characteristics of viruses, but morphologically are closer to bacteria. The typical *M. pneumoniae* infection produces an influenza-like respiratory illness characterized by headache, malaise, fever, and cough. If pneumonia occurs, physical exam can be relatively benign despite a grossly abnormal chest x-ray. (*Braunwald, p. 1073*)

740. (A) The x-ray shows a silhouette sign indicating right middle lobe pneumonia. The organism is most likely to be pneumococcus, but care must be taken to consider blockage of the right middle lobe bronchus. (*Braunwald, pp. 1477–1478*)

741. (A) The cause of cat scratch fever is a tiny gram-negative bacillus, *Bartonella henselae*. Cats acquire the organism from the soil and inoculate humans via scratches or bites. The disease is generally benign and self-limited, and is treated with analgesics and antipyretics. Encephalitis, seizures, coma, meningitis, and transiverse myelitis can occasionally occur even in immunocompetent patients. A variety of antibiotics have been used when severe disease is present but an optimal regimen has not been identified. (*Braunwald, p. 1003*)

742. (A) This is a typical case of measles. The Koplik's spots in the mouth are easily missed with poor illumination. Pneumonia is an infrequent complication but accounts for many measles deaths. Giant cell pneumonia is also seen, most commonly in children suffering with a severe disease such as leukemia or immunodeficiency. Aerosolized ribavirin has been used to treat severe pneumonia secondary to measles, but its efficacy is still unclear. The other potentially lethal complication of measles is encephalitis. *(Braunwald, p. 1143)*

743. **(E)** About half of all early-onset (< 60 days after surgery) prosthetic endocarditis is caused by staphylococcal infection, with *S. epidermidis* predominating. Early-onset prosthetic endocarditis is generally the result of intraoperative contamination of the prosthesis or a bacteremic postoperative complication. *(Braunwald, pp. 809–810)*

744. **(D)** *Staphylococcus* is the most common bacterial invader in pulmonary complications of influenza. Pneumonia is the leading cause of death and may also be due to *S. pneumoniae* and *H. influenzae*. Mixed viral and bacterial pneumonia is common; pure viral pneumonia in influenza is uncommon (but can be very severe). *(Braunwald, pp. 1128–1129)*

745. **(A)** Enteroviruses are not a prominent cause of gastroenteritis. They received their name because they multiply in the GI tract. Fever, sometimes associated with respiratory symptoms, is the most common sequela of enterovirus infection. There are about 70 enteroviruses that affect humans. These include polioviruses, coxsackieviruses, echoviruses, and others. The spectrum of disease includes paralytic disease, encephalitis, aseptic meningitis, pleurodynia, exanthems, pericarditis, myocarditis, and nonspecific febrile illnesses. They can on occasion cause fulminant disease in the newborn. The most important enteroviruses are the three poliovirus serotypes. *(Braunwald, p. 1139)*

746. **(A)** The incubation period of *C. botulinum* toxin is 18 to 36 hours but ranges from a few hours to days. There are no sensory symptoms. Foodborne botulinum is associated primarily with home-canned food. Severe foodborne botulinum can produce diplopia, dysarthria, and dysphagia; weakness then can progress rapidly to involve the neck, arms, thorax, and legs. There is usually no fever. Nausea, vomiting, and abdominal pain can precede the paralysis or come afterward. *(Braunwald, p. 921)*

747. **(D)** Heterophil antibody-negative mononucleosis syndrome is the most common manifestation of CMV infection in immunocompetent adults and is more common than the similar syndrome caused by toxoplasmosis. As of yet, no syndromes caused by HHV-7 have been identified in adults. *(Braunwald, p. 1113)*

748. **(E)** Coccidioidomycosis is the usual cause of pulmonary cavitation resulting from fungal infection. A rarefaction may be demonstrable in a pneumonic lesion within 10 days of onset. In the United States, most cases are acquired in California, Arizona, and western Texas. *(Braunwald, pp. 1172–1173)*

749. **(C)** In addition to otitis media—the most common complication of measles—other complications include mastoiditis, pneumonia, bronchitis, encephalitis, and lymphadenitis. The otitis media is usually a bacterial superinfection, and should be treated with antibiotics. *(Braunwald, p. 1143)*

750. **(D)** Subacute sclerosing panencephalitis causes involuntary spasmodic movements and progressive mental deterioration, frequently ending in death within a year. It usually occurs in children whose measles occurred at an early age (≤ 2 years). It occurs 6 to 8 years after the primary infection. It presents with nonspecific symptoms such as poor school performance or mood and personality changes. It then progresses to intellectual decline, seizures, myoclonus, ataxia, and visual disturbances. Continued deterioration results in inevitable death. *(Braunwald, p. 1140)*

751. **(A)** Rubella vaccination is usually given to children combined with measles and mumps vaccine between 12 and 15 months of age, and then repeated during childhood. It is given even to children with HIV infection. *(Braunwald, p. 1147)*

752. **(C)** Donovanosis or granuloma inguinale is a mildly contagious, chronic, indolent disease that can be sexually transmitted. *Calymmatobacterium granulomatis*, a gram-negative intra-

cellular bacterium, is felt to be the cause. It is endemic in many tropical areas. Daily doxycycline or weekly azithromycin until the lesions are healed are the usual treatments. Erythromycin is used in pregnant patients. *(Braunwald, pp. 1004–1005)*

753. (C) The patient is infected with *Pneumocystis* organisms invading an immunocompromised host. The treatment of choice is trimethoprim–sulfamethoxazole. Alternate therapies include pentamidine (highly toxic) and trimetrexate plus folinic acid. *(Braunwald, p. 1184)*

754. (A) Staphylococcal enterotoxin food poisoning is characterized by violent gastrointestinal (GI) upset with severe nausea, cramps, vomiting, and diarrhea. It occurs very rapidly after ingestion (1 to 6 hours) and usually resolves by 12 hours. *(Braunwald, p. 837)*

755. (C) The patient has tinea capitis, which may be caused by *Trichophyton* or *Microsporum* species. It may be successfully treated with topical Azole drugs (eg, clotrimazole). More severe infections are usually treated with systemic medications. *(Braunwald, p. 1180)*

756. (C) Coxsackie A viruses may cause a number of syndromes, including herpangina, exanthem, aseptic meningitis, common cold, paralysis, pneumonitis, and summer febrile illness. Basophilia in the blood is not seen. *(Braunwald, pp. 1141–1142)*

757. (E) Rabies is transmitted through the saliva of infected animals. Once clinical signs develop, the disease is almost 100% fatal. Symptoms of rabies may include apathy as well as hyperexcitability. Polymerase chain reaction for detection of viral material is another method of confirming the diagnosis. *(Braunwald, pp. 1149–1150)*

758. (C) EBV genetic material has been found in association with many malignancies. In Africa, about 90% of patients with Burkitt's lymphoma have an association with EBV, but in the United States, only 15% of cases are associated with EBV. In contrast, almost all

cases of anaplastic nasopharyngeal carcinoma and also HIV-related central nervous system (CNS) lymphomas are associated with EBV genetic material. *(Braunwald, p. 1110)*

759. (B) Coccidioidomycosis may present with a syndrome of erythema nodosum, fever, and conjunctivitis. Serious complications include cavitating lung lesions or meningitis. *(Braunwald, p. 1172)*

760. (D) Cytomegalovirus is probably transmitted in the leukocyte component of transfusions. The syndromes include fever and lymphocytosis. Screening donors for this virus reduces the incidence of transmission. *(Braunwald, p. 1113)*

761. (A) Toxic shock syndrome is most characteristically seen in females using vaginal tampons and is secondary to staphylococcal enterotoxins. Abrupt onset is characteristic. The clinical criteria for diagnosis include high fever, a diffuse rash that desquamates on the palms and soles over the subsequent 1 to 2 weeks, hypotension, and involvement in three or more organ systems. This involvement can include GI dysfunction (vomiting and diarrhea), renal insufficiency, hepatic insufficiency, thrombocytopenia, myalgias with elevated creatine kinase (CK) levels, and delirium. *(Braunwald, pp. 891–892)*

762. (A) Several antibiotic combinations could be used and may vary with the indigenous organisms. An aminoglycoside and a cephalosporin are commonly used in combination. The antibiotic combination must cover both gram-positive and gram-negative organisms. *(Braunwald, pp. 552–553)*

763. (A) Mixed infections are very common, and many anaerobes may grow on culture. Aerobic gram-negative rods are also frequently grown. *(Braunwald, p. 1013)*

764. (D) Legionnaire's disease is transmitted via infectious aerosols and may cause severe disease characterized by dry cough and fevers. Mild infections and asymptomatic seroconversion also occur. Natural reservoirs for the organisms include streams, hot springs, and stagnant lakes. Amplifiers are manmade water supplies that favor growth of *legionellae.* Common amplifiers are hot water systems and heat-exchange units. *(Braunwald, pp. 945–949)*

765. **(E)** Figure 10–2 illustrates Hutchinson's teeth, which is a manifestation of late congenital syphilis. This may be associated with cardiovascular and neurologic manifestations as well as "saddle nose" and "saber shins." *(Braunwald, pp. 1048–1049)*

766. **(B)** As many as 80% of patients with SBP will present with fever. Pre-existing ascites is almost always present, but only 10% of cirrhotics at most will develop SBP. The microbiology is characteristically that of a single organism (*E. coli* most commonly). Polymicrobial infection should suggest the possibility of peritonitis secondary to a perforation. More than 300 PMNs per microliter of ascitic fluid is said to be diagnostic. *(Braunwald, pp. 829–830)*

767. **(C)** Lyme disease is caused by the spirochete *Borrelia burgdorferi,* a fastidious microaerophilic bacterium. It is a tick-transmitted disease but is not caused by the tick. The incubation period is 3 to 32 days and is associated, initially, with minimal immune response. Perhaps as many as 25% of patients lack the characteristic skin lesion. *(Braunwald, p. 1061)*

768. **(C)** Infectious mononucleosis is an acute, self-limited infection of the lymphatic system, probably by the Epstein–Barr virus. Typical infectious mononucleosis has an incubation period of 4 to 8 weeks. The prodrome includes malaise, anorexia, and chills, and then the classic symptoms of pharyngitis, fever, and lymphadenopathy develop. Headache is also common. *(Braunwald, p. 1109)*

769. **(D)** The presence of IgG antibodies by the indirect immunofluorescence test indicates recent or prior EBV infection. IgM antibodies indicate recent infection only. Heterophil an-

tibodies are present in 50% of children and 90 to 95% of adolescents and adults with infectious mononucleosis. Mono spot tests are the best diagnostic tools but may not turn positive until the second or third week of the illness. Specific EBV antibodies and cultures are rarely used. *(Braunwald, pp. 1110–1111)*

770. **(B)** Adequate rest is the treatment of choice, but forced bedrest is not necessary. Glucocorticoids hasten defervescence and resolution of pharyngitis but are not routinely used. Acyclovir halts oropharyngeal shedding of EBV but has minimal effect on the clinical disease. Similarly alpha-interferon and ganciclovir have antiviral efficacy but have no role to play in uncomplicated infectious mononucleosis. Antibiotics are not helpful, and ampicillin is likely to cause a pruritic maculopapular rash in most patients. *(Braunwald, p. 1111)*

771. **(C)** Splenic rupture occurs during the second or third week of the illness and can be insidious or abrupt in presentation. Surgery is required. Hemorrhage is not a usual complication of infectious mononucleosis. Over 90% of cases are benign and uncomplicated, but liver involvement is clinical in 5 to 10%. Over 85% of EBV-associated neurologic problems resolve spontaneously. Although hemorrhage does not occur, autoimmune hemolytic anemia can occur. It is usually mediated by IgM antibodies with anti-i specificity. *(Braunwald, p. 1110)*

772. **(C)** The most common cause of non-Epstein–Barr virus is CMV. It is the most common presentation of CMV in non-neonates with normal immune function. *(Braunwald, p. 1113)*

773. **(E)** Mumps is an acute, communicable infection with localized swelling of one or more salivary glands. At times, gonads, meninges, pancreas, and other organs can be involved. Up to 25% of infections are inapparent clinically. The virus is transmitted in saliva but is also found in urine, and this might be another source of transmission. *(Braunwald, pp. 1147–1148)*

774. **(B)** Pain referring to either or both lower quadrants is common when oophoritis is present. Fever usually accompanies oophoritis. Sterility is not a consequence of mumps oophoritis. *(Braunwald, p. 1148)*

775. **(D)** Acute and convalescent titres of specific IgG antibodies will confirm the diagnosis of mumps. A single test revealing a specific IgM antibody can also confirm the disease. Urine, saliva, and throat swabs will grow the mumps virus, but blood does not. Salivary amylase is elevated but is relatively nonspecific. Of course, a typical presentation during an epidemic probably does not require any confirmatory tests. Sporadic cases require more active confirmation. Other causes of parotitis requiring specific treatment include calculi, bacterial infections, and drugs. Tumors, sarcoid, tuberculosis, leukemia, Hodgkin's disease, Sjögren syndrome, and lupus erythematosus can also cause parotid enlargement. *(Braunwald, p. 1148)*

776. **(A)** Antibiotics, sulfas, steroids, and mumps convalescent sera are of no value. Mouth care, analgesics, and a bland diet are usually recommended. Glucocorticoids are usually prescribed for orchitis, although definite evidence of their effectiveness is lacking. Prevention via vaccination is the preferred strategy for mumps. *(Braunwald, p. 1148)*

777. **(C)** Orchitis occurs in about 20% of males, but is usually unilateral, thus sterility is rare. The disease is caused by a paramyxovirus and one infection confers lifelong immunity. The incubation period is 14 to 18 days. Serum amylase is elevated in most cases of mumps because of parotitis, not pancreatitis. Other complications include thyroiditis, myocarditis, and polyarthritis. *(Braunwald, p. 1148)*

778. **(E)** The time course, clinical features, and stool examination are characteristic of intestinal amebiasis. It is very common in most developing countries in the tropics and infects about 10% of the world's population. It is the third most common cause of death from parasitic disease. *(Braunwald, pp. 1199–1200)*

779. **(E)** Demonstration of hematophagous trophozoites of *E. histolytica* in stool confirms the diagnosis. The trophozoites are rapidly killed by drying, so wet mounts of stool should be examined. *(Braunwald, p. 1200)*

780. **(D)** All the sites mentioned can be involved by amebiasis, but the liver is the most common. Most travelers who develop an amebic liver abscess will do so within a few months of their return. Pleuropulmonary and pericardial involvement results from extension from the liver. *(Braunwald, p. 1200)*

781. **(B)** In adults (age > 15), *S. pneumoniae* is the single most common organism, accounting for one third to one half of all cases. This pneumococcal predominance is even more pronounced in sporadic cases. *(Braunwald, pp. 884, 2462)*

782. **(B)** The source of pneumococcal meningitis is either direct extension from middle ear and sinus infections, or via seeding from a bacteremia. In the latter circumstance, bacteremia from a pneumonia would be more likely than from infective endocarditis. *(Braunwald, p. 884)*

783. **(B)** Since the introduction of *H. influenzae* type B vaccine, *S. pneumoniae* has become the most common type of meningitis in infants and toddlers. *(Braunwald, p. 884)*

784. **(A)** In epidemics, *N. meningitidis* is usually the cause, generally serotype A (sub-Saharan Africa) or C (North America). Serotype B is more common in sporadic outbreaks. *(Braunwald, p. 927)*

785. **(D)** Although only close contacts need chemoprophylaxis, it is sometimes given more widely than recommended because of community concern. Meningococcal vaccine is effective against serotype A and C, and will prevent late secondary infection in close contacts. Ciprofloxacin or ofloxacin are alternatives to Rifampin. *(Braunwald, p. 931)*

786. **(B)** The most common cause of travelers' diarrhea worldwide is toxigenic *E. coli*. In North Africa and Southeast Asia, *Campylobac-*

ter infections predominate. Other causative organisms include *Salmonella, Shigella,* rotavirus, and the Norwalk agent. The most common parasite causing travelers' diarrhea is *G. lamblia. (Braunwald, p. 836)*

787. **(B)** Current recommendations suggest that mild diarrhea be treated with oral rehydration alone, but when enteric symptoms such as cramps are bothersome, treatment with loperamide or bismuth subsalicylate is warranted. More severe infections with severe diarrhea, severe pain, or fever should be treated with antibiotics such as fluoroquinolones or trimethoprim–sulfamethoxazole. *(Braunwald, p. 838)*

788. **(E)** Prophylactic antibiotics can prevent enteric bacterial infections, but at the cost of drug side effects and the possibility of developing an infection with a drug-resistant organism. Bismuth subsalicylate at a dosage of 2 tablets (525 mg) four times a day is safe and effective for up to 3 weeks. *(Braunwald, p. 838)*

789. **(D)** *Histoplasma capsulatum* is a dimorphic fungus with worldwide distribution. In the United States, it is particularly common in southeastern, mid-Atlantic, and Central states. It is frequently found in soil enriched by droppings of certain birds and bats. Caves are common sites of infection. Most infections are asymptomatic or mild and require no therapy. *(Braunwald, pp. 1171–1172)*

790. **(B)** Acute disseminated infection usually occurs in patients with HIV infection or other immunocompromised states, but chronic dissemination can occur in immunocompetent patients. Findings may include hepatosplenomegaly, lymphadenopathy, anemia, and Addison's disease. *(Braunwald, pp. 1171–1172)*

791. **(E)** Mediastinal fibrosis can result in superior vena cava compression. Fibrosis can also involve the pulmonary arteries, esophagus, and pulmonary veins. Only rare nonviable organisms are found on pathologic examination in such cases. The prognosis is generally poor. *(Braunwald, p. 1171)*

792. **(C)** This woman likely has native valve endocarditis, probably in the setting of a previous valvular abnormality. Streptococci cause over half the cases of native valve endocarditis in nonintravenous drug abusers. Of these, 75% are viridans streptococci. *Streptococcus bovis* is the most common nonviridans streptococcus causing endocarditis and is usually found in an older population (60 years), particularly if bowel lesions are present. Staphylococcal endocarditis is the next most common type, but it is usually associated with a more acute presentation. Enterococci cause about 6% of cases in native valve endocarditis, but fungi are rare causes. *(Braunwald, pp. 809–811)*

793. **(A)** *S. aureus* causes more than 50% of cases of native valve endocarditis in drug abusers. The onset is usually acute, and the tricuspid valve is the most commonly affected. In staphylococcal tricuspid endocarditis, septic pulmonary emboli are common. Frequently, no murmur is heard. *(Braunwald, pp. 810–811)*

794. **(D)** Although enterococcal endocarditis is much less common than streptococcal infection, it is more resistant. Therefore, until microbiological identification of the infecting organism occurs, treatment should be directed against enterococci. A typical regimen would combine ampicillin and gentamicin, although high level resistance to aminoglycosides is becoming more common. In a more acute presentation, therapy should be directed against *S. aureus. (Braunwald, pp. 814–815)*

795. **(C)** The clinical manifestations of infective endocarditis are a result of three factors: (1) direct infection in the heart, (2) septic emboli, and (3) high levels of circulating immune complexes. Glomerulonephritis, arthritis, and many of the mucocutaneous lesions are secondary to circulating immune complexes. Renal emboli cause hematuria and flank pain, but rarely impair renal function. *(Braunwald, p. 811)*

796. **(E)** Cytotoxic chemotherapy frequently results in neutropenia and subsequently gram-

negative bacillary infection. *Pseudomonas, Staphylococcus, Candida,* and *Aspergillus* infections are also common. *(Braunwald, pp. 547–553)*

797. **(D)** Selective IgA deficiency predisposes to *G. lamblia* infection, hepatitis virus, and *S. pneumoniae. H. influenzae* infection occurs, but this is not as characteristic as *Giardia. (Braunwald, pp. 765, 1227)*

798. **(I)** Defects in the alternate pathway of complement (eg, sickle-cell disease) predispose to *Salmonella* infections, as well as *S. pneumonia. (Braunwald, p. 765)*

799. **(B)** All forms of T-lymphocyte deficiency/dysfunction are characterized by candidal infections. *Candida* species can cause thrush, skin lesions, esophagitis, and cystitis. Hematogenous spread can occur and disseminate the organism widely. *(Braunwald, pp. 765, 1176)*

800. **(A)** Microbicidal defects (chronic granulomatous disease, Chédiak–Higashi disease) predispose to staphylococcal infections. *(Braunwald, pp. 370–371)*

801. **(A)** The preformed toxin of *Staphylococcus* causes nausea within 1 to 6 hours of ingestion. Ham, poultry, potato and egg salad, mayonnaise, and cream pastries are common food sources. *(Braunwald, p. 837)*

802. **(D)** Enterotoxigenic *E. coli* causes 15 to 50% of travelers' diarrhea, depending on geographic location. The incubation period is more than 16 hours, and water and many foods can be the source. *(Braunwald, pp. 836–838)*

803. **(F)** *Shigella* causes an invasive diarrhea with blood and has an incubation period of more than 16 hours. Potato and egg salad, lettuce, and raw vegetables are common food sources. *(Braunwald, p. 837)*

804. **(C)** *V. cholerae* causes profuse watery diarrhea with an incubation period of more than 16 hours. Shellfish are a common source. *(Braunwald, p. 837)*

805. **(H)** *B. cereus* causes an early onset of food poisoning when found in fried rice. This occurs within 1 to 6 hours and, like staphylococcal food poisoning, is characterized by vomiting. The enteric form of *B. cereus* food poisoning is characterized by watery diarrhea and occurs 8 to 16 hours after ingestion of contaminated food such as meat, vegetables, dried beans, or cereals. *(Braunwald, p. 837)*

806. **(D)** The location of infection, the possibility of tick exposure, and the nonspecific nature of the presentation are consistent with a rickettsial infection, likely Rocky Mountain spotted fever. *(Braunwald, p. 1065)*

807. **(D)** Rocky Mountain spotted fever (RMSF) is the most severe of the rickettsial diseases and has been documented in 48 American states, Canada, and parts of Central and South America. The specific tick that is the vector for this rickettsial disease varies in the different geographical locations. *(Braunwald, p. 1065)*

808. **(A)** The pulmonary and systemic microcirculation are the primary targets of the disease. The resultant damage results in increased vascular permeability. This can cause edema, decreased plasma volume, decreased albumin, prerenal azotemia, and even hypotension. Involvement of the pulmonary microcirculation can result in noncardiogenic pulmonary edema. *(Braunwald, p. 1066)*

809. **(D)** Although all these can be manifestations of RMSF, encephalitis as manifested by confusion or lethargy is by far the most common CNS manifestation. It occurs in about one quarter of cases, and can progress to coma. *(Braunwald, p. 1066)*

810. **(E)** Doxycycline is the treatment of choice, with tetracycline as second choice. There is insufficient evidence to determine the exact role of fluoroquinolones in RMSF. Beta-lactam antibiotics, erythromycin, and aminoglycosides are of no value. Sulfa-containing drugs may actually exacerbate the condition. Glucocorticoids have not been shown to be helpful, but meticulous control of volume status is important. *(Braunwald, p. 1067)*

811. **(B)** The diagnosis is usually by proximal to distal "milking of the urethra" and showing evidence of a purulent or mucopurulent discharge. Other methods include examining a urethral swab or the sediment from the first 20 to 30 mL of voided urine (after the patient has not voided for several hours). Dysuria without inflammation may represent a functional problem and usually does not benefit from antibiotics. *(Braunwald, p. 841)*

812. **(B)** *C. trachomatis* causes 30 to 40% of cases in the United States. The exact prevalence depends on the effectiveness of *Chlamydial* control programs in the population. The other organisms can all cause urethritis in men. *(Braunwald, p. 840)*

813. **(E)** Even though gram stain is negative for *N. gonorrhoeae*, the test is only 50% sensitive and treatment should include coverage for both *Chlamydial* infection (with azithromycin) and *N. gonorrhoeae* infection. There are numerous alternatives for *N. gonorrhoeae* infection, such as oral cefixime, oral ciprofloxacin, or IM ceftriaxone. However, resistance to penicillin is too common to allow the routine use of this drug. *(Braunwald, pp. 841, 936)*

814. **(A)** HSV and *Candida albicans* are the common causes of vulvar infection. Although they can cause dysuria, it is of the "external" variety (ie, secondary to urine passing over the inflamed vulvar area). The other infections cause "internal dysuria" and/or vaginal discharge. *(Braunwald, p. 842)*

815. **(D)** There is no need to investigate or treat an asymptomatic male partner. If candidal dermatitis of the penis is present, topical azole therapy would be appropriate. *(Braunwald, pp. 840–843)*

816. **(D)** There is a definite midwinter spike in bacteremia in adults, but not in children. Invasive disease is highest in children under 2

years of age. Bacteremia is more common in certain groups (eg, Native Americans, Native Alaskans, African Americans), suggesting a genetic predisposition. Up to 40% of healthy children and 10% of healthy adults are asymptomatic carriers. In adults, the organism can persist in the nasopharynx for up to 6 months. *(Braunwald, p. 882)*

817. **(C)** The most specific immunological defense is directed at capsular antigens and is serotype specific. Antibodies are not naturally occurring, but are the result of prior colonization, infection, or vaccination. *(Braunwald, p. 883)*

818. **(B)** Infections of the middle ear, trachea, sinuses, bronchi, and lungs are caused by direct spread from nasopharyngeal colonization. Disease of the CNS, heart valves, bones, joints, and peritoneal are usually caused by hematogenous dissemination. *(Braunwald, pp. 883–884)*

819. **(B)** It is possible that such outbreaks can occur in people with no predisposing factors, unlike the vast majority of sporadic cases. However, the only common predisposing factor in a young healthy population such as this would be a previous viral respiratory infection. *(Braunwald, p. 884)*

820. **(B)** Approximately 2% of cases of pneumococcal pneumonia are complicated by empyema. However, not all pleural effusions in the setting of pneumococcal pneumonia represent pleural infection. Frank pus, a positive gram stain, or a pH $\leq$ 7.1 on thoracentesis suggest empyema and the need for aggressive drainage. *(Braunwald, p. 886)*

821. **(C)** The most common presentation is with cough and headache. Both can be quite severe. Cough becomes more prominent if a lower respiratory tract infection ensues, but sputum production is not usually prominent. Shaking chills and pleuritic chest pain are quite uncommon. *(Braunwald, p. 1073)*

822. **(B)** Although all the skin problems listed have been described with *M. pneumoniae* in-

fection, the only clearly linked entity is erythema multiforme. *(Braunwald, p. 1073)*

823. **(D)** Sulfonamides and trimethoprim competitively inhibit enzymes involved in folic acid biosynthesis. *(Braunwald, p. 870)*

824. **(E)** Ciprofloxacin, rifampin, and metronidazole inhibit DNA synthesis, albeit by different mechanisms. *(Braunwald, pp. 870–871)*

825. **(A)** Beta-lactams can be inactivated by beta-lactamase. *(Braunwald, p. 871)*

826. **(C)** Macrolides (clarithromycin, azithromycin, erythromycin), lincosamides (clindamycin), and chloramphenicol inhibit protein synthesis by binding to the 50S ribosomal subunit. Tetracyclines and aminoglycosides inhibit protein synthesis by binding to the 30S ribosomal subunit. *(Braunwald, pp. 869–870)*

827. **(E)** Some gram-negative bacteria acquire mutations in their outer-membrane pori, so they are no longer permeable to ciprofloxacin. Some gram-positive bacteria develop a mutation that allows them to actively pump the drug out. The most common form of resistance, however, is a mutation in the DNA gyrase, which is the target of ciprofloxacin action. *(Braunwald, p. 872)*

828. **(F)** Rifampin is an excellent inducer of many cytochrome P$_{450}$ enzymes and increases the hepatic clearance of a number of drugs, including oral contraceptives. *(Braunwald, p. 880)*

829. **(D)** Sulfonamides potentiate the effects of oral hypoglycemics through reduction in metabolism or displacement from serum protein. *(Braunwald, p. 880)*

830. **(E)** Metronidazole can cause a disulfiram-like syndrome when alcohol is ingested. Instructions to avoid alcohol should be given when this drug is prescribed. *(Braunwald, p. 880)*

831. **(F)** Rifampin's enzyme-induction properties can result in increased metabolism of cy-

closporine, with resultant organ rejection. In contrast, erythromycin inhibits the enzyme involved in cyclosporine metabolism and can result in enhanced toxicity. *(Braunwald, p. 880)*

832. **(D)** Sulfonamides may potentiate the effects of phenytoin through reduction in metabolism or displacement from serum protein. *(Braunwald, p. 880)*

833. **(C)** In histoplasmosis, oropharyngeal ulcerations begin as solitary indurated plaques with no pain present at first, although eventually pain becomes deep seated. These oropharyngeal manifestations are usually part of disseminated infection. *(Braunwald, p. 1171)*

834. **(B)** In coccidioidomycosis, hemoptysis may call attention to cavitations, or patients may complain of pain at the cavity site. Only half of the patients with a thin-wall pulmonary cavity secondary to coccidioidomycosis will have symptoms, however. *(Braunwald, p. 1172)*

835. **(G)** The intracutaneous tuberculin test with purified protein derivative (PPD) is read for evidence of delayed hypersensitivity at 48 hours. Although induration greater than 10 mm is felt to be positive, interpretation is really dependent on the population being studied. In an HIV-infected patient, any reaction should be considered significant. When testing household contacts, greater than 5 mm is probably enough to warrant prophylactic treatment. *(Braunwald, p. 1030)*

836. **(A)** In the United States, brucellosis is rare and found most commonly among farmers, meat-processing workers, and veterinarians. Transmission is by contact of *Brucella* organisms with abraded skin, through the conjunctiva, or by inhalation. Person-to-person transmission is rare or nonexistent. The disease can be acute, localized, or chronic. It requires prolonged antibiotic treatment. A typical treatment course would be doxycycline plus an aminoglycoside for 4 weeks followed by a further 4 weeks of doxycycline and rifampin. *(Braunwald, pp. 986–989)*

837. **(H)** Tularemia can be acquired through direct contact with an infected rabbit, which may occur in preparation or cooking inadequately. The incubation period is 2 to 5 days, and the syndrome includes fevers, chills, headaches, myalgias, and tender hepatosplenomegaly. In addition, specific syndromes such as ulceroglandular or oculoglandular tularemia can accompany the nonspecific syndrome. *(Braunwald, pp. 990–993)*

838. **(C)** On darkfield examination, *T. pallidum* (the spirochete that causes syphilis) is a thin, delicate organism with tapering ends and 6 to 14 spirals. When darkfield examination is not possible, direct fluorescent antibody tests are used. *(Braunwald, p. 1049)*

839. **(A)** Congenital toxoplasmosis is initiated in utero usually as a complication of a primary infection. Infants may be asymptomatic at birth but later can present with a multitude of signs and symptoms, including chorioretinitis, strabismus, epilepsy, and psychomotor retardation. The presence of hydrocephalus is a bad prognostic sign. *(Braunwald, pp. 1222–1226)*

840. **(G)** Salmonellosis is an acute infection resulting from ingestion of food containing bacteria and is characterized by abdominal pain and diarrhea. *Salmonella* gastroenteritis is not usually treated with antibiotics because the length of the illness is not shortened, but the length of time the organism is carried is increased. Antibiotics are used for more serious systemic *Salmonella* infections. *(Braunwald, p. 973)*

841. **(F)** Preventive measures are not used because smallpox is thought to be eradicated worldwide, and vaccination may be associated with serious side effects. As humans are the only reservoir for smallpox, there is no longer any risk of infection from natural sources. However, smallpox could be used in bioterrorism. *(Braunwald, pp. 763, 1115)*

842. **(B)** Patients with tetanus develop hypertonus, seizures, respiratory distress, and asphyxia unless they are treated with muscle relaxants. The treatment of tetanus requires muscle relaxants, antitoxin, respiratory care, and managing autonomic dysfunction. Antibiotics are given but are probably of little help. *(Braunwald, p. 919)*

CHAPTER 11

Immunology and Allergy
Questions

DIRECTIONS (Questions 843 through 862): Each of the numbered items or incomplete statements in this section is followed by answers or by completions of the statement. Select the ONE lettered answer or completion that is BEST in each case.

843. A 29-year-old woman is being treated with penicillin for "strep throat." She develops arthralgia, lymphadenopathy, urticaria, and an active urine sediment. This reaction is likely secondary to

   (A) immunoglobulin E (IgE) release
   (B) mast cell degranulation
   (C) immediate-type hypersensitivity
   (D) macrophage–endothelial cell interaction
   (E) circulating immune complexes

844. The body's major immunologic defense against histoplasmosis is mediated by

   (A) IgG antibodies
   (B) mononuclear leukocytes
   (C) complement
   (D) IgM antibody
   (E) neutrophils

845. Large, granular lymphoid cells that are mediators of antibody-dependent cellular cytotoxicity are known as

   (A) macrophages
   (B) natural killer (NK) cells
   (C) T lymphocytes, suppressor subset
   (D) B lymphocytes
   (E) granulocytes

846. A 9-year-old boy is diagnosed with hay fever. Which of the following statements about hay fever is correct?

   (A) Sufferers may develop asthma.
   (B) Symptoms are not improved by moving to different locations.
   (C) Sufferers are less prone to develop upper respiratory infections (URIs).
   (D) Sufferers are severely disturbed emotionally.
   (E) Hay fever can be improved symptomatically only with steroids.

847. A 19-year-old man has recurrent attacks of gastrointestinal colic and swelling of his face and legs. His father has a similar syndrome. Death in this disease is likely to result from

   (A) an unrelated condition
   (B) an anaphylactic shock reaction
   (C) edema of the glottis
   (D) overtreatment
   (E) a reaction

848. The peripheral blood cell counts in acquired immune deficiency syndrome (AIDS) are best characterized by

   (A) granulocytosis
   (B) lymphopenia
   (C) increased helper T cells
   (D) monocytosis
   (E) decreased NK cells

849. A 30-year-old woman with myasthenia gravis is found to have an autoimmune hemolytic anemia. Chest x-ray (CXR) reveals an anterior mediastinal mass. The most likely diagnosis is

(A) thymoma
(B) nodular sclerosing Hodgkin's disease
(C) small cleaved cell non-Hodgkin's lymphoma
(D) teratoma
(E) bronchogenic carcinoma, small cell undifferentiated type

850. Autoantibodies to basement membranes have been well demonstrated to play a role in the pathogenesis of

(A) thyroiditis
(B) myasthenia gravis
(C) Goodpasture syndrome
(D) thrombocytopenia
(E) hemolytic anemia

851. Antigen–antibody complex disease may play a part in the pathogenesis of renal disease in which of the following?

(A) acute tubular necrosis (ATN)
(B) Wegener's granulomatosis
(C) bacterial endocarditis
(D) hemolytic uremic syndrome (HUS)
(E) Goodpasture syndrome

852. A 25-year-old woman has been getting desensitization shots for an allergy for 1 year. Today, she developed diffuse urticaria 5 minutes after the injection. Proper therapy would include

(A) discontinuation of subsequent injections for 3 weeks
(B) application of a tourniquet distal to the injection site
(C) administration of steroids prior to the next injection
(D) administration of aminophylline subcutaneously
(E) administration of epinephrine (1:1000) subcutaneously

853. A 23-year-old man treated for strep throat with penicillin develops arthralgia, urticaria, and lymphadenopathy. Urinalysis reveals red cell casts. Which of the following is characteristic of the syndrome?

(A) It usually requires corticosteroids.
(B) Symptoms last several months.
(C) It may recur after apparent recovery.
(D) It may be transferred by leukocyte infusions.
(E) Most patients are children.

854. In a 22-year-old woman with suspected immunodeficiency secondary to impaired T-cell function, the most cost-effective screening test is

(A) quantification of serum IgA
(B) lymphocyte enumeration on a cell sorter
(C) lymphocyte responses to mitogens
(D) nitroblue tetrazolium assay
(E) intradermal skin test with *Candida albicans* extract

855. A 19-year-old female university student unwittingly eats shrimp in the dormitory dining room. Over the next 20 minutes, acute skin lesions consisting of erythematous, elevated wheals appear. These lesions

(A) are most common on the palms and soles
(B) are rarely itchy
(C) do not blanch on pressure
(D) are caused by a localized vasculitis
(E) are caused by an ongoing, immediate, hypersensitivity reaction

856. A 27-year-old man develops small (several mm) pruritic wheals when he goes jogging and when he takes very hot showers. Management will include

(A) discontinuation of all vigorous exercises
(B) counseling regarding recognition and treatment of anaphylactic reactions
(C) treatment with anticholinergic medications

(D) treatment with hydroxyzine

(E) cool baths rather than hot showers

857. A 42-year-old man develops angioedema after drug exposure. This syndrome is characterized by

(A) invariably severe itching

(B) prolonged nature of the edema

(C) fluid extravasation from subcutaneous and intradermal postcapillary venules

(D) involvement of lips, tongue, eyelids, genitalia, and dorsum of hands or feet

(E) fluid accumulation in the most dependent areas of the body

858. A 47-year-old woman with type 1 diabetes of 30 years' duration is in the hospital for assessment of atypical chest pain. While in the hospital she develops a true anaphylactic reaction. The most likely cause is

(A) radiographic contrast media

(B) erythromycin

(C) insulin

(D) folic acid supplement

(E) nuts

859. A 27-year-old long-time intravenous (IV) drug user has recurrent infections and a low CD4⁺ count. Which factor is true concerning this immunosuppression?

(A) Qualitative defects in T lymphocytes follow quantitative problems.

(B) The low CD4 count in advanced disease is secondary to the direct cytotoxic effects of virus infection.

(C) B-lymphocyte abnormalities do not occur early in the disease.

(D) Macrophages are important in viral dissemination.

(E) Circulating immune complexes are rarely present.

860. A 24-year-old man with known human immunodeficiency (HIV) infection presents with a left hemiparesis that developed over several days. Cognitive exam reveals global impairment and computed tomography (CT) scan reveals multiple cortical lesions that are spherical and ring enhancing. The likely diagnosis is

(A) glioblastoma multiforme

(B) toxoplasmosis

(C) lymphoma

(D) progressive multifocal leukoencephalopathy

(E) cytomegalovirus (CMV)

Questions 861 and 862

A 23-year-old woman has had several episodes of severe wheezing over several years. She is a nonsmoker and feels well inbetween episodes. The wheezing episodes are most likely to occur in the spring.

861. The major underlying factor in this woman is

(A) elevated IgE levels

(B) mast cell instability

(C) nonspecific hyperirritability of the tracheobronchial tree

(D) disordered immediate hypersensitivity

(E) disordered delayed hypersensitivity

862. The food most likely to precipitate an asthmatic reaction in this woman is

(A) red meat

(B) egg whites

(C) green salad

(D) gluten

(E) mayonnaise

DIRECTIONS (Questions 863 through 878): Each set of matching questions in this section consists of a list of lettered options followed by several numbered items. For each numbered item, select the appropriate lettered option(s). Each lettered option may be selected once, more than once, or not at all. EACH ITEM WILL STATE THE NUMBER OF OPTIONS TO SELECT. CHOOSE EXACTLY THIS NUMBER.

Questions 863 through 865

- (A) a true allergic reaction
- (B) may be mediated by drug effect on kinin system
- (C) skin rash is most likely manifestitation
- (D) predictive skin test available
- (E) final mediator of symptoms are leukotrienes
- (F) desensitization is feasible
- (G) may be more common in women and blacks
- (H) never fatal

863. A 23-year-old man has a reaction after being given oral penicillin for a sore throat (SELECT FOUR)

864. A 56-year-old woman is given an angiotensin-converting enzyme (ACE) inhibitor for control of hypertension and develops a reaction (SELECT TWO)

865. A 23-year-old man has an exacerbation of asthma when he takes aspirin for a headache (SELECT TWO)

Questions 866 through 872

Match the following diseases with the appropriate human lymphocyte antigen (HLA).

- (A) HLA B27
- (B) HLA DR4
- (C) HLA DR3
- (D) HLA B17
- (E) HLA B8

866. A 29-year-old man with severe back pain and a red eye (SELECT ONE)

867. A 24-year-old woman with skin lesions, thrombocytopenia, arthralgia, and pericarditis (SELECT ONE)

868. A 12-year-old child with deforming arthritis (SELECT ONE)

869. A 14-year-old girl with sudden onset of hyperglycemia (SELECT ONE)

870. A 22-year-old man with iritis, balanitis, urethritis, and arthritis (SELECT ONE)

871. A 27-year-old woman with severe symmetrical small joint arthritis (SELECT ONE)

872. A 33-year-old policeman who develops arthritis with a diarrheal illness (SELECT ONE)

Questions 873 through 878

- (A) B-cell deficiency/dysfunction
- (B) mixed T- and B-cell deficiency/dysfunction
- (C) T-lymphocyte deficiency/dysfunction
- (D) neutropenia
- (E) chemotaxis
- (F) C3 (complement 3) deficiency

873. A 73-year-old man with an IgG spike (SELECT ONE)

874. A 22-year-old woman with Hodgkin's disease (SELECT ONE)

875. A 73-year-old man with 30,000 mature lymphocytes on his blood film (SELECT ONE)

876. A 24-year-old woman with malar rash, thrombocytopenia, and arthralgia (SELECT ONE)

877. A 69-year-old man receiving chemotherapy for acute leukemia (SELECT ONE)

878. A young woman with ataxia–telangiectasia (SELECT ONE)

Answers and Explanations

843. **(E)** Drug hypersensitivity is the most common cause of serum sickness. It is believed that the drug acts as a hapten binding to a plasma protein. The resultant drug-protein complex induces an immune response. Common signs and symptoms include fever, skin rash (urticarial or morbilliform), arthralgias, lymphadenopathy, and albuminuria. Arthritis, nephritis, neuropathy, and vasculitis are less common. Primary sensitization requires 1 to 3 weeks, but symptoms can occur rapidly on re-exposure. *(Braunwald, p. 437)*

844. **(B)** The major reaction to fungal infections such as histoplasmosis is delayed-type hypersensitivity. This is a reaction of T cells, which have been stimulated by antigen to react against infectious agents, grafts, and tumors. A classic example is the response to the tuberculin skin test in a person previously exposed to *Mycobacterium tuberculosis* organisms which occurs between 48 to 72 hours after antigen exposure. *(Braunwald, pp. 1827–1828)*

845. **(B)** NK cells may be of T-cell lineage or monocyte–macrophage lineage. They appear to play an important role in surveillance mechanisms. *(Braunwald, pp. 1809–1811)*

846. **(A)** Allergic asthma is often associated with a personal and/or family history of allergic diseases. It is dependent on an IgE response controlled by T and B lymphocytes and activated when antigens interact with mast cell-bound IgE molecules. Most provoking allergens are airborne. Allergic asthma can be seasonal. *(Braunwald, pp. 1456–1459)*

847. **(C)** Hereditary angioedema is an autosomal dominant condition. The lesions are tense, rounded, nonpitting, and several centimeters in diameter. The edema, unlike urticaria, involves deeper tissue and is not pruritic. Edema of the glottis is the usual cause of death. *(Braunwald, pp. 1917–1918)*

848. **(B)** AIDS is characterized by lymphopenia, with a selective diminution of helper T cells. Likely infectious complications and their appropriate prophylaxis can be predicted by the CD4 T-lymphocyte count. Lymphocyte dysfunction can occur even when severe lymphopenia is not yet present. *(Braunwald, p. 1871)*

849. **(A)** Thymic tumors may be associated with myasthenia gravis, red cell aplasia, polymyositis, hemolytic anemia, pemphigus, and agranulocytosis. There is also an association with immunodeficiency and thymoma. These patients have B-lymphocyte deficiency and have bacterial infections and diarrhea. Erythroid aplasia may develop as well. *(Braunwald, pp. 1850, 2518)*

850. **(C)** Autoantibodies can be demonstrated by immunofluorescence or electron microscopy on the basement membranes of glomeruli and alveoli in Goodpasture syndrome. The disease is most common in young men but can strike at any age. The hemoptysis can be minimal or massive. The course of the hemoptysis is variable, but renal involvement is often progressive. Current therapy includes intensive plasma exchange, cytotoxic agents, and glucocorticoids. Other causes of lung–renal syndromes such as various vasculitides, Wegener's granulomatosis, mixed essential cryoglobulinemia, Henoch–Schönlein purpura, and systemic lupus erythematosus (SLE) are not characterized by antibodies to basement membranes. *(Braunwald, p. 1583)*

851. **(C)** Immune complexes are not detected in ATN, Wegener's, HUS, or Goodpasture syndrome. Immune complexes with low complement levels can be seen in idiopathic and postinfectious glomerulonephritis, lupus, cryoglobulinemia, shunt nephritis, and bacterial endocarditis. Immune complexes with normal complement levels are found in IgA nephropathy, and Henoch–Schönlein purpura. *(Braunwald, p. 1582)*

852. **(E)** These systemic reactions are uncommon and easily managed in the office if detected, but if the patient leaves too soon, it could be dangerous. The exact mechanism of benefit for hyposensitization therapy is unclear. No single measurement of immune function correlates well with clinical efficacy, suggesting a complex of effects that likely includes a reduction in T-cell cytokine production. This type of therapy is reserved for clearly seasonal diseases that cannot be adequately managed with drugs. *(Braunwald, pp. 1916, 1921)*

853. **(C)** The symptoms of serum sickness are usually self-limited and may recur after apparent recovery. The natural course is 1 to 3 weeks. Recurrence can occur rapidly (12 to 36 hours) if repeat exposure to the offending antigen occurs. *(Braunwald, pp. 437, 877)*

854. **(E)** A positive skin test with *C. albicans* extract (erythema and induration of 10 mm or more at 48 hours) excludes virtually all primary T-cell defects. Lymphocyte enumeration and responses to mitogens are much costlier tests. Serum IgA levels are a good screening test for agammaglobulinemia, and the nitroblue tetrazolium assay is useful to detect killing defects of phagocyte cells. *(Goldman, p. 1433)*

855. **(E)** Although urticaria can involve any epidermal or mucosal surface, the palms and soles are usually spared. The associated itching indicates stimulation of nociceptive nerves. The increased blood flow results in erythema that blanches on pressure. An ongoing, immediate hypersensitivity reaction in association with degranulation of mast cells is the most common cause. *(Goldman, pp. 1440–1441)*

856. **(D)** This represents a case of generalized heat urticaria or cholinergic urticaria rather than exercise-induced urticaria. The latter is characterized by larger lesions and possible anaphylactic reactions and is not triggered by hot showers. Although thought to be cholinergically mediated, atropine does not block symptoms in generalized heat urticaria. Because anaphylaxis does not occur and hydroxyzine is so effective, hot showers are not a great danger. *(Goldman, p. 1443)*

857. **(D)** Angioedema is often not itchy and, like urticaria, is transient; manifestation peaks in minutes to hours and disappears over hours to days. The fluid extravasates from deeper areas such as dermal and subdermal sites. Unlike other causes of edema, angioedema is not dependent and can involve all epidermal and submucosal surfaces, although the lips, tongue, eyelids, genitalia, hands, and feet are the most commonly involved. *(Goldman, p. 1441)*

858. **(E)** Anaphylaxis is characterized by an initial exposure followed by the formation of specific IgE antibody. Repeat exposure results in antigen combining with IgE bound to basophils and mast cells and subsequent degranulation. Anaphylactoid reactions, such as those to radiographic contrast media, are generally not immune mediated and do not require prior exposure. Insulin and folic acid rarely cause anaphylaxis. Similarly, erythromycin is not a common antibiotic to cause anaphylaxis. Nuts, eggs, seafood, and chocolate are among the many foods implicated in anaphylaxis. *(Goldman, pp. 1450–1451)*

859. **(D)** Even in advanced AIDS, only a minority of CD4+ lymphocytes are actually infected. Numerous other factors, including "innocent bystander destruction" and autoimmune phenomena, might be implicated. Impaired soluble antigen recognition by T lymphocytes can occur when absolute counts are still normal. Polyclonal activation of B cells, which occurs early in the disease, is unlikely to be triggered by direct HIV infection of B cells. Macrophages are felt to be particularly important in carrying the virus across the blood–brain barrier. Circulating immune complexes might help explain arthralgias, myalgias, renal disease, and vasculitis that occurs in infected individuals. (*Goldman, pp. 1890–1891*)

860. **(B)** The three most common causes of focal brain lesion in HIV disease are toxoplasmosis, primary central nervous system (CNS) lymphoma and progressive multifocal leukoencephalopathy (PML). Toxoplasmosis lesions are typically multiple, spherical, and ring-enhancing on CT scan. They are most likely located in the basal ganglia and the cortex. The symptoms develop characteristically over days and global brain dysfunction is common. Lymphoma presents with one or relatively few irregular, weakly enhancing lesions more commonly in the periventricular area. PML presents with multiple nonenhancing lesions in the white matter. CMV, herpes, and *Cryptococcus* generally cause diffuse brain disease. Glioblastoma multiforme is not characteristic of HIV disease. (*Goldman, pp. 1909–1910*)

861. **(C)** There is a constant state of hyperreactivity of the bronchi, during which exposure to an irritant precipitates an asthmatic attack. A following subacute phase has been described that can lead to late complications. The presence of inflammation in the airways has resulted in increased usage of inhaled corticosteroids for maintenance therapy. Many cases of asthma have no discernible allergic component. (*Braunwald, pp. 1456–1457*)

862. **(C)** Sulfites, used to keep salad greens fresh, can cause severe asthmatic reactions. Other sulfite-containing foods include fresh fruits, potatoes, shellfish, and wine. Aspirin, tartrazine (a coloring agent), and beta-adrenergic agonists also commonly provoke asthmatic attacks. (*Braunwald, p. 1458*)

863. **(A, C, D, F)** Penicillin can cause numerous allergic reactions, including anaphylaxis, interstitial nephritis, rashes (the most common manifestation), urticaria, fever, pneumonitis, dermatitis, and even asthma in workers exposed to airborne penicillin. Hemolytic anemia is often IgG mediated. Skin tests are reliable in predicting low risk (similar to general population) for those claiming previous penicillin reactions, and desensitization is feasible. The frequency of reactions to cephalosporins in penicillin-allergic patients is not definitely known. (*Goldman, p. 1465*)

864. **(B, G)** ACE inhibitors can cause angioedema of the face and oropharyngeal structures. This is felt to be a pseudoallergic reaction, possibly due to the drug's effect on the kinin system. It is thought that reactions may be more common in women, blacks, and those with idiopathic angioedema. If this occurs, therapy with alternate ACE inhibitors should not be attempted. (*Goldman, p. 1466*)

865. **(E, F)** Aspirin frequently can precipitate asthma in susceptible individuals. At highest risk are asthmatics with chronic rhinosinusitis and nasal polyps. This is probably a pseudoallergic reaction related to inhibition of cyclo-oxygenase with a resultant enhancement of leukotriene synthesis or effect. Densensitization regimens have been developed. (*Goldman, p. 1466*)

866. **(A)** Ankylosing spondylitis and HLA B27. (*Goldman, p. 1458*)

867. **(C)** SLE and HLA DR3. (*Goldman, p. 1458*)

868. **(B)** Juvenile rheumatoid arthritis and HLA DR4. (*Goldman, p. 1458*)

869. **(C)** Type 1 diabetes mellitus and HLA DR3. *(Goldman, p. 1458)*

870. **(A)** Reiter syndrome and HLA B27. *(Goldman, p. 1458)*

871. **(B)** Rheumatoid arthritis (RA) and HLA DR4. *(Goldman, p. 1458)*

872. **(A)** Reactive arthritis (eg, *Shigella* or *Yersinia*) and HLA B27. *(Goldman, pp. 1503–1504)*

The relationship between HLA antigens and diseases is not absolute, but rather one of increased relative risk. The presence of HLA B27 increases the relative risk of ankylosing spondylitis by a factor of about 80, of Reiter syndrome by a factor of 40, and also increases the likelihood of reactive arthritis. The presence of HLA DR4 increases the likelihood of juvenile RA by a factor of 7 and RA by a factor of 6. The presence of HLA DR3 increases the likelihood of both SLE and insulin-dependent diabetes mellitus by a factor of approximately 3.

873. **(A)** Multiple myeloma and B-cell deficiency/dysfunction. *(Goldman, p. 1574)*

874. **(C)** Hodgkin's disease and T-cell deficiency/dysfunction. *(Goldman, p. 1573)*

875. **(A)** Chronic lymphocytic leukemia and B-cell deficiency/dysfunction. *(Goldman, p. 1574)*

876. **(F)** SLE and complement deficiency. *(Goldman, p. 1432)*

877. **(D)** Therapy for hematologic malignancy and neutropenia. *(Goldman p. 1569)*

878. **(B)** Ataxia–telangiectasia and both T- and B-cell dysfunction. *(Goldman, p. 1574)*

Multiple myeloma and chronic lymphocytic leukemia are two of the more common causes of B-cell deficiency/dysfunction. Hodgkin's disease, AIDS, sarcoidosis, and thymic aplasia or hypoplasia result in T-lymphocyte depletion/dysfunction. SLE has been associated with C3 deficiency, but most severe complement deficiencies result from inherited disorders. Ataxia–telangiectasia, common variable hypogammaglobulinemia, severe combined immunodeficiency, and Wiskott–Aldrich syndrome have mixed T- and B-cell deficiency.

CHAPTER 12

Diseases of the Respiratory System
Questions

DIRECTIONS (Questions 879 through 930): Each of the numbered items or incomplete statements in this section is followed by answers or by completions of the statement. Select the ONE lettered answer or completion that is BEST in each case.

879. A 33-year-old farmer complains of recurrent episodes of wheezing after working in a barn where hay is stored. Which of the following is characteristic of this syndrome?

   (A) Symptoms appear a few days after exposure.
   (B) It is caused by exposure to oxides of nitrogen.
   (C) It is usually followed by complete recovery.
   (D) It usually progresses to diffuse fibrosis.
   (E) It usually progresses to diffuse obstructive emphysema.

880. Etiologic studies indicate that obstructive pulmonary emphysema is usually

   (A) caused by bronchial asthma
   (B) preceded by bronchitis
   (C) due to childhood mucoviscidosis
   (D) due to elastic tissue degeneration
   (E) a forerunner of pulmonary carcinoma

881. An agitated and nervous 24-year-old woman has had severe wheezing and shortness of breath for 2 days. She is hospitalized. Her treatment should avoid

   (A) theophylline
   (B) sedatives
   (C) corticosteroids

   (D) sympathomimetic amines
   (E) intravenous (IV) fluids

882. A 53-year-old man with a long respiratory history becomes sleepy in the hospital. A P_{CO_2} determination reveals severe hypercarbia. This syndrome

   (A) occurs only with CO_2 inhalation
   (B) does not occur in obstructive lung disease
   (C) does not occur in restrictive lung disease
   (D) may worsen with oxygen administration
   (E) occurs with chronic hypocapnia

883. A 63-year-old woman is seen in the emergency room with acute shortness of breath. A pulmonary embolism may be ruled out in the presence of a normal

   (A) chest x-ray (CXR)
   (B) electrocardiogram (ECG)
   (C) perfusion lung scan
   (D) computed tomography (CT) scan
   (E) magnetic resonance image (MRI)

Questions 884 and 885

884. A 23-year-old man has a long history of mild asthma. During a recent flare, infection was suspected and a CXR revealed pulmonary infiltrates. Blood work revealed an eosinophil count of 2000. The most likely cause is

   (A) ascaris infestation
   (B) allergic bronchopulmonary aspergillosis
   (C) Churg–Strauss allergic granulomatosis
   (D) Loeffler syndrome
   (E) hypereosinophilic syndrome

885. The treatment of this syndrome will likely require

(A) antihelminthic therapy
(B) a short course of systemic glucocorticoid therapy
(C) desensitization treatment
(D) high-dose glucocorticoids by puffer
(E) long-term systemic glucocorticoid therapy

886. A 63-year-old man has a P_{CO_2} of 60. This is indicative of

(A) ventilation–perfusion ratio inequality
(B) right-to-left shunt
(C) impaired diffusion
(D) hypoventilation
(E) carbon monoxide poisoning

887. The emphysematous type of chronic obstructive pulmonary disease (COPD) usually demonstrates

(A) copious, purulent sputum
(B) early cor pulmonale
(C) decreased total lung capacity
(D) normal or low arterial P_{CO_2}
(E) normal diffusing capacity

888. A 40-year-old man has a routine CXR, which reveals a posterior mediastinal mass. The most likely diagnosis is

(A) lipoma
(B) neurogenic tumor
(C) esophageal cyst
(D) fibroma
(E) bronchogenic cyst

889. A 35-year-old man is diagnosed with emphysema. Evaluation of his family reveals other affected individuals. This is most likely associated with

(A) alpha$_1$-antitrypsin deficiency
(B) beta-glycosidase deficiency
(C) glucose-6-phosphatase deficiency
(D) glucocerebrosides deficiency
(E) growth hormone deficiency

890. A 23-year-old man has a long history of back pain with prolonged morning stiffness. He has had an episode of iritis. The most likely pulmonary feature is

(A) fibrocavitary disease
(B) airflow obstruction
(C) bilateral lower lobe involvement
(D) pleural effusions
(E) hilar adenopathy

891. A patient with hypoxemia, hypercapnia, and polycythemia is able to restore his blood gases to normal by voluntary hyperventilation. The primary pathology is likely to be located in the

(A) cerebral cortex
(B) bone marrow
(C) ventricular septum
(D) respiratory center
(E) cerebellum

892. A diagnosis of idiosyncratic asthma is more likely with

(A) known antigenic stimulus
(B) adult onset
(C) history of atopy
(D) positive skin tests
(E) high immunoglobulin E (IgE) levels

893. A 74-year-old man with a history of smoking develops clubbing, and CXR reveals a mass. Which of the following suggests that the tumor is a small cell lung cancer?

(A) syndrome of inappropriate antidiuretic hormone (SIADH) secretion
(B) acanthosis nigricans
(C) Cushing syndrome
(D) leukemoid reaction
(E) Stevens–Johnson syndrome

894. Carbon dioxide retention is commonly seen in

(A) impaired diffusion syndromes
(B) right-to-left shunt
(C) hyperventilation

(D) ventilation–perfusion ratio inequality

(E) mechanical ventilation at fixed volume

895. A previously well 53-year-old man develops progressive shortness of breath. Pulmonary function tests reveal a restrictive defect and high-resolution CT suggests idiopathic pulmonary fibrosis (IPF). The role of transbronchial biopsy is to

(A) assess disease severity

(B) assess possible bronchiolar narrowing

(C) diagnose specific causes of IPF

(D) determine degree of inflammation

(E) diagnose possible cancer

896. Acute respiratory distress syndrome may be characterized by

(A) increased compliance

(B) responsiveness to antibiotics

(C) increased vascular permeability to proteins

(D) consolidation pattern on x-ray

(E) decreased ventilatory dead space

897. The treatment of chronic airway obstruction most likely includes

(A) long-term steroids

(B) calorie reduction

(C) intravenous aminophylline

(D) antibiotics for infection

(E) alpha-adrenergic blockage

898. Mediastinal emphysema is most likely to be caused by

(A) apical tuberculosis

(B) pericarditis

(C) alveolar rupture

(D) Hodgkin's disease

(E) aspergillosis

899. Cystic fibrosis in the adult patient is most likely to be associated with

(A) spontaneous remission

(B) good pancreatic exocrine function

(C) hemoptysis

(D) rectal polyps

(E) normal sweat chloride

900. Hypoxemia while receiving 100% oxygen indicates

(A) ventilation–perfusion ratio inequality

(B) right-to-left shunt

(C) hypoventilation

(D) impaired diffusion

(E) interstitial lung disease

901. A 50-year-old man with severe kyphoscoliosis is most likely to have

(A) enlarged overall lung volume

(B) alveolar hyperventilation

(C) left rather than right ventricular failure

(D) increased compliance

(E) recurrent pulmonary infections

902. Reduction of the ratio of forced expiratory volume to vital capacity (FEV/VC) is seen in

(A) emphysema

(B) ankylosing spondylitis

(C) pickwickian syndrome

(D) scleroderma of the chest wall

(E) lobar pneumonia

903. Which of the following statements concerning asbestosis is correct?

(A) The type of asbestos fiber is crucial in determining whether asbestos-related lung disease occurs.

(B) Moderate rather than severe obstruction to airflow is characteristic of asbestosis.

(C) Mesothelioma is the common malignancy associated with asbestosis.

(D) Pleural effusions are invariably associated with malignancy in asbestosis.

(E) Short-term (ie, 1 to 2 years) exposure can result in serious sequelae decades later.

904. Which of the following statements concerning pulmonary embolism is correct?

(A) Continuous IV heparin therapy is more effective than intermittent IV or intermittent subcutaneous therapy.

(B) The most common ECG change is that of acute pulmonary hypertension (rightward shift of the QRS axis; tall, peaked P wave)

(C) If symptoms occur, pleuritic chest pain is the most common symptom.

(D) Long delays in diagnosis and treatment of symptomatic pulmonary emboli are the major cause of death in this syndrome.

(E) It can be associated with petechiae.

905. A 50-year-old man presents with excessive daytime sleepiness and a history of snoring. He is obese and has moderate hypertension. The most common symptoms of this syndrome are

(A) related to cardiac dysfunction

(B) neuropsychiatric and behavioral

(C) pulmonary

(D) gastrointestinal (GI)

(E) musculoskeletal

906. Which of the following statements concerning hypoxemia in obstructive airways disease is correct?

(A) Erythrocytosis is an appropriate compensation for hypoxemia, and phlebotomy will worsen symptoms.

(B) Nocturnal oxygen therapy is effective in producing symptomatic and hemodynamic improvement in severe hypoxia.

(C) A PO_2 of 58 mm Hg is an indication for continuous oxygen therapy.

(D) A PO_2 of 65 mm Hg or below is an indication for supplemental oxygen during air travel.

(E) Continuous supplemental oxygen improves functional ability but does not alter the natural history of obstructive airways disease with severe hypoxemia.

907. A 58-year-old steampipe worker had a vague ache in the right chest and mild dyspnea of several months' duration. There was flatness on percussion of the right chest associated with diminished breath sounds. What is the most likely diagnosis (see Fig. 12–1)?

(A) pleural metastases

(B) Paget's disease

(C) mesothelioma and asbestosis

(D) pleural effusion

(E) multiple myeloma

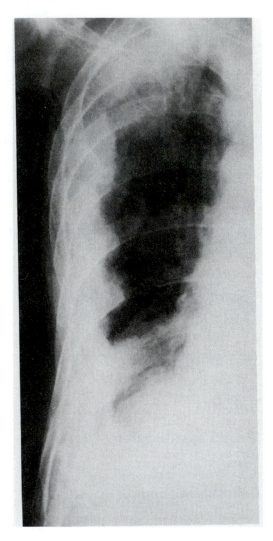

Figure 12–1.

908. Cough with blood-tinged sputum, chills, and fever of 2 days' duration brought a 24-year-old man to the hospital. Physical findings revealed dullness and moist rales in the left lower chest. What is the most likely diagnosis (see Fig. 12–2)?

(A) pneumonia, left lower lobe

(B) atelectasis, left lower lobe

(C) pulmonary embolism

(D) tuberculosis

(E) sarcoidosis

909. Figure 12–3 is a close-up view of a CXR from a 40-year-old man for an insurance checkup. What is the most likely diagnosis?

(A) hamartoma of the lung

(B) tuberculous granuloma of the left apex

(C) osteochondroma of the left fourth rib

(D) bronchogenic carcinoma

(E) pulmonary metastases

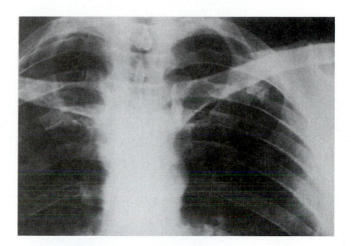

Figure 12–3.

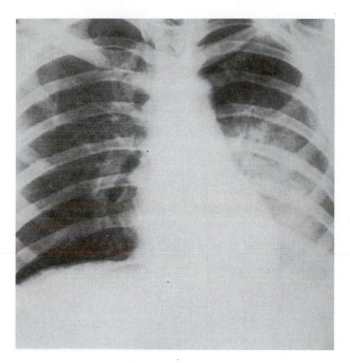

Figure 12–2.

910. A 17-year-old boy had slight tightness of the chest on heavy breathing of 2 days' duration. He had pain in the left arm, which showed a lytic lesion on x-ray. What is the most likely diagnosis (see Fig. 12–4)?

(A) eosinophilic granuloma

(B) cystic fibrosis

(C) pulmonary metastases

(D) bronchiectasis

(E) tuberculosis

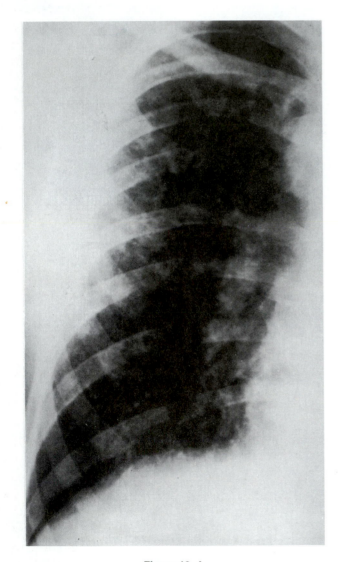

Figure 12–4.

911. The pulmonary function studies shown in Table 12–1 are of a 65-year-old man with severe dyspnea and cough. The most likely diagnosis is

(A) emphysema

(B) lobar pneumonia

(C) chronic bronchitis

(D) acute bronchitis

(E) congestive heart failure (CHF)

TABLE 12–1. PULMONARY FUNCTION STUDIES

Chronic Paco$_2$ mm Hg	35
Chronic Pao$_2$ mm Hg	70
Hematocrit %	35
Pulmonary hypertension	
Rest	None
Exercise	Moderate
Elastic recoil	Severely decreased
Resistance	Normal
Diffusing capacity	Decreased

912. A 33-year-old woman, otherwise perfectly well, presents with recurrent episodes of hemoptysis. Investigation is likely to reveal

(A) a peripheral lesion with "popcorn" calcification

(B) a benign lesion, centrally located on CXR

(C) ring shadows, tram lines, and cyst formation on the CXR

(D) significant airflow reduction on pulmonary function tests

(E) a large left atrium on CXR

Questions 913 through 916

A 34-year-old woman has been complaining of a 2-year history of increasing dyspnea and fatigue. Physical examination reveals increased jugular venous pressure and a reduced carotid pulse. Precordial examination reveals a left parasternal lift, loud P_2, and right-sided S_3 and S_4. There are no audible murmurs. CXR reveals clear lung fields and an ECG shows evidence of right ventricular hypertrophy. Pulmonary function tests show a slight restrictive pattern.

913. The most likely diagnosis is

   (A) asthma (without wheezing)
   (B) primary pulmonary hypertension
   (C) pulmonary veno-occlusive disease
   (D) pulmonary leiomyomatosis
   (E) "silent" tricuspid valve disease

914. Confirmation of the diagnosis usually requires

   (A) open lung biopsy
   (B) pulmonary angiography
   (C) cardiac catheterization
   (D) noninvasive exercise testing
   (E) electrophysiologic testing

915. The most common form of treatment is

   (A) anticoagulants
   (B) nitrates
   (C) alpha-adrenergic blockers
   (D) calcium channel blockers
   (E) angiotensin-converting enzyme (ACE) inhibitors

916. The most likely cause of death is

   (A) intractable left ventricular failure
   (B) intractable respiratory failure
   (C) massive pulmonary embolism
   (D) sudden death
   (E) myocardial infarction

Questions 917 and 918

An 83-year-old man with Parkinson's disease has had low-grade fever and cough for several weeks. A CXR reveals a probable lung abscess. The apical areas are clear.

917. The most likely bacteriologic diagnosis is

   (A) oropharyngeal flora
   (B) tuberculosis
   (C) *Staphylococcus aureus*
   (D) *Pseudomonas aeruginosa*
   (E) *Candida albicans*

918. The usual treatment regimen is

   (A) penicillin
   (B) clindamycin
   (C) ceftriaxone
   (D) penicillin plus aminoglycoside
   (E) penicillin plus metronidazole

Questions 919 and 920

A 69-year-old woman has recently returned on an overnight flight from Europe. She now complains of vague chest discomfort and shortness of breath.

919. Which is the correct statement concerning D-dimer assay done by the latex agglutination method?

   (A) It is sensitive but not specific.
   (B) It is specific but not sensitive.
   (C) It is neither specific nor sensitive.
   (D) A negative result suggests myocardial ischemia.
   (E) It is both sensitive and specific.

920. ECG reveals sinus tachycardia, and cardiac enzymes are negative. The lung scan is read as high probability. Which of the following tests is most likely to provide information that will guide therapy?

   (A) echocardiogram
   (B) CT scan
   (C) venous ultrasound of the legs
   (D) contrast phlebography
   (E) pulmonary function tests

Questions 921 through 925

A black woman presents with mild dyspnea on exertion, arthralgia, fever, and erythema nodosum. Physical examination reveals hepatosplenomegaly, generalized lymphadenopathy, and corneal opacities. CXR shows bilaterally symmetric hilar adenopathy.

921. The most likely diagnosis is

    (A) Hodgkin's disease
    (B) tuberculosis
    (C) rheumatic fever
    (D) sarcoidosis
    (E) rheumatoid arthritis (RA)

922. The most characteristic blood test is

    (A) hyperglobulinemia
    (B) elevated ACE
    (C) elevated sedimentation rate
    (D) low serum phosphorus
    (E) mild anemia

923. Which of the following laboratory tests would most likely be positive?

    (A) tuberculin test
    (B) alcohol tolerance test
    (C) latex fixation
    (D) antistreptolysin-O (ASLO) titer
    (E) Kveim test

924. The eye lesion is probably due to

    (A) uveitis
    (B) diabetic complications
    (C) steroids
    (D) congenital origin
    (E) infectious infiltration

925. This disease is best treated with

    (A) aspirin
    (B) isoniazid (INH) and streptomycin
    (C) steroids
    (D) nitrogen mustard
    (E) no therapy

Questions 926 through 930

A 30-year-old man presents with a history of recurrent pneumonias and a chronic cough productive of foul-smelling, occasionally blood-tinged, purulent sputum, which is worse in the morning and on lying down. On physical examination, the patient appears chronically ill with clubbing of the fingers. Wet inspiratory rales are heard at the lung bases posteriorly.

926. The most likely diagnosis is

    (A) bronchiectasis
    (B) chronic bronchitis
    (C) disseminated pulmonary tuberculosis
    (D) pulmonary neoplasm
    (E) chronic obstructive emphysema

927. This syndrome is most likely to be associated with

    (A) lung cancer
    (B) dextrocardia
    (C) fungal infection
    (D) carcinoid syndrome
    (E) Hodgkin's disease

928. The most likely precursor of the above condition was

    (A) bronchial asthma
    (B) endobronchial tuberculosis
    (C) pertussis
    (D) bronchopneumonia
    (E) influenza

929. The most important procedure necessary to define the extent of the disease would be

    (A) CT scan
    (B) bronchoscopy
    (C) bronchography
    (D) open thoracotomy
    (E) bronchoalveolar lavage

930. Therapy for this disease might include

    (A) antibiotics and postural drainage
    (B) steroids
    (C) radiotherapy

(D) aerosols

(E) INH

DIRECTIONS (Questions 931 through 940): Each set of matching questions in this section consists of a list of lettered options followed by several numbered items. For each numbered item, select the appropriate lettered option(s). Each lettered option may be selected once, more than once, or not at all. EACH ITEM WILL STATE THE NUMBER OF OPTIONS TO SELECT. CHOOSE EXACTLY THIS NUMBER.

Questions 931 through 935

(A) decreased fremitus, low diaphragms, prolonged expiration

(B) absent fremitus, hyperresonant, absent breath sounds

(C) decreased fremitus, tracheal shift away from affected side, flat percussion, absent breath sounds

(D) decreased fremitus, tracheal shift toward affected side, dull or flat percussion, absent breath sounds

(E) increased fremitus, dull to percussion, bronchophony

931. Atelectasis (SELECT ONE)

932. Complete pneumothorax (SELECT ONE)

933. Acute asthmatic attack (SELECT ONE)

934. Large pleural effusion (SELECT ONE)

935. Lobar pneumonia (SELECT ONE)

Questions 936 through 940

(A) epidermoid (squamous) carcinoma

(B) adenocarcinoma

(C) large cell carcinoma

(D) small cell carcinoma

(E) bronchioloalveolar carcinoma

936. The most common type of lung cancer associated with paraneoplastic hypercalcemia (SELECT ONE)

937. Most responsive to cytotoxic chemotherapy (SELECT ONE)

938. Can be cured by surgery (SELECT FOUR)

939. Most commonly associated with ectopic endocrine syndromes (SELECT ONE)

940. Most commonly associated with Pancoast syndrome (SELECT ONE)

Answers and Explanations

879. **(C)** When exposure to moldy hay is stopped, symptoms and signs of farmer's lung all tend to abate and complete recovery usually follows. In acute syndromes, the presentation is 4 to 8 hours after exposure. Symptoms include fever, chills, malaise, cough, and dyspnea without wheezing. The rate of disease depends on rainfall (which promotes fungal growth) and agricultural practices related to turning and stacking hay. *(Braunwald, pp. 1463–1465)*

880. **(B)** Emphysema and chronic bronchitis are closely related, and the term COPD is often used to encompass both. Chronic bronchitis is a clinical syndrome defined as excessive tracheobronchial mucous production severe enough to cause productive cough for at least 3 months of the year for at least 2 consecutive years. Emphysema is defined as distention of the air spaces distal to the terminale bronchiole, with destruction of alveolar septa. It is primarily a histologic diagnosis. Smoking is the usual antecedent for COPD. *(Braunwald, pp. 1491–1495)*

881. **(B)** Tranquilizers and sedatives should be avoided in prolonged asthma attacks. Bronchodilators, fluids, aminophylline, and steroids may be used. In acute situations, IV glucocorticoids are frequently used. Results of therapy should be monitored in an objective manner, with peak expiratory flow rates or FEV_1. In acute asthmatic attacks, hypocarbia is usual on blood gas analysis. Normal or elevated $PaCO_2$ is a bad sign and requires intensive monitoring and aggressive treatment. *(Braunwald, pp. 1460–1462)*

882. **(D)** Administration of oxygen may worsen the syndrome of carbon dioxide narcosis because the chief stimulus to ventilation is often hypoxia, and when this is suddenly relieved, the ventilation may drop quickly. Causes of the chronic hypoventilation syndrome include impaired respiratory drive (eg, prolonged hypoxia, central nervous system [CNS] disease), neuromuscular disorders (eg, motor neuron disease, myasthenia gravis), or impaired ventilatory apparatus (eg, kyphoscoliosis, COPD). *(Braunwald, pp. 1517–1518)*

883. **(C)** The perfusion lung scan is most valuable in ruling out a pulmonary embolism. If properly performed early in the course of symptoms, a normal scan rules out the diagnosis. High-probability scans are usually considered enough evidence of pulmonary embolism to warrant definitive treatment. Intermediate- or low-probability scans may require further investigation (eg, with pulmonary angiography), depending on the prior probability of disease. *(Braunwald, p. 1510)*

884. **(B)** Allergic bronchopulmonary aspergillosis (in asthmatics), parasitic reactions, and drugs are known causes of pulmonary eosinophilia. Idiopathic causes include Loeffler syndrome (benign, acute eosinophilic pneumonia), chronic eosinophilic pneumonia, hypereosinophilic syndrome, and Churg–Strauss allergic granulomatosis. *(Braunwald, pp. 1466–1467)*

885. (E) Allergic bronchopulmonary aspergillus usually requires long-term treatment with glucocorticoids. The major diagnostic criteria are bronchial asthma, pulmonary infiltrates, eosinophilia greater than 1000, immediate wheal and flare response to *Aspergillus fumigans*, serum precipitins to *A. fumigans*, elevated serum IgE, and central bronchiectasis. *(Braunwald, p. 1466)*

886. (D) Hypoventilation always causes both hypoxemia and hypercapnia. If the hypoventilation syndrome is caused exclusively by impaired respiratory drive (eg, drug overdose), then the alveolar–arterial PaO_2 gradient remains normal. Often, hypoventilation results from more than one disorder in the respiratory system (eg, COPD plus metabolic alkalosis secondary to diuretics and glucocorticoids). *(Braunwald, pp. 1517–1519)*

887. (D) Emphysematous COPD usually demonstrates scanty mucoid sputum, late onset of heart failure, increased total lung capacity, and markedly reduced diffusing capacity. Hypercarbia and hypoxemia are not as marked as in the chronic bronchitic type. The cough is not very productive and follows the onset of dyspnea. The body build is thin, usually with evidence of weight loss. However, in most patients, emphysema and chronic bronchitis coexist. *(Braunwald, p. 1495)*

888. (B) Neurogenic tumors are the most common posterior mediastinal masses. Other posterior mediastinal masses include meningoceles, meningomyeloceles, gastroenteric cysts, and esophageal diverticula. Common anterior mediastinal masses include thymomas, lymphomas, teratomas, and thyroid masses. Middle mediastinal masses include vascular lesions, lymph nodes, and pleuropericardial and bronchogenic cysts. *(Braunwald, p. 1516)*

889. (A) Most people have two MM genes and a resultant alpha$_1$-antitrypsin level in excess of 2.5 g/L. Homozygotes with ZZ or SS genotypes have severe alpha$_1$-antitrypsin deficiency and develop severe panacinar emphy-

sema in the third or fourth decade of life. Smoking is an important cofactor in the development of disease. Heterozygotes (MZ or MS) have intermediate levels of alpha$_1$-antitrypsin (ie, genetic expression is that of an autosomal codominant allele). This heterozygous state is common (5 to 14% of general population), but it is unclear whether it is associated with lung function abnormalities. *(Braunwald, p. 1492)*

890. (A) Ankylosing spondylitis is characterized by bilateral upper lobe fibrosis, which may be complicated by fibrocavitary disease. The pulmonary involvement is rare and is usually very slowly progressive. The cavities can be colonized by *Aspergillus. (Braunwald, p. 1501)*

891. (D) The primary pathology is likely to be located in the respiratory center. Cyanosis, especially when asleep, is caused by a combination of polycythemia and hypoxia. The symptoms of alveolar hypoventilation are caused by both hypercarbia and hypoxemia. *(Braunwald, p. 1517)*

892. (B) A significant portion of asthmatics have no known personal or family history of atopy and have normal IgE levels. Idiosyncratic asthma is more likely to have its onset in adult life. Upper respiratory infections can serve as triggers for idiosyncratic asthma. *(Braunwald, p. 1456)*

893. (A) Paraneoplastic syndromes are classified as metabolic, neuromuscular, connective tissue, dermatologic, and vascular. Stevens–Johnson syndrome usually follows drug allergy. Acanthosis nigricans and other cutaneous manifestations (eg, dermatomyositis) are rare (< 1%). Clubbing is common and occurs in up to 30% of non–small cell lung cancers. The various endocrine syndromes occur in 12% of cases. At times, paraneoplastic syndromes may be the presenting finding in lung cancer or be the first sign of recurrence. Most occur with non–small cell lung cancer, but SIADH is more characteristic of small cell lung cancer. *(Braunwald, pp. 632–642)*

894. **(D)** Carbon dioxide retention is seen in right-to-left shunt only with exercise and is uncommon in impaired diffusion syndromes. Disorders of the chest wall, lower airways, and lungs can cause an increased $Paco_2$ because of severe ventilation–perfusion mismatching despite normal or increased minute volume of ventilation. *(Braunwald, pp. 1517–1518)*

895. **(C)** Transbronchial biopsy helps differentiate IPF from similar syndromes with specific treatments. These include chronic hypersensitivity pneumonitis, cryptogenic organizing pneumonia, and sarcoidosis. *(Braunwald, pp. 1501–1502)*

896. **(C)** The increased vascular permeability is the hallmark of the disease. Diagnostic criteria include acute onset, $Pao_2/FIo_2 \leq 200$ mm Hg (regardless of PEEP level), bilateral infiltrate on frontal CXR, and pulmonary artery occlusion pressure ≤ 18 mm Hg (or if not measured, no evidence of left atrial hypertension). *(Braunwald, pp. 1524–1525)*

897. **(D)** Treatment includes antibiotics such as trimethoprim-sulfa or doxycycline or amoxicillin. Some patients respond to steroids, but these are used only in strictly controlled circumstances. Steroid use is usually confined to acute exacerbations. Dietary support to prevent malnutrition and improve muscle strength can be helpful. Exercise programs seem to provide subjective improvement as well. Obviously, stopping smoking is crucial. *(Braunwald, pp. 1495–1499)*

898. **(C)** Mediastinal emphysema may also result from thoracocentesis, trauma to the trachea or esophagus, or dissection of the retroperitoneum. Clinical presentation may include substernal chest pain, subcutaneous emphysema, and Hamman's signs, a crunching or clicking noise synchronous with the heartbeat. *(Braunwald, p. 1516)*

899. **(C)** Hemoptysis suggests infection in a patient with advanced lung disease. Pancreatic exocrine function is poor. Nasal polyps are common, but not rectal polyps. About 7% of cases of cystic fibrosis are diagnosed after age

18. Because of improved therapy, cystic fibrosis is no longer just a pediatric disease. Median survival is now 32 years for men and 29 years for women. *(Braunwald, pp. 1487–1489)*

900. **(B)** Hypoxemia while receiving 100% oxygen indicates right-to-left shunt. Shunts permit circulation of blood that never passes through the ventilated lung. Shunting can occur within the lung (atelectasis, vascular abnormalities) or outside the lung (congenital cardiac malformations). The hypoxemia of ventilation–perfusion mismatch is more easily correctable by 100% oxygen. *(Braunwald, p. 1452)*

901. **(E)** Bony deformities of the chest can lead to respiratory failure with raised Pco_2, as well as recurrent pulmonary infection. The pattern on pulmonary function testing is usually that of a restrictive pattern. *(Braunwald, pp. 1449, 1517)*

902. **(A)** The vital capacity is reduced in emphysema, but the FEV_1 is grossly reduced because of high airway resistance. In predominant emphysema, diffusing capacity is more profoundly decreased than in predominant bronchitis. *(Braunwald, pp. 1493–1494)*

903. **(E)** All forms of asbestos fiber have been associated with lung disease. Restrictive, not obstructive, disease is characteristic. Lung cancer, either squamous cell or adenocarcinoma, is the most common malignancy and the risk is greatly increased by smoking. Benign pleural effusions can occur in both symptomatic and asymptomatic individuals. Reports of mesothelioma 30 to 35 years after brief exposure to asbestos emphasize the importance of a complete occupational/environmental history. *(Braunwald, p. 1469)*

904. **(E)** Pulmonary embolism secondary to fat emboli is characterized by petechiae on the upper thorax and arms. Although continuous heparin therapy with an infusion pump is the most popular method of acute treatment, other methods can also be effective. The common ECG change is tachycardia. Sudden onset of dyspnea is the most common symptom of pulmonary embolism. Pleuritic pain (and hemoptysis) occur only when infarction, an uncommon event, occurs. Some 90% of deaths related to pulmonary embolism occur in the first hour or two, too quickly to allow effective diagnosis and therapy. The thrust of management is therefore prevention. *(Braunwald, pp. 329, 1508–1512)*

905. **(B)** The description of a middle-aged man with daytime sleepiness, obesity, hypertension, and snoring suggests obstructive sleep apnea. Although nasal continuous positive airway pressure is effective treatment, simple O_2 therapy is not. Stopping sedative medications and avoiding alcohol improves symptoms. Restless sleep and sudden death have been described as part of the syndrome and surgery (uvulopalatopharyngoplasty or tracheostomy) has been used in severe cases. A wide variety of symptoms can occur, but neuropsychiatric and behavioral manifestations secondary to sleep disturbance are the most common. *(Braunwald, p. 1521)*

906. **(B)** Nocturnal oxygen supplementation improves symptoms but is not as effective as continuous supplementation in prolonging life and decreasing hospitalization. Some symptoms of erythrocytosis, headaches, and fullness can be relieved by phlebotomy. In prolonged air travel, even those with a PO_2 in the mid-70s should be considered for oxygen therapy. A PO_2 below 55 mm Hg is an indication for oxygen therapy, but between 55 and 60 mm Hg, associated evidence of right heart dysfunction should also be present before therapy is commenced. *(Braunwald, pp. 1496–1497)*

907. **(C)** In asbestosis there is moderate pleural thickening, with scalloped margins from apex to base. There is a similar finding in the mediastinal and diaphragmatic pleura. Furthermore, there is a plaque of pleural calcification in the base. The association of asbestosis with mesothelioma has long been known. As the neoplasm progresses, it may envelop the thorax. *(Braunwald, p. 1469)*

908. **(A)** The diagnosis is pneumonia. There is consolidation of the left lower lobe. The increased density, presence of air bronchogram, and the silhouetting of the left diaphragm point to a parenchymal lesion. Pneumococcal infection, as in this patient, is still the most common etiology, although other bacterial infections such as *Klebsiella*, *Streptococcus*, or *Staphylococcus* are often encountered. Viral and arthropod-borne diseases are also seen. *(Braunwald, pp. 1477–1479)*

909. **(B)** There is a calcified nodule in the left apex. Obviously, a calcified tuberculous granuloma is the most common lesion. This may be from reinfection tuberculosis, where its preference for the apicoposterior segment is well known. It is also possible that it may be a calcified Ghon's lesion. *(Braunwald, p. 1027)*

910. **(A)** Eosinophilic granuloma is the diagnosis. There is a coarse, reticular pattern in the whole lung—somewhat more prominent in the upper lobes—suggesting a honeycomb appearance. It is the density here that is abnormal and not the lucency. *(Braunwald, p. 1505)*

911. **(A)** Because of the maintained increase in minute volume and the maintenance of arterial Pa_{O_2}, patients with emphysema are referred to as *pink puffers*. The relatively high Pa_{O_2} and relatively low hemoglobin, as compared to chronic bronchitis, make cyanosis unusual in emphysema. *(Braunwald, pp. 1493–1494)*

912. **(B)** This history suggests a benign bronchial adenoma. These are usually centrally located on CXR. A peripheral lesion with "popcorn" calcification suggests a hamartoma, not an adenoma, and does not usually present with hemoptysis. Bronchiectasis (tram line, cysts), COPD (airflow reduction), and mitral stenosis (enlarged left atrium), although potential causes of hemoptysis, rarely present without other symptoms as well. *(Braunwald, pp. 205–207)*

913. **(B)** This presentation is characteristic of primary pulmonary hypertension. Pulmonary veno-occlusive disease is much less common.

The predominant pathology, plexogenic arteriopathy, is characterized by medial hypertrophy associated with laminar intimal fibrosis and plexiform lesions. The thrombotic arteriopathy is characterized by eccentric intimal fibrosis with medial hypertrophy, fibroelastic intimal pads in the arteries and arterioles, and evidence of old recanalized thrombi. There is a female predominance, and the third or fourth decade is the most common age at presentation. By the time of diagnosis, the pulmonary hypertension is usually severe. (Braunwald, pp. 1506–1507)

914. **(C)** Open lung biopsy is not required. Pulmonary angiography is usually performed only if a lung scan suggests thromboembolic disease. Cardiac catheterization is useful to exclude an underlying cardiac shunt as the cause of the pulmonary hypertension. The pulmonary capillary wedge pressure is normal but can be difficult to obtain. (Braunwald, p. 1507)

915. **(D)** Patients frequently are subjected to test doses of short-acting vasodilators such as IV prostacyclin or adenosine, or inhaled nitric oxide. About half of these responders will then respond to high oral doses of nifedipine or diltiazem. Prostacyclin is also available as a treatment, but its applicability is limited by the necessity to administer it as a continuous IV infusion. (Braunwald, pp. 1507–1508)

916. **(D)** The natural history of the disease is unclear because the disease is asymptomatic for a long period. Survival from diagnosis is dependent on the functional class of the patient. Functional class IV dyspnea suggests a mean survival of only 6 months. Death is usually the result of either intractable right heart failure or sudden death. (Braunwald, p. 1507)

917. **(A)** Most lung abscesses and all anaerobic abscesses involve the normal flora of the oropharynx. Septic embolic usually contain *S. aureus*. Factors that predispose to gram-negative colonization of the oropharynx include hospitalization, debility, severe under-

lying diseases, alcoholism, diabetes, and advanced age. Impaired consciousness, neurologic disease, swallowing disorders, and nasogastric or endotracheal tubes all increase the likelihood of aspiration. (Braunwald, pp. 1013–1014, 1476–1477)

918. **(E)** Traditionally, penicillin has been the treatment of choice for lung disease. However, clindamycin or penicillin plus metronidazole has a better spectrum of activity against oral anaerobes. Generally, the combination of penicillin and metronidazole is preferred, but clindamycin alone is also acceptable therapy. (Braunwald, p. 1016)

919. **(C)** Elevated D-dimer levels suggests thromboembolic disease. When done by the enzyme-linked immunosorbent assay (ELISA) technique, it is relatively specific (ie, a negative result helps rule out pulmonary embolism). However, when done by the latex agglutination method, it is neither specific nor sensitive enough to guide therapy. (Braunwald, p. 1510)

920. **(A)** In most circumstances, treatment is anticoagulation to prevent further pulmonary emboli. However, hemodynamic instability may warrant primary therapy for the embolus (eg, thrombolysis). Evidence of right ventricular hypokinesis on echocardiogram can be an indication for such primary therapy. (Braunwald, pp. 1511–1512)

921. **(D)** Sarcoidosis is the most likely diagnosis. Granulomatous inflammatory changes of sarcoidosis may occur in almost any organ. About 90% of patients with sarcoid will have an abnormal CXR at some point. (Braunwald, pp. 1970–1971)

922. **(B)** There is no diagnostic blood test, but two thirds of patients with sarcoidosis will have an elevated level of ACE. Five percent of positive tests are false positives. (Braunwald, p. 1973)

923. **(E)** The Kveim test requires 6 weeks' incubation and must be biopsied to be interpreted.

The material for the test is not widely available, and with easy availability of transbronchial biopsy, the test is rarely used. It is positive only in 70 to 80% of people with sarcoid, and has a 5% false-positive rate. *(Braunwald, p. 1973)*

924. (A) Acute granulomatous uveitis may be the initial manifestation of sarcoidosis. It can cause blindness. About 25% of patients with sarcoid have eye involvement; three quarters have anterior uveitis, and one quarter have posterior uveitis. Involvement of lacrimal glands can lead to dry, sore eyes. *(Braunwald, p. 1972)*

925. (C) Relatively asymptomatic patients often require no treatment. Steroids are used with ocular (as in this case), CNS, or other serious complications. Although 50% of patients are left with permanent organ impairment, these are usually not symptomatic or significant. Only in 15 to 20% of cases does the disease remain active or recur. Glucocorticoids are the treatment of choice, but numerous other agents have been used. *(Braunwald, pp. 1973–1974)*

926. (A) Bronchiectasis is defined as a permanent abnormal dilatation of large bronchi due to destruction of the wall. It is a consequence of inflammation, usually an infection. Other causes include toxins or immune response. Persistent cough and purulent sputum production are the hallmark symptoms. *(Braunwald, pp. 1485–1487)*

927. (B) Kartagener's syndrome consists of situs inversus (with dextrocardia), bronchiectasis, and nasal polyps. The bronchiectasis results from impaired ciliary function. *(Braunwald, p. 1486)*

928. (E) In the pre–antibiotic era, bacterial bronchopneumonia was the most common cause of bronchiectasis. Now it is felt that influenza and adenoviruses are the most common causes. Of the bacterial causes, *S. aureus, Klebsiella*, and anaerobes are the most common. *(Braunwald, pp. 1486–1487)*

929. (A) Bronchography has been superseded by CT scan in defining the extent of bronchiectasis. Occasionally, advanced cases of saccular bronchiectasis can be diagnosed by routine CXR. The use of high-resolution CT scanning, in which the images are 1.5 mm thick, has resulted in excellent diagnostic accuracy. *(Braunwald, p. 1486)*

930. (A) Antibiotics and postural drainage might be included in therapy. The choice of antimicrobial agents is guided by the sputum culture, but ampicillin and tetracycline are used if normal flora are found. The general principles of therapy include eliminating underlying problems, improved clearance of secretions, control of infections, and reversal of airflow obstruction. *(Braunwald, p. 1487)*

931. (D)

932. (B)

933. (A)

934. (C)

935. (E)

Careful physical examination can be very useful in diagnosing many common pulmonary disorders. Atelectasis and large pleural effusions both can present with decreased fremitus, dullness or flatness to percussion, and absent breath sounds. In atelectasis, tracheal shift, if present, is toward the affected side, and the opposite for a large pleural effusion. Asthma's most typical manifestations are prolonged expiration and diffuse wheezing. However, impaired expansion, decreased fremitus, hyperresonance, and low diaphragms can also be found. A complete pneumothorax results in absent fremitus, hyperresonance or tympany, and absent breath sounds. Lobar pneumonia is characterized by consolidation with increased fremitus, dullness, and auscultatory findings of bronchial breathing, bronchophony, pectoriloquy, and crackles. *(Braunwald, p. 1444)*

936. (A) Hypercalcemia may be due to metastatic destruction of bone, ectopic formation of parathyroid hormone, or formation of other osteolytic substances. *(Braunwald, pp. 562–570)*

937. **(D)** Combination chemotherapy has produced promising results in lung cancer, particularly of the small cell anaplastic type. Alkylating agents and anthracyclines are active among other agents. *(Braunwald, p. 569)*

938. **(A, B, C, E)** Early stage non–small cell lung cancer can be cured by surgery. However, 70% present with disseminated disease. *(Braunwald, p. 567)*

939. **(D)** The most commonly encountered syndromes are SIADH, Cushing syndrome, and gynecomastia. *(Braunwald, pp. 564–565)*

940. **(A)** Pancoast syndrome (or superior sulcus syndrome) is found in apical lung tumors, usually epidermoid. Shoulder pain secondary to involvement of the eighth cervical and first and second thoracic nerves is characteristic. Horner syndrome frequently coexists. *(Braunwald, p. 564)*

CHAPTER 13

Clinical Pharmacology
Questions

DIRECTIONS (Questions 941 through 983): Each of the numbered items or incomplete statements in this section is followed by answers or by completions of the statement. Select the ONE lettered answer or completion that is BEST in each case.

941. A 72-year-old man is prescribed hydrochlorothiazide for hypertension. The most likely symptomatic side effect is

   (A) increased serum potassium
   (B) metabolic acidosis
   (C) sexual impotence
   (D) respiratory alkalosis
   (E) hypernatremia

942. A 73-year-old man with gastroesophageal reflux is prescribed ranitidine. Its most profound effect is on

   (A) stimulated acid secretion
   (B) H_1 receptors
   (C) columnar epithelium of the esophagus
   (D) bicarbonate production
   (E) basal acid secretion

943. A 58-year-old man with a lung lesion develops hyponatremia. The likely mechanism involved in the low sodium is

   (A) increased permeability of the proximal renal tubule to water
   (B) increased permeability of the distal renal tubule to water
   (C) decreased glomerular filtration rate
   (D) increased sodium excretion
   (E) active reabsorption of water from the loop of Henle

944. A 38-year-old woman develops palpitations, weight loss, and mild tremor. After evaluation, she is started on methimazole. This drug works by

   (A) inhibition of iodine uptake
   (B) inhibition of thyroidal organic binding and coupling reactions
   (C) lowering serum calcium
   (D) adrenal suppression
   (E) the same mechanism as perchlorate

945. A 69-year-old man develops exertional chest pain. He is also hypertensive, and is prescribed nifedipine. This medication works by

   (A) beta-adrenergic stimulation
   (B) interfering with calcium flux
   (C) inhibition of angiotensin 1
   (D) alpha-adrenergic blockade
   (E) direct smooth muscle relaxation

946. A 48-year-old man develops pneumococcal pneumonia. Oral treatment with ampicillin rather than penicillin might be preferred because

   (A) penicillin is not effective orally
   (B) ampicillin is not inactivated by penicillinase
   (C) ampicillin is acid stable
   (D) ampicillin is not effective against coliform organisms and therefore has a narrower spectrum
   (E) ampicillin is not allergenic

947. A 69-year-old man develops renal failure. Which of the following drugs requires a major adjustment in dosage?

(A) tetracycline
(B) methicillin
(C) erythromycin
(D) chloramphenicol
(E) ampicillin

948. Thiocyanate and perchlorate are examples of agents that

(A) inhibit thyroglobulin release
(B) increase basal metabolic rate (BMR)
(C) inhibit iodide transport
(D) inhibit thyroid organic binding
(E) increase thyroxin synthesis

949. A 63-year-old woman with hypertension is started on a beta blocker. Extreme care must be taken in prescribing this medication if she has

(A) migraine headaches
(B) hypertrophic subaortic stenosis
(C) Marfan syndrome
(D) AV node dysfunction
(E) intermittent claudication

950. A 69-year-old woman with poor dietary habits and alcoholism is found to have a macrocytic anemia with hypersegmented neutrophils. Diagnosis will most likely be made via

(A) red blood cell vitamin levels
(B) plasma vitamin levels
(C) bone marrow
(D) Schilling test
(E) therapeutic trial

951. A 69-year-old man is given a multivitamin containing B_{12}. Absorption is characteristically

(A) totally dependent on the intrinsic factor
(B) best in the duodenum
(C) improved in folic acid deficiency

(D) best in the distal ileum
(E) prevented by anti–parietal cell antibodies

952. A 19-year-old man takes an overdose of lysergic acid diethylamide (LSD). This is most likely to be associated with

(A) pupillary dilatation
(B) pupillary constriction
(C) bradycardia
(D) blindness
(E) deafness

953. A 15-year-old boy is given tetracycline for acne. The most likely side effect is

(A) neutropenia
(B) allergic reactions
(C) hepatitis
(D) gastrointestinal (GI) symptoms
(E) polyuria

954. A 79-year-old man on quinidine develops thrombocytopenia. In this syndrome, it is likely that

(A) there is a relation of dose to thrombocytopenia
(B) there is a more common incidence in males
(C) thrombocytopenia lasts 3 weeks following cessation of the drug
(D) it is immunologically mediated
(E) there is cross-reactivity with penicillin

955. A 28-year-old psychiatric patient has a lithium level of 2.3 mEq/L. This can result in

(A) mania
(B) depression
(C) tremor
(D) hyponatremia
(E) leukopenia

956. A 69-year-old man with stable angina is given nitroglycerin. The drug works by

(A) dilating coronary arteries
(B) increasing cardiac venous return

(C)   increasing cardiac output

(D)   constricting peripheral veins and capillaries

(E)   decreasing cardiac work

957.   A 74-year-old man with gout is given allopurinol. The medication works by

(A)   increasing uric acid production

(B)   blocking excretion of uric acid by renal tubular mechanism

(C)   inhibiting xanthine oxidase

(D)   diminishing inflammation of acute gouty arthritis

(E)   stabilizing lysozymes

958.   A 29-year-old woman develops deep vein thrombosis (DVT) in the third trimester. Heparin therapy

(A)   is active by mouth

(B)   affects hepatic synthesis of factors

(C)   is monitored by prothrombin time (PT)

(D)   is contraindicated in pregnancy

(E)   may be neutralized by protamine

959.   A 19-year-old college student smokes cannabis very heavily. Evaluation an hour after inhalation might reveal

(A)   a decrease in heart rate

(B)   an increase in intraocular pressure

(C)   prolonged reaction time

(D)   peripheral vasoconstriction

(E)   an increase in intelligence quotient (IQ)

960.   An 83-year-old woman has a grade IV ventricle and requires 80 mg of furosemide per day. This may lead to

(A)   acidosis

(B)   edema

(C)   alkalosis

(D)   hyperkalemia

(E)   hypernatremia

961.   Three teenaged high school students develop meningitis. A classmate is concerned and comes to see you. Appropriate management includes

(A)   penicillin

(B)   sulfonamides

(C)   only reassurance and observation

(D)   rifampin

(E)   doxycycline

962.   A 69-year-old man's dyspepsia is improved with cimetidine. The beneficial result occurs because it

(A)   almost totally abolishes acid secretion

(B)   blocks histamine-H_1 receptors

(C)   is well absorbed in the stomach

(D)   must be taken four times per day

(E)   has no neurologic side effects

963.   A 68-year-old man with heart failure might not be given furosemide if he

(A)   has hypoalbuminemia

(B)   is oliguric

(C)   has an acidosis

(D)   had a rash with trimethoprim–sulfamethoxazole

(E)   is on anticoagulants

964.   A 43-year-old woman with breast cancer is being treated with doxorubicin. Therapy is likely to be limited by

(A)   neurologic toxicity

(B)   severe nausea

(C)   cystitis

(D)   neutropenia

(E)   heart failure

965.   A 23-year-old homeless man is found to have consumed alcohol adulterated with methanol. The standard treatment is effective because it

(A)   enhances renal excretion

(B)   prevents biotransformation

(C)   combines to form a nontoxic polymer

(D)   changes the toxin's volume of distribution

(E)   sedates, thus preventing neurologic damage

966. A 69-year-old man with heart failure and ventricular premature beats is prescribed amiodarone. This drug is known to have

(A) excellent oral absorption
(B) a short half-life
(C) an active metabolite
(D) few drug interactions
(E) a small volume of distribution

967. Coma from barbiturate intoxication

(A) requires at least 20 to 30 times the full sedative dose
(B) is increasing in frequency
(C) is characterized by an initial period of hyperventilation
(D) causes death by depression of the cardiovascular system
(E) causes death by pulmonary complications

968. Which of the following stimulates insulin secretion?

(A) hypoxia
(B) hypothermia
(C) severe burns
(D) beta$_2$-adrenergic receptor antagonists
(E) ketones

969. The most prominent effect of epinephrine infusion on cardiac function in humans is

(A) increased heart rate
(B) increased stroke volume
(C) increased cardiac output
(D) arrhythmias
(E) increased coronary blood flow

970. The most striking difference in the cardiac actions of epinephrine and norepinephrine is on

(A) heart rate
(B) stroke volume
(C) cardiac output
(D) arrhythmias
(E) coronary blood flow

971. Which of the following statements concerning the relative effects of epinephrine and norepinephrine infusion on peripheral circulation is correct?

(A) Both drugs increase total peripheral resistance.
(B) Neither drug increases total peripheral resistance.
(C) Neither drug increases renal blood flow.
(D) Both drugs increase cutaneous blood flow.
(E) Both drugs increase muscle blood flow.

972. Which of the following statements concerning the use of isoproterenol and dobutamine for shock is correct?

(A) Isoproterenol is preferred because of its short half life.
(B) Neither drug will potentiate cardiac ischemia.
(C) Dobutamine has a more prominent inotropic effect than chronotropic effect compared with isoproterenol.
(D) Neither drug affects smooth muscle.
(E) Isoproterenol raises blood pressure more than dobutamine.

973. Beta$_2$-selective adrenergic agonists are preferred to nonselective beta-adrenergic agonists in the treatment of asthma because they

(A) relax bronchial smooth muscle and thus decrease airway resistance
(B) improve mucociliary function
(C) suppress the release of leukotrienes and histamine from mast cells in lung
(D) decrease microvascular permeability
(E) have fewer side effects

974. Which of the following statements concerning innate tolerance to alcohol is correct?

(A) It develops over many years of even moderate drinking.
(B) High levels of innate tolerance protect against the development of alcoholism.

(C) This is likely a result of polygenic inheritance.

(D) Pharmacokinetic factors are not involved.

(E) It is not a factor in the development of alcoholism.

975. Pharmacokinetic tolerance is usually caused by

(A) changes in absorption
(B) changes in distribution
(C) changes specific to that drug
(D) changes in metabolism
(E) renal adaptation

976. An example of learned tolerance would be

(A) avoiding alcohol when feeling unsteady
(B) drinking alcohol only with food
(C) walking a straight line when intoxicated
(D) not driving when drunk
(E) using vitamins to prevent alcohol damage

977. Sensitization to a drug can best be described as

(A) an allergic response
(B) a purely behavioral effect
(C) a shift to the right of a dose response curve
(D) reverse tolerance
(E) a response to an acute binge

978. The administration of which of the following drugs is most likely to result in sterilization?

(A) heroin
(B) cocaine
(C) tobacco
(D) alcohol
(E) diazepam

979. The drug most likely to result in addiction among those who have ever used it is

(A) alcohol
(B) tobacco

(C) cocaine
(D) heroin
(E) cannabis

980. Which of the following is a symptom of withdrawal from prolonged moderate dose benzodiazepine usage?

(A) delirium
(B) somnolence
(C) seizures
(D) decreased hearing
(E) muscle cramps

981. Which of the following statements concerning heroin withdrawal is correct?

(A) It is frequently life threatening.
(B) It starts about 24 hours after the last dose.
(C) Pupillary constriction is present.
(D) Piloerection ("gooseflesh") occurs.
(E) Blood pressure is lowered.

982. The opioid analgesic most likely to cause central nervous system (CNS) disturbance is

(A) heroin
(B) morphine
(C) meperidine
(D) fentanyl
(E) codeine

983. Fentanyl does not disturb cardiovascular stability as much as morphine because it

(A) is water soluble
(B) is lipid soluble
(C) does not stimulate histamine release
(D) is long acting
(E) is not as potent as morphine

DIRECTIONS (Questions 984 through 1006): Each set of matching questions in this section consists of a list of lettered options followed by several numbered items. For each numbered item, select the appropriate lettered option(s). Each lettered option may be selected once, more than once, or not at all. EACH ITEM WILL STATE THE NUMBER OF OPTIONS TO SELECT. CHOOSE EXACTLY THIS NUMBER.

Questions 984 through 988

    (A) this "prodrug" requires activation in an acid environment

    (B) works by binding to cysteine

    (C) can cause myopathy

    (D) irreversible H_2-receptor blockade

    (E) synthetic analogue of prostaglandin E

    (F) inhibits acid secretion

    (G) prevents hydrolysis of mucosal proteins by pepsin

    (H) can enhance gastric secretion

    (I) cannot be taken with other drugs

Match the following drugs often used in acid peptic disorders with the appropriate answer(s) above.

984. Calcium carbonate (SELECT ONE)

985. Ranitidine (SELECT ONE)

986. Sucralfate (SELECT TWO)

987. Misoprostol (SELECT TWO)

988. Anticholinergic drugs (SELECT ONE)

Questions 989 through 993

    (A) combines with cytochromes and catalase to block hydrogen and electron transport, thus producing tissue asphyxia

    (B) methemoglobinemia

    (C) vertigo, hyperventilation, tinnitus, and deafness

    (D) bone marrow depression

    (E) acute hepatic insufficiency

    (F) severe renal injury

989. A 43-year-old man works in a factory where industrial solvents are frequently used (SELECT ONE)

990. A 75-year-old woman with rheumatoid arthritis (RA) who is adjusting her own medications (SELECT ONE)

991. A young child ingests silver polish (SELECT ONE)

992. A troubled youth with a long history of gasoline sniffing (SELECT ONE)

993. A skid-row alcoholic ingests antifreeze (SELECT ONE)

Questions 994 through 997

    (A) digitalis

    (B) verapamil

    (C) diltiazem

    (D) beta blockers

    (E) methyldopa

    (F) quinidine

    (G) flecainide

    (H) propafenone

    (I) theophylline

    (J) sotalol

    (K) procainamide

    (L) disopyramide

    (M) amiodarone

Match the drug induced arrhythmia below with the drug(s) that can cause it.

994. Increased ventricular rate in atrial fibulation in patients with Wolf–Parkinson–White (WPW) syndrome (SELECT TWO)

995. Polymorphic VT with increased QT interval (torsades de pointes) (SELECT FIVE)

996. Multifocal atrial tachycardia (SELECT ONE)

997. Atrial tachycardia with atrioventricular (AV) block (SELECT ONE)

Questions 998 through 1001

(A) Hodgkin's disease
(B) acute lymphocytic leukemia
(C) multiple myeloma
(D) chronic lymphocytic leukemia
(E) chronic granulocytic leukemia
(F) malignant melanoma
(G) breast cancer
(H) colon cancer
(I) hairy cell leukemia
(J) choriocarcinoma
(K) prostate cancer
(L) ovarian cancer
(M) Kaposi's sarcoma

Match the chemotherapeutic agent below with the diseases it is used in above.

998. Melphalan (SELECT THREE)

999. Methotrexate (SELECT THREE)

1000. Bleomycin (SELECT ONE)

1001. Flutamide (SELECT ONE)

Questions 1002 and 1003

(A) sensory loss
(B) prolonged QT interval
(C) Parkinson-like symptoms
(D) action tremor
(E) insomnia
(F) increased refractory period
(G) dystonic movements

1002. A 74-year-old woman with Alzheimer's disease is treated with haloperidol (SELECT TWO)

1003. A 69-year-old woman being treated for dysrhythmias with quinidine (SELECT TWO)

Questions 1004 through 1006

(A) albuterol
(B) ethanol
(C) atropine
(D) ipratroprium bromide
(E) nonsteroidal anti-inflammatory drugs (NSAIDs)
(F) caffeine
(G) gingivitis
(H) potassium iodide
(I) propranolol

1004. A 29-year-old woman has asthma. Which of the above may cause bronchodilation? (SELECT THREE)

1005. A 69-year-old man suffers from acid-peptic disease. Which of the above may increase gastric secretion? (SELECT TWO)

1006. A 79-year-old woman complains of dry mouth. Which of the above may be a factor? (SELECT ONE)

Answers and Explanations

941. **(C)** The most common symptomatic side effect in men is impotence, and it should be specifically looked for. The most serious complications relate to fluid and electrolyte imbalance and include hyponatremia, hypokalemia, and volume contraction. *(Hardman, p. 776)*

942. **(E)** Ranitidine is an H_2 blocker that reversibly competes with histamine for binding to H_2 receptors on gastric parietal cells. Its effect is profound on basal acid secretion, but it also has a significant effect on stimulated (eg, food, hypoglycemia, vagal stimulation) acid production. *(Hardman, p. 1009)*

943. **(B)** The mediator of the hyponatremia is likely antidiuretic hormone (ADH). Although controlling water permeability is the main function under ADH control, there is some evidence that ADH influences sodium transport in the cortical collecting duct. ADH can also act as a neurotransmitter. Autonomic effects of ADH in the CNS include bradycardia, increase in respiratory rate, suppression of fever, and alteration of sleep patterns. *(Hardman, pp. 802–803)*

944. **(B)** Methimazole is an effective treatment for hyperthyroidism. Methimazole interferes with thyroid function mainly by inhibition of thyroidal organic binding and coupling reactions. In contrast to other agents such as perchlorate, the action of thioamides is not prevented by large doses of iodide. *(Hardman, p. 1581)*

945. **(B)** Nifedipine is a synthetic agent that is a potent, long-acting systemic vasodilator for treatment of coronary vasospasm. It is also effective for hypertension. At doses used clinically, nifedipine does not block transmission through the AV node. The vasodilatation can result in a reflex increase in heart rate. *(Hardman, pp. 853–856)*

946. **(C)** Polar side chains added to penicillin molecules made these compounds acid stable and, therefore, improved absorption. Intake of food prior to ingestion of ampicillin will decrease absorption. In cases of severe renal impairment, the dose should be adjusted downward. *(Hardman, pp. 1201–1202)*

947. **(A)** Tetracycline requires a major adjustment in dosage in the presence of renal disease. An injection may accentuate azotemia by its catabolic effect in increasing nitrogen turnover. Doxycycline, however, is different from other tetracyclines in that blood levels are not affected by renal failure. Thus, it is the safest member of the tetracycline family for use in patients with renal failure. Ampicillin needs to be adjusted only with severe renal failure. *(Hardman, p. 1242)*

948. **(C)** Because of their toxicity, neither drug is widely used in treatment, but both are effective in inhibiting iodide transport. They work by preventing the thyroid gland from concentrating iodide. Thiocyanate is produced following enzymatic hydrolysis of certain plant glycosides (eg, cabbage) and may be a contributing factor to endemic goiter in certain parts of the world where iodide intake is low. *(Hardman, p. 1579)*

949. **(D)** Beta blockers are frequently used in the treatment of hypertrophic cardiomyopathy and for migraine prophylaxis and might prevent aortic dilatation in Marfan syndrome. It rarely causes clinical problems in patients with claudication, but if AV conduction defects are present (either by disease or use of other drugs) life-threatening bradyarrhythmias can occur. *(Hardman, pp. 257–260)*

950. **(A)** Folate deficiency can be secondary to small bowel disease, alcoholism, inadequate intake, disease states with high cell turnover (hemolytic anemia), drugs (methotrexate), and pregnancy. The concentration of folate in plasma changes rapidly with changes in food intake, so the diagnosis of anemia secondary to folate deficiency is made more reliable by measuring red blood cell folate. *(Hardman, pp. 1511–1512)*

951. **(D)** Vitamin B_{12} absorption is best in the distal ileum. Receptors for the intrinsic factor are present in the distal ileum, but mass action absorption also occurs with large doses. However, the oral route is still felt to be unreliable if hematologic or neurologic effects are present. The Schilling test, with and without intrinsic factor, can help diagnose the exact cause of B_{12} deficiency. *(Hardman, pp. 1506–1508)*

952. **(A)** Sympathomimetic effects such as pupillary dilatation, piloerection, hyperthermia, and tachycardia are common in an overdosage of LSD. Other symptoms include dizziness, weakness, drowsiness, nausea, and parasthesias. The hallucinogenic effects can last for hours and are mainly visual. *(Hardman, pp. 638–639)*

953. **(D)** GI symptoms are the major side effects of tetracycline. Stomatitis, glossitis, and diarrhea are seen and may be related to superinfections. Hepatic toxicity has been reported but is rare except in massive doses or during pregnancy. Tetracyclines can cause discoloration of teeth in children and in fetuses of mothers given the drug during pregnancy. *(Hardman, p. 1245)*

954. **(D)** Thrombocytopenia usually occurs after weeks or months of therapy. It is due to formation of drug–platelet complexes that evoke a circulating antibody. Thrombocytopenia and bleeding can be severe but resolve rapidly on discontinuing the drug. The antibody is long lasting, and reintroduction of quinidine, even in a small dose, can rapidly cause thrombocytopenia. Other hypersensitivity reactions to quinidine include hepatitis, bone marrow suppression, and a lupus syndrome. The most common side effects of quinidine, however, are gastrointestinal and include nausea, vomiting, and diarrhea. *(Hardman, pp. 965–966)*

955. **(C)** Lithium is used primarily for bipolar affective disorder, either to treat mania or prevent recurrences of the bipolar disorder. It has also been used in severe unipolar depression. Acute intoxication can result in vomiting, diarrhea, tremor, ataxia, coma, and convulsions. Leukocytosis is also a side effect of lithium therapy. Polyuria and polydipsia secondary to acquired nephrogenic diabetes insipidus is a common side effect. Both acute and chronic intoxication can be lethal. The toxic and therapeutic levels of lithium are very close, and patients on lithium require close medical observation, including measurement of serum lithium levels. *(Hardman, pp. 509–510)*

956. **(E)** The benefit of nitroglycerin is probably due to diminution in cardiac output and work of the heart. Nitroglycerin generally dilates most veins and arteries, and this results in both a decreased preload and a decreased afterload for the heart. This leads to decreased myocardial oxygen requirements. Although coronary artery dilation also occurs, it is probably not as important in relieving anginal pain. *(Hardman, p. 848)*

957. **(C)** Allopurinol effectively blocks uric acid production by inhibiting xanthine oxidase. Allopurinol is indicated in patients with a history of uric acid calculi of the urinary tract. In addition, it is often used in patients with malignancy (eg, leukemia, lymphoma), particularly when chemotherapy or radiation therapy is being used. (*Hardman, pp. 721–722*)

958. **(E)** Heparin must be given parenterally (usually intravenously or subcutaneously) to be active, and its activity is monitored by the partial thromboplastin time (PTT), not the PT. It is safer than oral anticoagulants in pregnancy and does not deplete clotting factors as its mode of action. Rather, it potentiates the effect of antithrombin III on the clotting cascade. It can be neutralized by administration of protamine. Because protamine can cause a bleeding tendency by its own actions, it is used only when bleeding is severe, and in the lowest possible dose. When low-molecular-weight heparin is used, it has a more predictable pharmacokinetic profile which allows for weight-adjusted dosage without laboratory follow up. (*Hardman, pp. 1522–1523*)

959. **(C)** The most common therapeutic use of cannabis is as an antiemetic during cancer chemotherapy. It might have some analgesic and anticonvulsant properties. Its ability to lower intraocular pressure has not been therapeutically useful in glaucoma. However, all the possible therapeutic effects of cannabis are accompanied by psychoactive effects, which include impaired cognition and perception, prolonged reaction time, and impaired memory and learning. (*Hardman, p. 637*)

960. **(C)** In addition to dehydration, hypokalemia, hypochloremia, and alkalosis also result from excessive use of furosemide. Loop diuretics such as furosemide act primarily to inhibit electrolyte reabsorption in the thick ascending limb of the loop of Henle. The degree of diuresis is greater than in other classes of diuretics. (*Hardman, pp. 772–773*)

961. **(D)** This is likely an outbreak of meningitis secondary to *Neisseria meningitidis*. The first line of drugs used for treatment of acute disease include cefixime, levofloxacin, and ceftriaxone. For prophylaxis, rifampin is the preferred agent. (*Hardman, pp. 1150, 1278*)

962. **(A)** Cimetidine blocks histamine-H_2 to receptors and is well absorbed in the small intestine. Initially, it was thought to require administration four times per day, but has now been shown to be effective if given twice a day, or even once at night. It decreases all gastric secretion, not just acid, and is helpful in short bowel syndromes, whereas omeprazole is not. (*Hardman, pp. 1009–1010*)

963. **(D)** Furosemide is effective despite gross electrolyte disturbances or hypoalbuminemia. Excretion of large volumes of bicarbonate-poor urine leads to alkalosis, so an acidosis is not a contradiction in severe fluid and electrolyte depletion; a trial in oliguric states is often appropriate. Furosemide is related to sulfonamide, and severe allergic reactions can occur. (*Hardman, pp. 769, 773*)

964. **(E)** Anthracyclines include daunorubicin and doxorubicin. The major site of metabolism is the liver, and the mechanism of action includes inhibition of deoxyribonucleic acid (DNA)-dependent ribonucleic acid (RNA) metabolism. The cardiomyopathy is characteristic of these drugs and is characterized by arrhythmias and cumulative dose-related congestive heart failure (CHF). (*Hardman, pp. 1428–1429*)

965. **(B)** Ethanol is the standard antidote for methanol. It inhibits the conversion of methanol to its toxic metabolite, formic acid, by alcohol dehydrogenase. (*Hardman, p. 78*)

966. **(C)** With prolonged treatment, the active desethyl derivative of amiodarone accumulates in plasma, and its concentration may exceed that of the parent compound. Amiodarone is poorly (approximately 30%) absorbed and there is marked interindividual variability. The half-life is long, 25 to 60 days, presumably because it is extensively bound to tissues, resulting in a large volume of distribution and a reservoir of drug. (*Hardman, pp. 954, 956*)

967. **(E)** Most deaths from barbiturate-induced coma are caused by pulmonary complica-

tions (atelectasis, edema, bronchopneumonia) or renal failure. Hypoventilation is characteristic, and only ten times the full reactive dose can cause severe poisoning. This low toxic–therapeutic ratio is one reason why barbiturate use (hence barbiturate coma) is declining. *(Hardman, p. 418)*

968. **(E)** Ketones, glucose amino acids, and fatty acids promote insulin secretion. Stimulation of $alpha_2$-adrenergic receptors inhibits insulin secretion, whereas $beta_2$-adrenergic receptor stimulation enhances release of insulin. As a result, $beta_2$-adrenergic receptor antagonists decrease insulin levels. Activation of the autonomic nervous system (hypoxia, hypothermia, severe burns, surgery) will also suppress insulin secretion. *(Hardman, p. 1682)*

969. **(D)** All the changes listed are correct, but the increased automaticity of the heart with the development of ventricular premature beats (or more serious ventricular arrhythmias) is the most prominent change. *(Hardman, p. 222)*

970. **(C)** Epinephrine results in a more rapid heart rate and more powerful systolic contraction resulting in increased cardiac output. Norepinephrine results in an unchanged or even decreased cardiac output. *(Hardman, pp. 222, 226)*

971. **(C)** Both epinephrine and norepinephrine decrease renal blood flow. Epinephrine decreases total peripheral resistance whereas norepinephrine increases total peripheral resistance. Both drugs decrease cutaneous blood flow and only epinephrine increases muscle blood flow. *(Hardman, p. 222)*

972. **(C)** The preferential effect of dobutamine on contractility makes it useful in low cardiac output states. Both drugs are very short acting, can potentiate cardiac ischemia, and affect smooth muscle. Unlike isoproterenol, dobutamine frequently increases blood pressure quite significantly thus requiring dosage adjustment. *(Braunwald, pp. 228–229)*

973. **(E)** Most of the side effects from the use of beta-adrenergic agonists in asthma come from stimulation of the $beta_1$ receptors in the heart. Thus, $beta_2$-selective agonists, which act primarily in the lung, are safer to use. Both selective and nonselective beta agonists will decrease airway resistance. This is their major therapeutic effect. The effects on mucociliary transit, mast cells, and microvascular permeability occur with both nonselective and selective agonists, but the clinical importance of these effects is unclear. *(Hardman, pp. 229–230)*

974. **(C)** It is felt that innate tolerance is a polygenic characteristic. Frequently, variation in pharmacokinetic variables (absorption, metabolism, excretion), which can be inherited, are the cause of different levels of innate tolerance. Those who have high levels of innate tolerance are more likely to become addicted to alcohol. There is a higher concordance rate for alcoholism among identical twins than fraternal twins, but it is not 100%. *(Hardman, p. 623)*

975. **(D)** The most common cause of pharmacokinetic tolerance is an increase in the metabolism of the drug. Since these same enzymes can then metabolize other drugs, this kind of tolerance is not necessarily specific to the drug that induced it. *(Hardman, p. 625)*

976. **(C)** Learned tolerance refers to the reduction of the effect of a drug due to compensatory mechanisms that are learned. An example is walking a straight line despite the motor impairment caused by alcohol. This likely represents both acquisition of motor skills and the learned awareness of one's deficit, thus the person walks more carefully. *(Hardman, p. 625)*

977. **(D)** Sensitization is the reverse of tolerance. It refers to an increase in effect of the drug with repetition of the same dose. It does not occur during an acute binge. The dose response curve would be shifted to the left. *(Hardman, p. 625)*

978. **(B)** Cocaine and amphetamines are the drugs most likely to cause sensitization. It is poorly

studied in humans, but it is thought that stimulant psychosis results from sensitization after prolonged use. *(Hardman, pp. 625–626)*

979. **(B)** Almost one third of people who have tried tobacco become addicted. In comparison, about 15% become addicted to alcohol. Heroin is also highly addictive (23% of users become addicted), but since so few people even try heroin, the addiction rate in society as a whole is quite low (0.4%). *(Hardman, p. 623)*

980. **(E)** Muscle cramps, anxiety, insomnia, and dizziness are among the common side effects of withdrawal from moderate dose usage. Withdrawal seizures and delirium occur usually in withdrawal from high dosage. Withdrawal should be done gradually, often over many months. *(Hardman, pp. 628–629)*

981. **(D)** Piloerection, pupillary dilatation, sweating, tachycardia, and blood pressure elevation are frequently seen in heroin withdrawal. It starts within 6 to 12 hours of the last dose and is quite unpleasant, but not life threatening. *(Hardman, p. 633)*

982. **(C)** Meperidine has a half-life of 3 hours, but it has an active metabolite, normeperidine, which has a half-life of 15 to 20 hours. Therefore, accumulation of normeperidine with toxicity is common. The drug should not be used for prolonged periods (over 48 hours), and probably should not be used at all in those susceptible to delirium (eg, the elderly). *(Hardman, p. 594)*

983. **(C)** Morphine releases histamine and can cause cardiovascular instability. Fentanyl does not release histamine, and causes only mild decreases in heart rate and blood pressure. Fentanyl, a lipid-soluble drug, has an elimination half-life between 3 and 4 hours. It is 100 times more potent than morphine. *(Hardman, p. 595)*

984. **(H)** Although doctors seldom prescribe antacids because of the availability of superior medications, patients still use them extensively. As well as neutralizing acid, calcium carbonate enhances secretion in the stomach. The release of CO_2 from bicarbonate can result in belching, nausea, and abdominal distension. Belching can exacerbate gastroesophageal reflex. *(Hardman, p. 1013)*

985. **(F)** Ranitidine inhibits acid production by reversibly competing with histamine for binding to H_2 receptors on parietal cells. Ranitidine's most prominent effect is on basal acid secretion, but it still significantly suppresses stimulated (feeding, gastrin, etc.) acid production. *(Hardman, p. 1009)*

986. **(G, I)** After the mucosa is damaged by acid, further damage is caused by pepsin-mediated hydrolysis of mucosal proteins. Sucralfate, in an acid environment, forms a sticky protective gel over epithelial tissues and ulcer craters to prevent further damage by pepsin. This viscous layer can inhibit absorption of many drugs, so patients should wait for at least 2 hours after taking other medications before taking sucralfate. *(Hardman, p. 1012)*

987. **(E, F)** Prostaglandins have two effects on gastric mucosa: they inhibit acid secretion by binding to the EP_3 receptor on parietal cells, and they have a cytoprotective effect by stimulating mucin and bicarbonate secretion and local mucosal blood flow. Misoprostol is a synthetic prostaglandin analogue, and has both an acid suppression and cytoprotective effect. *(Hardman, p. 1011)*

988. **(F)** Anticholinergic drugs can decrease acid production by 40 to 50%. This is far less than proton pump inhibitors or even H_2 blockers. As well, side effects are common, and the drugs are no longer used specifically for acid-peptic disorders. *(Hardman, p. 1014)*

989. **(E)** In chronically poisoned patients, neurologic symptoms and evidence of liver damage may develop. Many industrial solvents are chlorinated hydrocarbons and have been implicated in several deaths. Carbon tetrachloride was once used widely for medical

purposes and as a cleaning agent. It has been replaced by safer alternatives. Hepatotoxicity of these compounds is exacerbated by concurrent ethanol ingestion. In lethal cases, death is usually due to deep narcosis, aspiration of vomitus, or cardiac arrhythmias. *(Hardman, pp. 1884–1886)*

990. **(C)** Salicylates are associated with vertigo, hyperventilation, tinnitus, and deafness. Excretion of salicylates is renal, and in the presence of normal renal function, about 50% will be excreted in 24 hours. Severe toxicity can cause severe acid–base abnormalities. It can be difficult to diagnose when the toxicity is secondary to a therapeutic regimen. *(Hardman, pp. 697–700)*

991. **(A)** Cyanide is contained in silver polish, insecticides, rodenticides, and some plants. Inhalation of hydrogen cyanide may cause death within a minute; oral doses act more slowly, requiring several minutes to hours. Cyanide combines with cytochromes and catalase to produce tissue asphyxia. The treatment for cyanide poisoning includes the administration of intravenous sodium thiosulfate, which hastens the transformation of the cyanide to thiocyanate, which is excreted in the urine. *(Hardman, pp. 1892–1893)*

992. **(D)** Benzene is associated with bone marrow depression. Benzene is present to some extent in most gasolines, and poisoning may result from ingestion or from vapors. Acute benzene poisoning can cause severe CNS symptoms such as blurred vision, tremors, shallow and rapid respiration, ventricular irregularities, paralysis, and loss of consciousness. *(Hardman, p. 1888)*

993. **(F)** Ethylene glycol is widely used as antifreeze. It causes CNS depression and renal toxicity characterized by oxalate crystals in the tubules. As in methanol poisoning, ethanol is used as a competitive substance for alcohol dehydrogenase to decrease the rate of formation of toxic metabolites. *(Hardman, p. 1887)*

994. **(A, B)** Digitalis and verapamil decrease the refractoriness of the accessory pathways in WPW syndrome, and the ventricular rate can exceed 300/min. This can be life threatening and is treated with IV procainamide or cardioversion. *(Hardman, p. 939)*

995. **(F, J, K, L, M)** Numerous cardiac and noncardiac medications can cause torsades de pointes. Although it has been described with amiodarone, this is quite rare. The arrhythmia can result in sudden death. *(Hardman, p. 939)*

996. **(I)** This usually occurs in the setting of advanced lung disease. Treatment involves withdrawing theophylline and improving lung function. There may be some role for treatment with verapamil. *(Hardman, p. 939)*

997. **(A)** Digitalis causes numerous arrhythmias. Usual treatment is drug withdrawal, but in life-threatening occurrences antidigitalis antibodies have been used. *(Hardman, p. 939)*

998. **(C, G, L)** Melphalan is an alkylating agent of the nitrogen mustard type. Although not curative therapy, it is particularly useful in the management of multiple myeloma. *(Hardman, p. 1383)*

999. **(B, G, J)** Methotrexate is classified as an antimetabolite, and is a folic acid analogue. Other tumors where methotrexate has an effect include osteogenic sarcoma, mycosis fungoides, and lung cancer. *(Hardman, p. 1383)*

1000. **(A)** Bleomycin, a naturally occurring antibiotic, is useful in Hodgkin's disease, non-Hodgkin's lymphoma, and cancers of the testes, head and neck, skin, esophagus, lungs, and genitourinary tract. *(Hardman, p. 1384)*

1001. **(K)** Flutamide is an antiandrogen that is useful in prostate cancer. Leuprolide, a gonadotropin-releasing hormone analogue, and various estrogen compounds are the other hormonal type agents used in prostate cancer therapy. *(Hardman, p. 1385)*

1002. (C, G) Sensory loss is not a side effect of phenothiazines. Parkinson-like symptoms disappear when phenothiazine is withdrawn. Dystonic movements involve the mouth, tongue, and shoulder girdle. As well as having useful antipsychotic effects, phenothiazines are useful as antiemetics and antinausea agents. They can also potentiate the effects of sedatives, analgesics, and general anesthetics. Some phenothiazines are intrinsically sedating, but none of them commonly interfere with sleep. *(Hardman, pp. 490–493)*

1003. (B, F) The increased refractory period increase accounts for the effect on tachycardia. Similar effects are seen with procainamide. The slowed repolarization can result in a prolonged QT interval. Life-threatening polymorphic ventricular tachycardias (Torsade de pointes) can be provoked by quinidine. It is rarely used in modern practice. *(Hardman, pp. 965–966)*

1004. (A, C, D) Potassium iodide is not a bronchodilator. It assists in the liquefaction of sputum, as does glyceryl guaiacolate. Potassium iodide is also used to treat the lymphocutaneous form of sporotrichosis. It has been used for treatment of erythema nodosum and nodular vasculitis as well. In susceptible individuals, the beta$_2$-adrenergic blocking effect of propranolol can cause life-threatening bronchoconstriction. Ephedrine, isoproterenol, and albuterol are beta-adrenergic agonists. Ipratropium bromide results in bronchodilatation by its anticholinergic effect. Atropine does as well but is too toxic for routine asthma therapy. *(Hardman, pp. 736–747, 1310)*

1005. (B, F) Caffeine and other methylxanthines also stimulate acid production. Vagal cholinergic stimulation is a major stimulus for gastric secretion. Alcohol may increase secretion by stimulating gastrin and histamine release, as well as psychically. *(Hardman, p. 433)*

1006. (C) Xerostomia does not result from gingivitis. Radiation of salivary glands may cause permanent dryness secondary to gland atrophy. Atropine is a muscarinic cholinergic blocking agent. Besides depression of salivary and bronchial secretions, atropine causes dilation of the pupil, tachycardia, and numerous other signs and symptoms of parasympathetic blockade. *(Hardman, pp. 162–171)*

CHAPTER 14

Comprehensive Review
Questions

DIRECTIONS (Questions 1 through 100): Each of the numbered items or incomplete statements in this section is followed by answers or by completions of the statement. Select the ONE lettered answer or completion that is BEST in each case.

1. A 28-year-old man has purulent urethritis. A swab reveals gram-negative diplocci within neutrophils. The appropriate treatment is

   (A) intramuscular ceftriaxone plus oral doxycycline
   (B) oral penicillin G
   (C) intramuscular penicillin V
   (D) intramuscular ampicillin and oral penicillin V
   (E) intravenous (IV) tobramycin

2. Which of the following best characterizes a feature of geriatric patients compared to younger patients?

   (A) Medical problems are less complex.
   (B) They spend less money on housing.
   (C) Homeostasis is impaired.
   (D) Hepatic enzyme deterioration is a result of aging.
   (E) Senile dementia is a result of aging.

3. In patients suspected of having Alzheimer's disease, an initial search for reversible causes of dementia might include

   (A) electroencephalogram (EEG)
   (B) urine tests for heavy metals
   (C) thyroid function tests
   (D) red blood cell (RBC) folate
   (E) urinary and plasma amino acids

4. A 74-year-old woman develops atrial fibrillation. Her thyroid-stimulating hormone (TSH) level is very low. Other cardiac findings might include

   (A) aortic regurgitation
   (B) hypotension
   (C) soft S_1
   (D) systolic murmurs
   (E) soft S_2

5. A 74-year-old woman has metastatic bone disease on x-ray. The mediator least likely to be involved is

   (A) interleukin-6 (IL-6)
   (B) ectopic parathyroid hormone (PTH)
   (C) tumor necrosis factor (TNF)
   (D) interleukin-1 (IL-1)
   (E) prostaglandins

6. A 30-year-old woman develops acute onset of erythema nodosum, fever, malaise, and anorexia. Chest x-ray (CXR) reveals bilateral hilar lymphadenopathy and a left paratracheal lymph node. The most likely diagnosis is

   (A) acquired immune deficiency syndrome (AIDS)
   (B) rheumatic fever
   (C) sarcoidosis
   (D) tuberculosis
   (E) bronchogenic carcinoma

7. The imaging technique that is best able to measure regional brain substrate uptake and metabolic kinetics is

(A) magnetic resonance imaging (MRI)
(B) computed tomography (CT)
(C) positron emission tomography (PET)
(D) serial thallium scintigrams
(E) Doppler ultrasound

8. A 47-year-old man suddenly develops high fever and hypotension. He has a generalized erythematous macular rash and over the next day develops gangrene of his left leg. The most likely organism is

(A) *Corynebacterium diphtheriae*
(B) *Streptococcus* group C
(C) *Neisseria gonorrhoeae*
(D) *Streptococcus* group A
(E) *Salmonella enteritidis*

9. In malignant hypertension, the agent that reduces blood pressure immediately and is the easiest to administer is

(A) hydralazine
(B) labetalol
(C) methyldopa
(D) diazoxide
(E) nifedipine

10. Vacuolization of proximal tubular epithelium and loss of urinary concentrating ability is most likely to be associated with

(A) severe potassium depletion
(B) hypercalcemia
(C) gouty nephropathy
(D) diabetic nephropathy
(E) rheumatoid arthritis (RA)

11. A 13-year-old boy has periods when he seems to be unresponsive, associated with blinking of his eyes. These are momentary, and he seems normal thereafter. The most effective treatment would be

(A) phenytoin
(B) carbamazepine

(C) phenobarbital
(D) gabapentin
(E) ethosuximide

12. Which of the following lymphoid malignancies is invariably of B-cell origin?

(A) chronic lymphocytic leukemia (CLL)
(B) hairy cell leukemia
(C) Burkitt's lymphoma
(D) mycosis fungoides
(E) angioimmunoblastic lymphadenopathy

13. A patient with human immunodeficiency virus (HIV) infection may be considered to have progressed to category C with the presence of

(A) antibodies to HIV
(B) palpable lymphadenopathy
(C) invasive cervical cancer
(D) fever
(E) urticaria

14. Which of the following is more characteristic of ulcerative colitis when compared to regional enteritis?

(A) segmental involvement
(B) granulomas
(C) lymph node involvement
(D) rectal bleeding
(E) palpable abdominal mass

15. A 28-year-old pregnant woman develops sudden onset of dyspnea and tachycardia with no other physical findings. The most likely explanation is

(A) pulmonary emphysema
(B) pulmonary embolism
(C) myocardial infarction
(D) ventricular tachycardia
(E) lobar pneumonia

16. A 60-year-old man from a poor socioeconomic environment is admitted with an acute illness characterized by mental disturbances, bilateral sixth nerve palsy, and ataxic gait. He may require emergency treatment with

(A) thiamine
(B) lecithin
(C) vitamin D
(D) phenytoin
(E) diazepam

17. Which of the following is most characteristic of calcitonin?

(A) It increases bone resorption.
(B) It decreases renal calcium clearance.
(C) It is produced by hepatocytes.
(D) It raises blood phosphate.
(E) It binds to osteoclasts.

18. Following a severe sore throat, a 15-year-old boy feels unwell. He has had pain and swelling in his elbows and knees, and cardiac exam reveals new mitral regurgitation and tachycardia. Further examination might reveal

(A) chronic arthritis
(B) involvement of spinal joints
(C) subcutaneous nodules
(D) erythema nodosum
(E) meningeal irritation

19. A home parenteral nutrition program is most likely to be useful for patients with

(A) an untreatable disease
(B) a 4-day requirement for nutrition
(C) severe radiation enteritis
(D) neoplasms with bowel obstruction
(E) anorexia nervosa

20. The most important factor in selecting a patient as a potential heart transplant recipient is

(A) absence of long-standing pulmonary hypertension
(B) survival on mechanical assistance devices
(C) availability of a human lymphocyte antigen (HLA)-compatible donor
(D) age under 20 years
(E) ventricular ejection fraction over 80%

21. CLL can be best characterized as

(A) usually a T-cell disorder
(B) a disease of children
(C) responsive to splenectomy
(D) frequently asymptomatic
(E) most common in Orientals

22. A 69-year-old man with alcoholic cirrhosis develops confusion and sleep disturbance. The most likely cause is

(A) digoxin
(B) furosemide
(C) penicillin
(D) gastrointestinal (GI) bleeding
(E) stroke

23. An asymptomatic patient with glomerular hematuria is most likely to have

(A) diabetes mellitus
(B) amyloidosis
(C) immunoglobulin A (IgA) nephropathy (Berger's disease)
(D) focal glomerulosclerosis
(E) thalassemia minor

24. A 63-year-old man with a 60 pack/year history of smoking has been previously diagnosed as having emphysema. The most likely finding would be

(A) mild dyspnea
(B) copious purulent sputum
(C) hematocrit over 55%
(D) severe pulmonary hypertension at rest
(E) decreasing diffusing capacity

25. Muscle weakness in RA is best characterized as

(A) occurring after several months of pain and immobility
(B) showing a neutrophilic infiltrate on muscle biopsy
(C) secondary to vasculitis
(D) showing heavy mononuclear cell infiltrate on muscle biopsy
(E) showing type II fiber atrophy and muscle fiber necrosis on muscle biopsy

a-thalassemia leads to increased forma-
of hemoglobin

(A) H
(B) A
(C) F
(D) A$_2$
(E) C

27. Which of the following is most characteristic of diabetic neuropathy?

(A) It is usually bilateral.
(B) Pain is not a feature.
(C) It most commonly affects the brain.
(D) It spares the autonomic system.
(E) It responds to meticulous control of blood glucose.

28. A 57-year-old man, previously asymptomatic and on no medications, develops acute poda-gra. It is so painful that even the weight of his sheets is excruciating. Which of the following medications is relatively contraindi-cated?

(A) indomethacin
(B) colchicine
(C) ibuprofen
(D) allopurinol
(E) naproxen

29. Of the following, the most common cause of ischemic stroke is

(A) cerebral haemorrhage
(B) cerebral embolism
(C) arteritis
(D) dissecting aneurysm
(E) hemorrhage into atherosclerosis

30. Transfusion-related hepatitis that is not due to hepatitis B is most likely due to

(A) hepatitis A
(B) Epstein–Barr hepatitis
(C) hepatitis C
(D) hepatitis D
(E) enteric hepatitis

31. A 20-year-old man with abrupt onset of hematuria and proteinuria, accompanied by azotemia and salt and water retention, most likely has

(A) nephrotic syndrome
(B) multiple myeloma
(C) diabetic nephropathy
(D) nephrolithiasis
(E) acute glomerulonephritis

32. The most common symptom of duodenal ul-cer is

(A) epigastric pain
(B) nausea
(C) melena
(D) anorexia
(E) midback pain

33. An elderly patient receiving a blood transfu-sion for myelodysplastic syndrome develops tachypnea, lumbar pain, tachycardia, and nausea. The most likely explanation is

(A) anxiety
(B) fluid overload
(C) hemolysis
(D) pulmonary embolism
(E) acute leukemia

34. A 23-year-old pregnant woman in her first trimester develops hyperthyroidism. Which treatment is contraindicated?

(A) thyroid surgery
(B) propylthiouracil (PTU)
(C) drugs that cross the placenta
(D) radioactive iodine
(E) glucocorticoids

35. A 78-year-old woman is treated for depres-sion with nortriptyline. The most likely side effects are related to

(A) impaired cardiac contractility
(B) heart block
(C) weight loss
(D) anticholinergic side effects
(E) diarrhea

36. Mitral valve prolapse is most likely to be characterized by

    (A) a pansystolic murmur
    (B) a lifelong benign course
    (C) sudden death
    (D) infective endocarditis
    (E) highest incidence in men over age 50

37. A 14-year-old boy develops nephrotic syndrome. A renal biopsy shows foot process fusion and no deposits on the membranes under electron microscopy. The most likely lesion is

    (A) mesangial proliferative glomerulonephritis
    (B) minimal change disease
    (C) focal glomerulosclerosis
    (D) membranous glomerulonephritis
    (E) Goodpasture syndrome

38. A 65-year-old man with positive sputum cytology for malignant cells, but a normal CXR is best managed with

    (A) annual CXR
    (B) unilateral pneumonectomy
    (C) blind percutaneous needle biopsies
    (D) bronchoscopic brushings and biopsies
    (E) mediastinoscopy and biopsy

39. A dyspneic patient manifests a 20 mm Hg decrease in systolic arterial pressure during slow inspiration. The most likely cause is

    (A) cardiac tamponade
    (B) pulmonary hypertension
    (C) ventricular septal defect
    (D) coarctation of the aorta
    (E) malignant hypertension

40. Suppression of immune rejection of the transplanted kidney is best accomplished with

    (A) splenectomy and irradiation
    (B) plasmapheresis and steroids
    (C) cyclosporine and steroids
    (D) azathioprine and plasmapheresis
    (E) steroids and thymectomy

41. A 42-year-old woman has a history of loss of vision and eye pain that spontaneously reversed. She now has diplopia and weakness and spasticity in her right leg. The most likely diagnosis is

    (A) cerebral emboli
    (B) subclavian steal syndrome
    (C) Guillain–Barré syndrome
    (D) recurrent transient ischemic attacks (TIAs)
    (E) multiple sclerosis

42. A 16-year-old female presents with abdominal pain and purpuric spots on the skin. Laboratory investigation reveals a normal platelet count, with hematuria and proteinuria. The most likely diagnosis is

    (A) hemolytic–uremic syndrome
    (B) thrombotic thrombocytopenic purpura
    (C) heavy metal poisoning
    (D) subacute bacterial endocarditis (SBE)
    (E) Henoch–Schönlein purpura

43. Which of the following drugs causes an increase in the effective refractory period of the atrioventricular (AV) node?

    (A) bretylium
    (B) amiodarone
    (C) procainamide
    (D) quinidine
    (E) disopyramide

44. Postmenopausal women with hyperparathyroidism, who are unable to undergo surgery, may benefit from

    (A) estrogen therapy
    (B) androgen therapy
    (C) calcium therapy
    (D) radioiodine
    (E) IV phosphate

45. A 23-year-old man of African descent is treated for malaria contracted on a recent trip. He develops hemolysis after treatment is started. The most likely diagnosis is

    (A) fulminant malaria
    (B) paroxysmal nocturnal hemoglobinuria
    (C) hereditary spherocytosis
    (D) glucose-6-phosphatase dehydrogenase (G6PD) deficiency
    (E) microangiopathic hemolysis

46. Community-acquired pneumonia in a previously healthy 20-year-old woman is best initially treated with

    (A) carbenicillin
    (B) tobramycin
    (C) levofloxacin
    (D) methicillin
    (E) tetracycline

47. A 60-year-old man with polyuria, nocturia, and renal transport defects is most likely to have

    (A) acute nephritis
    (B) acute renal failure
    (C) renal tubular defects
    (D) nephrolithiasis
    (E) systolic hypertension

48. A 62-year-old man is found to have severe erosive esophagitis on endoscopy. The most effective treatment will work because it

    (A) binds to the ulcer bed
    (B) antagonizes H_2 receptors
    (C) inhibits acetylcholine
    (D) stimulates mucin secretion
    (E) inhibits parietal cell proton pump

49. A 70-year-old woman, previously in good health, is found to have an asymptomatic monoclonal immunoglobulin peak on serum electrophoresis. The most likely diagnosis is

    (A) monoclonal gammopathy of uncertain significance (MGUS)
    (B) multiple myeloma

    (C) Waldenström's macroglobulinemia
    (D) amyloidosis
    (E) non-Hodgkin's lymphoma

50. A 30-year-old woman with dryness of the mouth and cutaneous palpable purpura probably has

    (A) ankylosing spondylitis
    (B) mixed connective tissue disease
    (C) systemic sclerosis
    (D) thrombotic thrombocytopenic purpura
    (E) Sjögren syndrome

51. In an extreme emergency, patients may be transfused with unmatched blood from a donor who is

    (A) type AB
    (B) polycythemic
    (C) a sibling of the recipient
    (D) type O
    (E) Lewis A positive

52. In mild mitral stenosis, the earliest change on CXR is

    (A) general enlargement of the heart
    (B) Kerley B lines
    (C) attenuation of pulmonary arteries
    (D) straightening of the left heart border
    (E) diffuse modulation of the lower lung fields

53. A 25-year-old woman with diplopia, ptosis, weakness, and fatigability of muscles on repeated use is most likely to have

    (A) myasthenia gravis
    (B) multiple sclerosis
    (C) TIAs
    (D) muscular dystrophy
    (E) cerebral palsy

54. The group of women with the highest risk of developing breast cancer are

    (A) cousins of breast cancer patients
    (B) those receiving CXRs as children
    (C) those with late onset menarche

(D) multiparous

(E) those who have already had one breast cancer

55. Patients with cystic fibrosis are more likely to be diagnosed for the first time as adults if

(A) the reproductive system is not involved

(B) heatstroke occurs

(C) pulmonary hypertension is avoided

(D) GI disease is mild

(E) hypersplenism is prominent

56. A 25-year-old nonsmoking man has a 2-cm solitary pulmonary nodule in the left lower lobe, with a "popcorn ball" calcification. The best management would be

(A) left lower lobe resection

(B) serial CXRs

(C) needle aspiration biopsy

(D) left pneumonectomy

(E) mediastinoscopy

57. A 60-year-old man with unstable angina pectoris fails to respond to heparin, nitroglycerin, beta-adrenergic blockers, and calcium channel antagonists. The best management includes

(A) IV streptokinase

(B) coronary angiography

(C) exercise testing

(D) oral aspirin

(E) antihypertensive therapy

58. The major effect of glucocorticoids in asthma is

(A) anti-inflammatory

(B) bronchodilatory

(C) sedative

(D) mucus dissolving

(E) antibacterial

59. Immunofluorescence studies of focal glomerulosclerosis demonstrate

(A) nodular deposits of immunoglobulin M (IgM) and C_3

(B) linear deposits of immunoglobulin G (IgG)

(C) nothing

(D) granular deposits of IgG and C_4

(E) extensive fibrin strands

60. Burning retrosternal chest pain, radiating to the sides of the chest and aggravated by bending forward, is most likely to arise from the

(A) heart

(B) lumbar spine

(C) intercostal nerves

(D) pancreas

(E) esophagus

61. Raynaud's phenomenon associated with systemic sclerosis is best managed with

(A) amphetamines

(B) ergotamines

(C) beta-blocking drugs

(D) warmth

(E) surgical sympathectomy

62. The most common presentation of hemophilia A is

(A) hematuria

(B) melena

(C) hemarthrosis

(D) pressure neuropathy

(E) intracerebral haemorrhage

63. Three weeks after surgery to implant a mechanical aortic valve, a 70-year-old man develops chest pain, fever, leukocytosis, and increased jugular venous pressure. The most likely diagnosis is

(A) infection in the aortic valve

(B) postpericardiotomy syndrome

(C) cytomegalovirus (CMV) infection

(D) pulmonary embolism

(E) acute myocardial infarction

64. Which of the following typically causes a macrocytic anemia?

    (A) blind loop syndrome
    (B) iron deficiency
    (C) thalassemia
    (D) chronic inflammation
    (E) sideroblastic anemia

65. An 18-year-old woman develops weakness, weight gain, amenorrhea, abdominal striae, and behavioral abnormalities. Physical examination reveals lateral visual field loss. The most likely diagnosis is

    (A) a functional pituitary tumor
    (B) adrenal hyperplasia
    (C) anorexia nervosa with bulimia
    (D) glioblastoma multiforme
    (E) multiple sclerosis

66. Lipoprotein measurements in diabetes mellitus (DM) are likely to demonstrate

    (A) marked increase in chylomicrons
    (B) increase in intermediate-density lipoproteins (IDLs)
    (C) increase in low-density lipoproteins (LDLs)
    (D) lipoprotein lipase deficiency
    (E) an abnormal ratio of lipoproteins

67. A previously asymptomatic 62-year-old woman presents with sudden onset of severe midback pain. X-rays reveal an anterior compression fracture of T10. Other vertebral bodies show decreased density and prominent vertical striations. The most likely diagnosis is

    (A) multiple myeloma
    (B) metastatic breast cancer
    (C) vitamin D deficiency
    (D) osteoporosis
    (E) Paget's disease of bone

68. A 70-year-old man, with no evidence of heart disease, develops TIAs, and investigations suggest carotid artery involvement. The best

nonsurgical management would include long-term

    (A) heparin
    (B) aspirin
    (C) beta blockers
    (D) nonsteroidal anti-inflammatory drugs (NSAIDs)
    (E) calcium channel antagonists

69. A 60-year-old woman being investigated for menorrhagia is found, on history, to have lethargy, constipation, cold intolerance, and muscle stiffness. The most likely diagnosis is

    (A) uterine carcinoma
    (B) systemic lupus
    (C) hypothyroidism
    (D) severe iron deficiency
    (E) hypercalcemia

70. A 20-year-old patient with asymptomatic lymphadenopathy in the right supraclavicular area is found to have nodular sclerosing Hodgkin's disease on biopsy. There is no other evidence of disease. The best management is

    (A) combination chemotherapy with MOPP (mechlorethamine, vincristine [Oncovin], procarbazine, prednisone)
    (B) wide surgical excision following radiotherapy
    (C) combination chemotherapy with ABVD (Adriamycin [doxorubicin], bleomycin, vinblastine, dacarbazine)
    (D) radiotherapy alone
    (E) observation until symptoms occur

71. A 45-year-old man presents with weakness, fever, weight loss, and abdominal pain, and is found to be hypertensive and in renal failure. While being investigated, he has a focal seizure. Laboratory studies show a high erythrocyte sedimentation rate (ESR), anemia, and a positive test for hepatitis B surface antigen. The most likely diagnosis is

    (A) polyarteritis nodosa (PAN)
    (B) acute hepatitis B

(C) SBE

(D) multiple staphylococcal abscesses

(E) chronic active hepatitis

72. Patients with AIDS can have chorioretinitis with blindness, enteritis with intractable diarrhea, interstitial pneumonitis, and adrenalitis, all caused by infection with

(A) cryptosporidium

(B) herpes zoster

(C) *Toxoplasma*

(D) pneumocystis carinii pneumonia

(E) CMV

73. A patient with extrahepatic biliary obstruction is most likely to have

(A) negative urine bilirubin

(B) marked increase in conjugated bilirubin

(C) normal unconjugated bilirubin

(D) painless jaundice

(E) decrease in glucuronyl transferase

74. A 19-year-old man has a pigmented skin lesion. Which of the following characteristics suggests a dysplastic nevus (atypical mole) rather than a benign acquired nevus?

(A) uniform tan color

(B) located on buttock

(C) 4 mm in diameter

(D) 20 similar lesions on body

(E) located on back

75. In distinguishing prerenal azotemia from acute renal failure (ARF), the urine findings in prerenal azotemia should show

(A) urine osmolality less than 400

(B) brown granular casts

(C) urine creatinine less than 20

(D) a high fractional excretion of filtered sodium

(E) urine sodium of less than 20

76. Which of the following results of blood gas analysis is most likely in a patient with hyperventilation caused by anxiety?

(A) increased P_{CO_2}

(B) decreased P_{O_2}

(C) decreased pH

(D) decreased P_{CO_2}

(E) increased P_{O_2}

77. Following an acute myocardial infarct, the early injury pattern on electrocardiogram (ECG) is likely to show

(A) tall P waves

(B) prominent U waves

(C) small QRS complex

(D) elevated ST segments

(E) widened QRS complex

78. An emergency room patient with extreme lethargy admits to taking a large number of phenobarbital tablets. Management is likely to include

(A) acidification of urine to pH 3.0

(B) repetitive administration of activated charcoal

(C) ipecac to induce vomiting

(D) hemoperfusion

(E) hemodialysis

79. Five years after exposure to radiation from a nuclear reactor accident, the exposed population is in the greatest danger from

(A) aplastic anemia

(B) radiation dermatitis

(C) lung cancer

(D) multiple myeloma

(E) leukemia

80. Which of the following statements concerning progressive supranuclear palsy is correct?

(A) Tremor is the usual presenting symptom.

(B) Superior gaze impairment is the most common gaze abnormality.

(C) Dementia is a rare consequence.

(D) Men are more frequently affected.

(E) Response to L-dopa therapy is usually dramatic.

81. Which of the following diuretics will continue to induce significant diuresis after return of blood volume to normal levels?

    (A) hydrochlorothiazide
    (B) spironolactone
    (C) triamterene
    (D) furosemide
    (E) metolazone

82. The polyneuropathy that occurs in association with isoniazid (INH) can best be described as

    (A) acute
    (B) demyelinating
    (C) pure sensory
    (D) vitamin sensitive
    (E) pure motor

83. A patient with recurrent arthritis of the knees recalls an acute illness with fever and severe dermatitis 1 year earlier. The most likely diagnosis is

    (A) RA
    (B) Lyme disease
    (C) syphilis
    (D) PAN
    (E) systemic lupus erythematosus (SLE)

84. Zidovudine (AZT) is indicated for treatment of

    (A) retroviral infection
    (B) pneumocystis carinii pneumonia
    (C) Kaposi's sarcoma
    (D) toxoplasmosis
    (E) herpes simplex of the genitals

85. Which of the following statements concerning women's health issues is correct?

    (A) Breast cancer is the leading cause of death in U.S. women.
    (B) Men benefit more from thrombolytic therapy than women.
    (C) The mortality from acute myocardial infarction is greater in women than men.
    (D) Estrogen therapy decreases mortality in postmenopausal women primarily by its ability to prevent osteoporosis-related fractures.
    (E) Immune-related disorders are less common in women

86. Which of the following statements concerning hypertension during pregnancy is correct?

    (A) Pre-eclampsia becomes manifest during the end of the middle trimester.
    (B) Angiotensin-converting enzyme (ACE) inhibitors are useful antihypertensives in pregnant woman.
    (C) Pregnancy increases the risk for future renal impairment in the woman with essential hypertension.
    (D) Alpha-methyldopa is a useful antihypertensive in the pregnant woman.
    (E) Gestational hypertension infrequently recurs in subsequent pregnancies.

87. Which of the following statements concerning pregnancy and infection is correct?

    (A) Cytomegalovirus is the most common cause of congenital viral infection.
    (B) Postpartum infections are the most common cause of maternal mortality in the United States.
    (C) *N. gonorrhoeae* infection is transmitted to the child only during delivery.
    (D) Asymptomatic bacteriuria is common but unimportant in pregnant women.
    (E) HIV infection in newborns is invariably contracted during the first trimester

88. A 35-year-old man presents with left-sided periorbital headaches of severe intensity. He has been awakened from sleep for three nights in a row. He had similar headaches a year ago. These headaches

    (A) are likely tension headaches
    (B) are typical of common migraine (without an aura)
    (C) may be relieved by the vasodilation of alcohol

(D) usually recur in cycles lasting several months to years

(E) can be relieved by administration of oxygen

89. A 75-year-old woman presents with sudden onset of a communication disorder. She speaks fluently but in a series of incomprehensible syllables. She cannot read or repeat sounds or words. This syndrome is

(A) unlikely to improve with time

(B) usually associated with hemiparesis of the dominant side

(C) usually associated with hemiparesis of the nondominant side

(D) usually in the distribution of the posterior cerebral artery

(E) frequently associated with parietal lobe sensory defects

90. A 38-year-old man acutely develops severe retrosternal chest pain radiating to the back. It is aggravated by breathing and movement. He has always been in perfect health but did have a mild upper respiratory tract infection 1 week ago. His cardiogram is pictured in Figure 14–1. The syndrome is likely caused by

(A) occlusion of left anterior descending artery

(B) occlusion of circumflex artery

(C) a viral infection

(D) dissection of the aortic artery

(E) pneumococcal infection

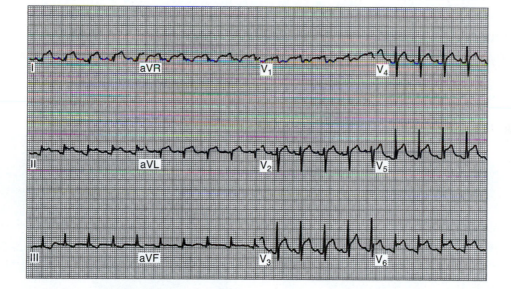

Figure 14–1.

91. A 27-year-old woman develops cough and fever with some sputum production. She is a nonsmoker and, although ill, is deemed to not require hospitalization. Her CXR is revealed in Figure 14–2. Her management will include

    (A) a repeat CXR in 2 weeks
    (B) a repeat CXR in 6 weeks
    (C) antibiotic coverage for *Legionella* infection
    (D) antibiotic coverage for *Mycoplasma* infection
    (E) antibiotic coverage for gram-negative infection

92. A 63-year-old man has had significant shortness of breath for 2 years. His CXR is revealed in Figure 14–3. The most likely diagnosis is

    (A) primary pulmonary hypertension
    (B) right ventricular dysfunction
    (C) left ventricular dysfunction
    (D) emphysema
    (E) mitral stenosis

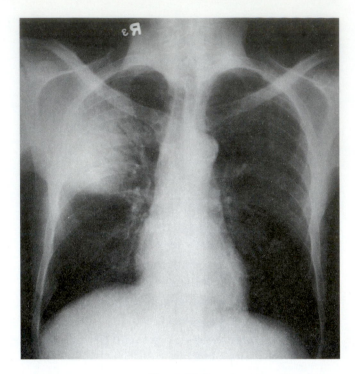

Figure 14–2.

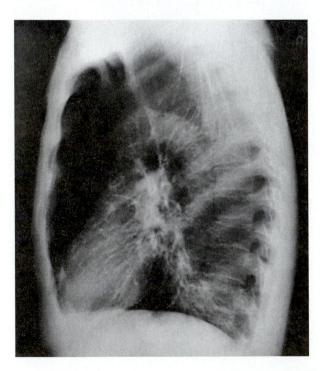
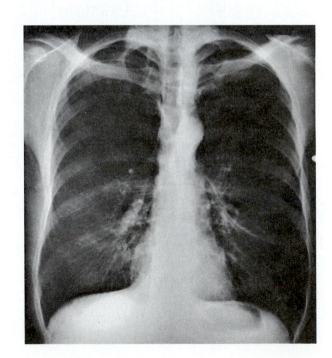

Figure 14–3.

93. A 42-year-old woman presents with fever, weight loss, and malaise. Physical examination reveals hypertension of 190/100 (normal 1 year earlier). Her ESR is 105, and urinalysis reveals numerous RBCs. Her abdominal angiogram is revealed in Figure 14–4. The most likely diagnosis is

(A) Wegener's granulomatosis

(B) rapidly progressive glomerulonephritis

(C) renal artery stenosis

(D) hypernephroma

(E) PAN

94. A 29-year-old man complains of back pain for several months. It takes him over 2 hours to limber up in the morning. His x-ray is shown in Figure 14–5. The most likely diagnosis is

(A) RA

(B) spondylolithiasis

(C) osteomalacia

(D) ankylosing spondylitis

(E) bone involvement with Hodgkin's disease

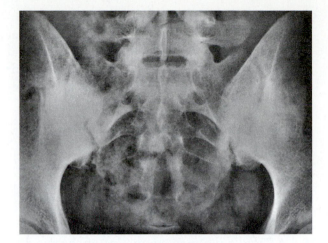

Figure 14–5.

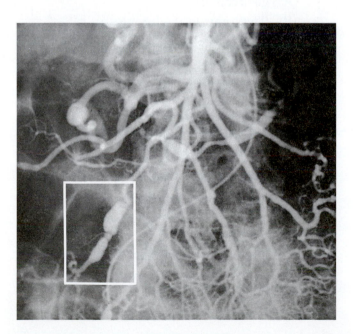

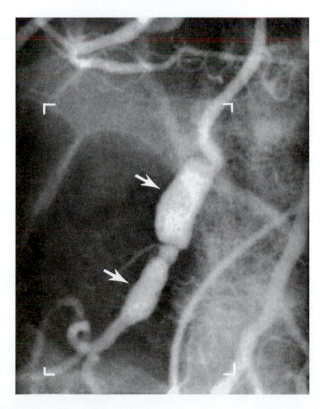

Figure 14–4.

95. A 69-year-old man has had mild arthritis involving many joints for several years. Over 1 or 2 days, he develops severe pain and swelling of his knee. His x-ray reveals calcifications in his articular cartilage. The most likely diagnosis is

    (A) acute gout
    (B) RA
    (C) pseudogout
    (D) infectious arthritis
    (E) torn ligament

96. A 75-year-old man complains of chronic dysphagia to fluids and solids. On occasion, he regurgitates food he has eaten 1 or 2 days before. Last year, he was hospitalized for pneumonia, but he is otherwise well. His x-ray is shown in Figure 14–6. The most likely definitive treatment is

    (A) endoscopic dilatation
    (B) myotomy

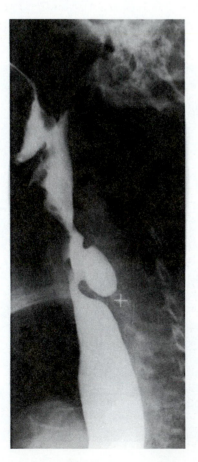

Figure 14–6.

(C) balloon dilatation of lower esophageal sphincter
(D) surgical excision
(E) vigorous antireflux therapy with surgery if medical management fails

97. A 69-year-old woman is feeling fatigued. Blood work reveals a hemoglobin of 90 g/L (14 g/L 1 year earlier). She has no other symptoms. Her blood film is shown in Figure 14–7. The most likely next investigation is

    (A) serum B_{12} level
    (B) hemoglobin electrophoresis
    (C) colonoscopy
    (D) bone marrow aspiration
    (E) sickle-cell preparation

98. A 94-year-old female nursing home resident is referred for evaluation of anemia of 8 g/L. She is demented, and adequate documentation of her past medical history is not available. She eats well and is cooperative. Examination reveals evidence of cognitive impairment, primitive reflexes, and a well-healed midline abdominal scar, likely many years old. Her blood film is shown in Figure 14–8. Presuming a relationship with the anemia, the most likely kind of surgery she received is

    (A) gastrectomy
    (B) vagotomy and pyloroplasty
    (C) cholecystectomy
    (D) right hemicolectomy
    (E) common bile duct exploration

99. A 42-year-old man suffers a myocardial infarction during coronary angiography. The physician who testifies as an expert witness

    (A) must be the defendant's physician
    (B) must be the plaintiff's physician
    (C) will have seen the claimant after the incident
    (D) might never have seen the claimant
    (E) may not review a hospital record

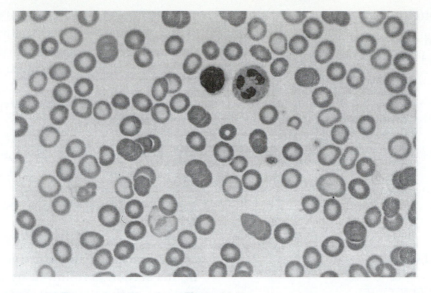

Figure 14–7.

100. An asymptomatic 59-year-old man treated with oral anticoagulants for atrial fibrillation suffers a cerebral hemorrhage. Under actions in tort in common law, recovery of damages requires that the injured party show the

(A) plaintiff owed the defendant a duty
(B) plaintiff suffered injuries
(C) plaintiff's conduct breached a duty
(D) victim's negligence contributed to the injury
(E) plaintiff neglected the defendant

DIRECTIONS (Questions 101 through 113): Each set of matching questions in this section consists of a list of lettered options followed by several numbered items. For each numbered item, select the appropriate lettered option(s). Each lettered option may be selected once, more than once, or not at all. EACH ITEM WILL STATE THE NUMBER OF OPTIONS TO SELECT. CHOOSE EXACTLY THIS NUMBER.

Match the appropriate statement about pharmacology with each of the following medications.

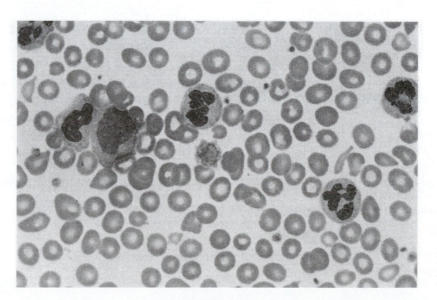

Figure 14–8.

Questions 101 through 105

    (A) increased sensitivity with aging

    (B) decreased sensitivity with aging

    (C) altered excretion with aging

    (D) altered metabolism with aging

    (E) altered distribution with aging

101. Beta blockers (SELECT ONE)

102. Nitrazepam (SELECT ONE)

103. Warfarin (SELECT ONE)

104. Lithium (SELECT ONE)

105. Fentanyl (SELECT ONE)

Questions 106 through 110

    (A) selective serotonin reuptake inhibitors (SSRIs)

    (B) mineral oil

    (C) diuretics

    (D) INH

    (E) phenytoin and phenobarbital

    (F) salicylates

    (G) corticosteroids

    (H) L-dopa

106. Disinterest in food with protein/calorie malnutrition (SELECT ONE)

107. Zinc deficiency (SELECT ONE)

108. Vitamin B_6 deficiency (SELECT ONE)

109. Impaired calcium absorption (SELECT ONE)

110. Altered vitamin D metabolism (SELECT ONE)

Questions 111 through 113

    (A) sleep more than younger adults

    (B) increased arousals during the night

    (C) increased slow-wave sleep

    (D) sleep improved with alcohol

    (E) most common cause of excessive daytime sleepiness in the elderly

    (F) breakdown of normal temporal organization of sleep–wake cycling

111. A common change in sleep as people age (SELECT ONE)

112. Common in a 73-year-old woman with Alzheimer's disease (SELECT TWO)

113. Sleep apnea syndrome (SELECT ONE)

DIRECTIONS (Questions 114 through 118): Each of the numbered items or incomplete statements in this section is followed by answers or by completions of the statement. Select the ONE lettered answer or completion that is BEST in each case.

A 73-year-old man is brought into the hospital by his family. He is very confused, but collateral history reveals that this is new. Physical examination reveals crackles in his lungs, some abdominal distension, and bilateral asterixis.

114. The first urgent radiological examination would be

    (A) CT scan of head

    (B) CT scan of head with enhancement

    (C) chest x-ray

    (D) MRI of head

    (E) spiral CT of chest

115. Extensive investigation does not reveal a specific cause of confusion in this man, and the medical service wonders whether the true diagnosis is dementia. Which of the following cognitive or behavioral impairments is more typical of delirium than dementia?

    (A) impaired long-term memory

    (B) paranoid behavior

    (C) language impairment

    (D) impaired attention

    (E) fluctuating performance

116. Further investigations reveal a urinary tract infection, and the man improves somewhat after treatment, but still exhibits poor judgement and bizarre behavior. Pressing the family for information, the intern unearths a history of 8 years of progressive bizarre behavior. The man has undressed himself and made sexual advances to young female relatives, has urinated in hallways, and pushes food into his mouth with alarming speed. The likely diagnosis is

    (A) Alzheimer's disease
    (B) frontotemporal dementia
    (C) dementia with diffuse Lewy bodies
    (D) vascular dementia
    (E) benign frontal tumor

117. The most common reason for institutionalization for this man who lives with a supportive family would be

    (A) inability to perform instrumental activities of daily living (IADLs)
    (B) immobility
    (C) forgetfulness
    (D) intolerable behavior
    (E) incontinence

118. At death, pathological examination is likely to reveal

    (A) amyloid plaques
    (B) lacunar infarcts
    (C) diffuse Lewy bodies
    (D) pigmentary degeneration
    (E) neurofibrillary tangles

Answers and Explanations

1. **(A)** Since 1986, increasing penicillin resistance has meant that penicillin/ampicillin are no longer drugs of choice. Alternatives to ceftriaxone include ciprofloxacin, ofloxacin, or cefixime given orally, with 7 days of doxycycline or a single 1 gram dose of azithromycin in case of coinfection with *Chlamydia*. In pregnant women, erythromycin replaces doxycycline. Disseminated gonococcal infection should be treated in a hospital with IV antibiotics. *(Braunwald, pp. 936–937)*

2. **(C)** The impaired physiologic reserve of every organ system is characteristic of aging. The term *homeostenosis* has been used to describe this phenomenon. Decline in most systems starts in the third decade and is gradual and progressive. Decrements in each organ system seem independent of other systems and are influenced by diet, environment, personal habits (eg, exercise), and genetic factors, as well as just chronological age. At times, it can be difficult to differentiate between age-related physiologic change and age-related diseases. *(Braunwald, p. 37)*

3. **(C)** Other tests to rule out reversible disease might include serum electrolytes, B_{12} levels, complete blood count (CBC), Venereal Disease Research Laboratory (VDRL), and CT or MRI. Diagnosis of Alzheimer's disease remains a diagnosis of exclusion. However, the insidious and subtle onset, with few focal signs (except for higher mental functioning) and a slowly progressive course are characteristic. Careful attention to the pattern of cognitive defects also improves diagnostic accuracy. The intensity of investigation will depend on numerous factors, including age, presence of atypical findings, and the timing of presentation. There is as yet no definite consensus on the most appropriate plan of investigation. *(Braunwald, pp. 150, 2392)*

4. **(D)** Cardiac complications are more common in the elderly patient and may dominate the clinical presentation. There is often a wide pulse pressure, systolic murmurs, increased intensity of the first heart sound, and cardiomegaly. Sinus tachycardia and atrial fibrillation are the most common arrhythmias. A to-and-fro high-pitched sound in the pulmonic area (Means–Lerman scratch) can mimic a pericardial friction rub. *(Braunwald, p. 1375)*

5. **(B)** A whole host of locally produced hormones and cytokines, as well as ectopically produced hormones, are implicated in local osteoclastic hypercalcemia. Parathormone-related protein is often elevated in malignant hypercalcemia (with or without bony metastases), but ectopic PTH production in malignancy is quite rare. *(Braunwald, pp. 646–647)*

6. **(C)** Sarcoidosis presents as an asymptomatic CXR in at least 10 to 20% of cases in the United States, but more frequently in countries where pre-employment CXRs are mandatory. At least 40% of patients present with acute symptoms and hilar lymphadenopathy. Approximately 90% will have an abnormal CXR at some point in their illness. Only a small proportion develop progressive disease. *(Braunwald, pp. 1970–1971)*

7. **(C)** PET scans use glucose analogues to demonstrate metabolic activity. They are rarely available, however, and functional MRI scans are now being used extensively to assess areas of brain activity. *(Braunwald, p. 2340)*

8. **(D)** *Streptococcus* group A can cause a toxic shock–like syndrome, and has been increasing in frequency in North America. Streptococcal toxic shock–like syndrome was so named because of its similarity to staphylococcal toxic shock syndrome. The illness includes fever, hypotension, renal impairment, and the respiratory distress syndrome. It is usually caused by strains that produce exotoxin. It may be associated with localized infection as well; the most common associated infection is a soft tissue infection such as necrotizing fasciitis. The mortality is high (up to 30%), usually secondary to shock and respiratory failure. The rapid progression of the disease and its high mortality demand early recognition and aggressive treatment. Management includes fluid resuscitation, pressor agents, mechanical ventilation, antibodies, and, if necrotizing fasciitis is present, surgical débridement. *(Braunwald, pp. 905–906)*

9. **(D)** Diazoxide acts immediately in malignant hypertension and is the easiest to administer for no individual titration of dosage is required. Nitroprusside is more effective, but requires an intravenous infusion. Labetalol is also useful but has more contraindications. It is particularly useful in the setting of angina or myocardial infarction. Regardless of which drug is selected, early administration of medications for long-term control is mandatory. *(Braunwald, p. 1429)*

10. **(A)** Hypokalemia, if severe and protracted, leads to tubular vacuolization and ultimately glomerular loss. Early changes are reversible with potassium repletion. Nocturia, polyuria, and polydipsia are common symptoms in hypokalemic nephropathy. Urinalysis is not remarkable, and urea and creatinine are not remarkable. After correction of hypokalemia, maximal urinary concentrating ability might not return to normal for several months. *(Braunwald, p. 1609)*

11. **(E)** Ethosuximide and valproic acid are common medications used to treat petit mal epilepsy. Side effects of ethosuximide include GI irritation, skin rash, and bone marrow suppression. *(Braunwald, pp. 2364–2365)*

12. **(B)** Hairy cell leukemia is a B-cell malignancy. Burkitt's lymphoma is of T-cell origin 5% of the time. CLL can be of T- or B-cell origin. Mycosis fungoides and angioimmunoblastic lymphadenopathy are of T-cell origin. *(Braunwald, p. 724)*

13. **(C)** The current case definition of AIDS in a patient with HIV infection is done by symptoms and $CD4^+$ T-lymphocyte cell count. Any category C symptoms (eg, cervical cancer, mycobacterium avium infection, CMV, retinitis, etc.) indicates frank AIDS as does a $CD4^+$ T-cell count less than 200 per microliter regardless of symptoms. *(Braunwald, pp. 1852–1853)*

14. **(D)** Rectal bleeding is more characteristic of ulcerative colitis, as is malignancy with long-standing disease, but both can occur in regional enteritis. Transmural involvement, lymph node involvement, skip lesions, granulomas, and anorectal complications (abscesses, fistulas, fissures) are characteristic of Crohn's disease. *(Braunwald, pp. 1682–1683)*

15. **(B)** Sudden onset of unexplained dyspnea is the most common and often the only symptom of pulmonary embolism. Findings on physical examination may be deceptively normal, but tachycardia is a consistent finding. Pleuritic chest pain and hemoptysis suggest a peripheral embolism adjacent to the pleura. *(Braunwald, p. 1509)*

16. **(A)** The patient has Wernicke's encephalopathy and requires treatment with thiamine. A delay of a few hours may permit progression to psychosis. The eye findings in Wernicke's encephalopathy include bilateral (but not necessarily symmetrical) abductor weakness

or paralysis, horizontal diplopia, strabismus, and nystagmus. The nystagmus is most frequently horizontal or vertical gaze-evoked nystagmus. *(Braunwald, p. 2496)*

17. **(E)** Calcitonin is secreted by cells in the thyroid. Calcitonin reduces bone resorption and increases renal calcium clearance. The inhibition of osteoclast-mediated bone resorption and the stimulation of renal calcium clearance are mediated by receptors on osteoclasts and renal tubular cells. Other receptors to calcitonin are present in the brain, GI tract, and immune system. *(Braunwald, pp. 2208–2209)*

18. **(C)** Major manifestations of rheumatic fever include carditis, migratory polyarthritis, chorea, erythema marginatum, and subcutaneous nodules. Minor manifestations include arthralgia, fever, elevated acute phase reactants (ESR, C-reactive protein), and prolonged P-R interval. The diagnosis is made with two major or one major and two minor criteria, and evidence of group A streptococcal infection (positive throat culture or rapid streptococcal antigen test, or rising antibody titers). *(Braunwald, p. 1341)*

19. **(C)** Home parenteral nutrition is usually helpful in extreme short-bowel syndrome, chronic obstruction due to adhesions, and severe radiation enteritis. Placement of a central venous catheter, careful calculation of fluid and nutritional requirements, and meticulous monitoring are required in a long-term parenteral nutrition program. *(Braunwald, p. 474)*

20. **(A)** In selecting a heart for transplantation, size, ABO match, negative lymphocyte cross-match, and other disease states, are important factors. The presence of severe pulmonary hypertension can result in intraoperative death. In the United States, it is estimated that only 2000 potential donor hearts become available each year for 20,000 potential recipients. This means that careful recipient selection is very important. The optimal candidates will have a high likelihood of return to a high level of function, to be mentally vigorous and medically compliant. *(Braunwald, p. 1329)*

21. **(D)** CLL is frequently discovered on routine evaluation of elderly patients and may not require treatment for several years. Splenomegaly, when present, rarely leads to symptoms. It is usually a disorder of B cells and is very indolent in its course. Most therapeutic regimens are designed for symptom control, not cure. Common reasons for treatment include hemolytic anemia, cytopenias, disfiguring lymphadenopathy, symptomatic organomegaly, or systemic symptoms. Chlorambucil is easy to administer, but fludarabine is considerably more effective. It requires intravenous administration. Maintenance therapy is not helpful. *(Braunwald, p. 720)*

22. **(D)** GI bleeding is the most common precipitating factor for hepatic encephalopathy. Furosemide, by causing hypokalemia, is another common cause. Narcotics and sedatives are also frequently implicated. *(Braunwald, p. 1765)*

23. **(C)** Other causes of asymptomatic hematuria, with or without proteinuria, include sickle-cell disease, Alport syndrome, resolving glomerulonephritis, and thin basement disease. Berger's disease is characterized by IgA deposits in the mesangium. It most commonly affects older children and young adults, and is more common in blacks than whites. Macroscopic hematuria may occur with intercurrent illness or vigorous exercise. The prognosis is variable but tends to progress slowly. Spontaneous remissions are more common in children than in adults. About 20 to 50% of patients develop end-stage renal disease within 20 years of diagnosis. *(Braunwald, p. 1588)*

24. **(E)** Chronic obstructive pulmonary disease (COPD) due to emphysema usually demonstrates severe dyspnea, scanty mucoid sputum, and normal hematocrit. Chronic bronchitis is characterized by milder dyspnea, greater sputum production, more frequent hypercarbia and polycythemia, and more evidence of cor pulmonale and pulmonary hypertension. *(Braunwald, p. 1495)*

25. (E) Muscle weakness in RA is common and can occur within weeks of onset of RA. It is most apparent in muscles adjacent to involved joints. There is not usually a vasculitis present, although a mononuclear infiltrate may be present. The most common finding on biopsy is type II fiber atrophy and muscle fiber necrosis. *(Braunwald, p. 1932)*

26. (A) Alpha-thalassemia involves a decrease in alpha-chain production and leads to the formation of beta-globin tetramers known as hemoglobin H. Individuals normally inherit four alpha-chain genes. The clinical syndrome depends on how many genes are deleted. Deletion of one gene results in a silent carrier state. Deletion of all four is the most severe and presents as hydrops fetalis. This condition is incompatible with life. *(Braunwald, p. 672)*

27. (A) Diabetic neuropathy usually presents as peripheral polyneuropathy, usually bilateral, including symptoms of numbness, paresthesia, severe hyperesthesia, and pain. Impairment of proprioceptive fibers can lead to gait abnormalities and Charcot joints. Mononeuropathy is less common and is often spontaneously reversible. Common syndromes include wrist or foot drop and third, fourth, or sixth cranial nerve palsies. Autonomic neuropathy may cause gastroesophageal dysfunction, bladder dysfunction, and orthostatic hypotension. *(Braunwald, pp. 2122–2123)*

28. (D) Uricosuric drugs and allopurinol have no role in the treatment of acute gouty arthritis. Salicylates are also not used in the treatment of gout. The treatments of choice are colchicine, NSAIDs, and intra-articular steroid injection. Response is best when initiated early in the disease. Colchicine can be given intravenously to avoid GI distress. A short course of systemic corticosteroids is also quite effective therapy. Allopurinol is started only when all inflammation is gone and colchicine prophylaxis has been started. It is not always required. *(Braunwald, p. 1995)*

29. (B) The two broad categories of ischemic stroke are embolic and thrombotic. Emboli can originate from an arterial atheroma (eg, common carotid bifurcation) or from the heart. In the latter case, anticoagulants are often indicated. On occasion emboli occur without obvious source (eg, hypercoagulable states, malignancy, eclampsia). *(Braunwald, pp. 2369–2371)*

30. (C) Screening for antibodies to hepatitis C has reduced the incidence of this infection, but numerous chronic cases remain. Treatment options include interferon and ribavirin. The hepatitis C virus is a linear, single-stranded ribonucleic acid (RNA) virus. There are at least six distinct genotypes. *(Braunwald, pp. 1729, 1746)*

31. (E) Causes of acute glomerulonephritis include infectious diseases, especially *Streptococcus*, vasculitides, and primary glomerular disease. The acute nephritic syndrome consists of the abrupt onset of hematuria and proteinuria, often accompanied by azotemia and renal salt and water retention. Oliguria may be present. *(Braunwald, pp. 1580–1584)*

32. (A) The pain may be described as sharp, burning, or gnawing, usually 90 minutes to 3 hours after eating, relieved by food or antacids. The pain frequently awakens the patient at night. Symptoms are usually episodic and recurrent. Periods of remission are usually longer than periods with pain. The ulcer crater can recur or persist in the absence of pain. Only a minority of patients with dyspepsia are found to have an ulcer on endoscopy. *(Braunwald, p. 1654)*

33. (C) Intravascular hemolysis from blood transfusion is usually due to ABO incompatibility, often from human error. Symptoms of intravascular hemolysis include flushing, pain at the infusion site, chest or back pain, restlessness, anxiety, nausea, and diarrhea. Signs include fever and chills, shock, and renal failure. In comatose patients, hemoglobulinuria or bleeding from disseminated intravascular coagulation can be the first sign. Management is supportive. Acute hemolysis can also result from antibodies directed against other red blood cell antigens such as Rh, Kell, or Duffy. *(Braunwald, p. 736)*

34. **(D)** Radioactive iodine is contraindicated both in scanning and treatment as it damages the fetal thyroid. Propylthiouracil crosses the placenta, but is safe and effective in pregnancy. The lowest effective dose should be used. Hyperthyroidism is hardest to control in the first trimester and easiest in the third trimester. *(Braunwald, pp. 28, 2073)*

35. **(D)** Antihistamine side effects (sedation) and anticholinergic side effects (dry mouth, constipation, urinary hesitancy, blurred vision) are the most common side effects. Orthostasis is probably the most common serious side effect and is difficult to manage. Severe cardiac toxicity is uncommon and diarrhea and weight loss are associated with SSRI antidepressants. *(Braunwald, p. 2544)*

36. **(B)** The most common pathogenic mechanism is thought to be excessive or redundant mitral leaflet tissue, with the posterior leaflet more commonly involved. Myxomatous degeneration can also be seen on pathological examination. Reassurance regarding the benign nature of the disease is the mainstay of management. When a murmur is present, antibiotic prophylaxis for endocarditis is warranted. *(Braunwald, p. 1348)*

37. **(B)** Little or no changes are seen on light microscopy in this syndrome. The disease is most common in children. Spontaneous remission is common in children and is enhanced by steroid therapy. Over 95% of children achieve remission within 8 weeks of institution of prednisone therapy. Therefore, in children with nephrotic syndrome, empiric therapy is frequently employed, rather than initial renal biopsy. Only 50% of adults will remit, and thus biopsy is more frequently required. Relapse is common in both children and adults. *(Braunwald, p. 1585)*

38. **(D)** Over 90% of lesions can be localized by fiberoptic bronchoscope in the sedated, but awake, patient and collection of a series of differential brushings and biopsies. When lesions are found, conservative resection is usually performed. Five-year cure rates in such lesions approach 60%, but second primaries are common (5% per patient per year). There is no evidence that screening programs based on sputum examination will decrease mortality. *(Braunwald, pp. 502, 1455)*

39. **(A)** This is an important clue to cardiac tamponade, called paradoxical pulse. When severe, the arterial pulse may weaken on palpation during inspiration. Pulsus paradoxus is uncommon in constrictive pericarditis and rare in restrictive cardiomyopathy. It is commonly found in severe asthma as well. *(Braunwald, p. 1256)*

40. **(C)** Cyclosporine A blocks production of interleukin-2 (IL-2) by helper–inducer (CD4$^+$) T cells. It works alone but is more effective in combination with glucocorticoids. The use of cyclosporine has improved 1-year cadaveric survival rates to the 80 to 85% range. Side effects include hepatotoxicity, hirsutism, tremor, and gingival hyperplasia, but only the nephrotoxicity presents a serious management problem. *(Braunwald, pp. 1567–1571)*

41. **(E)** Typically, multiple sclerosis presents with optic neuritis. There is usually a history of at least two episodes of neurologic deficit at more than one site. Other common presenting symptoms include weakness, sensory loss, and parasthesias. *(Braunwald, pp. 2454–2455)*

42. **(E)** Other symptoms include arthralgia and GI function abnormalities. Renal biopsy shows immunoglobulin deposits. There is an underlying vasculitis. The prognosis is generally good, although relapses can occur before the final remission. *(Braunwald, p. 1965)*

43. **(B)** Amiodarone causes a decrease in the sinus rate and an increase in the effective re-

fractory period in the atrium, the AV node, and the ventricle. The pharmacology of amiodarone is complex and incompletely understood. *(Fuster, p. 914)*

44. **(A)** Estrogen therapy may retard demineralization of the skeleton and may also reduce blood and urinary calcium levels. However, there is insufficient evidence for a formal recommendation. There is no clear consensus on when asymptomatic hyperparathyroidism requires surgery. Many experts will elect to follow elderly patients with mild hyperparathyroidism who are asymptomatic and have normal renal function and bone mass. *(Braunwald, p. 2212)*

45. **(D)** Other drugs, besides antimalarials, that precipitate hemolysis in G6PD deficiency include dapsone, phenacetin, doxorubicin, and nalidixic acid. The disease is sex linked and thus most common in males. About 11% of people of African descent have an abnormal allele. Female heterozygotes have a dual population of red cells and, depending on the proportion, may develop symptoms. During hemolysis, older red cells with the lowest enzyme levels are destroyed, and diagnostic tests done at this time may be falsely normal. They should be repeated some time after the hemolysis has resolved. *(Braunwald, pp. 433, 437, 685–686)*

46. **(C)** Levofloxacin would be effective for most strains of *Streptococcus pneumoniae, Legionella pneumophila,* and other likely pathogens. Other commonly used drugs for community-acquired pneumonia are amoxicillin, cefuroxime, trimethoprim-sulfamethoxazole, and doxycycline. Theoretically, empiric therapy should be guided by knowledge of local resistance patterns. *(Braunwald, pp. 1481–1482)*

47. **(C)** Other clues to renal tubule defects include electrolyte disorders, renal osteodystrophy, large kidneys, and proteinuria. Categories of tubulointerstitial kidney disease include toxins (exogenous and metabolic), neoplasia, immune diseases, vascular disorders, infections, and hereditary renal dis-

eases. Defects in urinary acidification and concentrating ability are frequently the most troublesome manifestations of tubulointerstitial kidney disease. *(Braunwald, p. 1606)*

48. **(E)** Proton pump inhibitors (eg, omeprazole and lansoprazole) are the most effective treatments for ulcerative esophagitis. Antacids, sulcalfrate, and H_2 blockers are all useful in less severe reflux disease. *(Braunwald, p. 240)*

49. **(A)** MGUS is vastly more common than multiple myeloma, occurring in 1% of the population over age 50. Patients with MGUS have smaller M components (usually < 20 g/L); no urinary Bence Jones protein; less than 5% marrow plasmacytosis; and no anemia, renal failure, lytic bone lesions, or hypercalcemia. About 25% of patients with MGUS will go on to develop multiple myeloma. *(Braunwald, p. 730)*

50. **(E)** Sjögren syndrome is an immunologic disorder characterized by progressive destruction of the exocrine glands leading to mucosal dryness. Pathology reveals lymphocytic infiltration. About one third develop systemic (nonglandular) symptoms. The most common systemic manifestation is arthritis or arthralgia. If vasculitis occurs, purpura, urticaria, skin ulcers, and mononeuropathy are its most common manifestations. *(Braunwald, pp. 1947–1949)*

51. **(D)** The type O donor may contain sufficient anti-A or anti-B to destroy some of the patient's RBCs, but this is seldom clinically significant. Generally, however, crystalloid or colloid solutions are sufficient for volume replacement until properly matched blood is available. *(Braunwald, p. 734)*

52. **(D)** Other early changes in mitral stenosis include prominence of the main pulmonary arteries and backward displacement of the esophagus. The CXR changes are caused by enlargement of the left atrium. Severe disease can cause pulmonary congestion (Kerley B lines) and enlargement of the right ventricle, right atrium, and superior vena cava. *(Braunwald, p. 1345)*

53. **(A)** The distribution of muscle weakness is characteristic with early involvement of the cranial nerves, especially the lids and extraocular muscles. Women are more frequently affected than men (3:2 ratio), and the age for peak incidence in women is in the third or fourth decade. *(Braunwald, p. 2516)*

54. **(E)** History of one breast cancer is a risk factor for a second tumor. Risk of breast cancer is increased in women with a family history, early menarche, late menopause, nulliparity, and late age at first pregnancy. Obesity, alcohol, and dietary fat are other possible risk factors. *(Braunwald, p. 572)*

55. **(D)** Patients with minimal or absent GI symptoms and atypical respiratory symptoms may be diagnosed as adults. This accounts for 7% of cases. Moreover, because of modern therapy, about 36% of CF patients in the United States are over 18 years of age, and 12% are over 30. *(Braunwald, pp. 1487–1490)*

56. **(B)** Signs of benignity of a solitary pulmonary nodule are lack of growth over a prolonged period and certain patterns of calcification. "Popcorn" calcification does suggest a benign hamartoma. A search for previous CXRs can provide a definitive diagnosis. In nonsmokers under age 35 more than 1% of solitary pulmonary nodules are malignant. *(Braunwald, p. 568)*

57. **(B)** A period of 24 to 48 hours is usually allowed to attempt medical therapy. Cardiac catheterization and angiography may be followed by bypass surgery or angioplasty. For those who do settle down, some form of subsequent risk stratification (eg, exercise ECG) is indicated. *(Braunwald, p. 1406)*

58. **(A)** Glucocorticoids are not bronchodilators, and their major use is in reducing airway inflammation. It is difficult to provide precise recommendations for their use, and a wide range of systemic and inhaled doses are used. *(Braunwald, p. 1461)*

59. **(C)** Immunofluorescence is usually negative. By electron microscopy, focal basement membrane collapse and denudation of epithelial surfaces are noted. The course is generally progressive in adults. It is believed that remission of proteinuria with steroid therapy will improve the prognosis. Cytotoxic drugs and cyclosporine have also been used in treatment. The degree of proteinuria correlates with the likelihood of developing renal failure. The disease recurs rapidly in transplanted kidneys, suggesting a humoral factor in pathogenesis. *(Braunwald, p. 1586)*

60. **(E)** Heartburn is a characteristic symptom of reflux esophagitis and may be associated with regurgitation. Odynophagia and atypical chest pain also occur in esophageal disease. *(Braunwald, p. 239)*

61. **(D)** Surgical sympathectomy usually provides only temporary improvement and does not prevent progression of the vascular lesion. Nifedipine is now the drug of choice for treating symptoms not responding to local warming measures (gloves, mitts) and avoidance of smoking and cold. Reserpine, alphamethyldopa, and prazosin may also be useful. *(Braunwald, p. 1439)*

62. **(C)** The most common presentation is with pain in a weight-bearing joint such as the hip, knee, or ankle. Hematuria is also common. Bleeding can occur at almost any site without prior trauma. *(Braunwald, p. 751)*

63. **(B)** The principal symptom is the pain of acute pericarditis that usually develops 1 to 4 weeks following the cardiac surgery but could appear after months. It can also occur after myocardial infarction (Dressler syndrome) or after trauma to the heart (stab wound, blunt trauma). The syndrome can remit and recur for up to 2 years. The acute symptoms usually subside in 1 or 2 weeks. *(Braunwald, p. 1369)*

64. **(A)** Blind loop syndrome leads to megaloblastic anemia and macrocytosis because of B_{12} deficiency. The deficiency is caused by colonization with bacteria that takes up ingested cobalamin before it can be absorbed.

The other conditions generally cause microcytic or normocytic anemias. *(Beutler, p. 426)*

65. **(A)** The patient has Cushing syndrome secondary to an adrenocorticotropic hormone (ACTH)-secreting pituitary tumor. Relatively few of such patients have a large pituitary tumor that affects the visual pathways. Over 50% have a microadenoma which is under 5 mm in diameter. *(Braunwald, p. 2091)*

66. **(E)** Elevated triglycerides are the most common dyslipidemia in diabetes mellitus. However, the LDL particles in DM are more atherogenic than in nondiabetics, even though they are not elevated by DM alone. DM frequently results in lower high-density lipoprotien (HDL) levels as well. *(Braunwald, pp. 2124–2125)*

67. **(D)** The vertebral bodies in osteoporosis may become increasingly biconcave because of weakening of the subchondral plates. This results in "codfish" vertebra. When vertebral collapse occurs, the anterior height of the vertebra is usually decreased. Plain x-rays are insensitive diagnostic tools because up to 30% of bone mass can be lost without any apparent x-ray changes. Dual-energy x-ray absorptiometry (DEXA) and CT scan are more sensitive tests for bone loss, but their exact clinical role has not been clearly established. *(Braunwald, pp. 84, 2231)*

68. **(B)** Aspirin is given in low doses such as 300 mg a day, although the initial studies were done with higher doses. Carotid endarterectomy is the best treatment for stenoses of 70% or more. *(Braunwald, pp. 2383–2385)*

69. **(C)** Later symptoms of hypothyroidism include loss of intellectual and motor activity, declining appetite, dry hair and skin, and deepening voice. In the elderly, hypothyroidism can be misdiagnosed as due to aging or to other diseases such as Parkinson's disease, Alzheimer's disease, or depression. *(Braunwald, p. 2067)*

70. **(D)** Radiation therapy in stage lA Hodgkin's disease has a very high cure rate. Patients must be followed for hypothyroidism. The long-term disease-free survival is 80%. Mantle irradiation can result acutely in transient dry mouth, pharyngitis, fatigue, and weight loss. The most common long-term effect is hypothyroidism (in 30% of cases), but radiation pneumonitis and fibrosis or pericardial disease can occur. Although radiotherapy alone would be acceptable in this case, there is a trend to add chemotherapy as well. *(Braunwald, p. 726)*

71. **(A)** PAN may be associated with hepatitis B antigenemia in 30% of cases, suggesting immunologic phenomena in the pathogenesis of the disease. Aneurysmal dilatations along involved arteries are characteristic and their presence in small and medium-sized arteries in renal, hepatic, and visceral vasculature is diagnostic. Biopsy of involved areas can also be diagnostic. *(Braunwald, pp. 1959–1960)*

72. **(E)** CMV can also cause neurologic complications from CNS infection. Treatment is with ganciclovir, foscarnet, or cidofavir. Relapse rates are high with both drugs, and therefore maintenance therapy is mandatory. *(Braunwald, pp. 1112–1114)*

73. **(B)** Most patients have fever, pain, and chills, as well as elevated alkaline phosphatase. Mechanical obstruction is most commonly due to stones, tumors, or strictures. For reasons that are unclear, the serum bilirubin tends to plateau and rarely exceeds levels of 600 mmol/L (25 mg/dL). *(Braunwald, pp. 256–257)*

74. **(B)** Dysplastic nevi and benign acquired nevi are both most common on sun-exposed areas such as the back. Atypical moles can occur on the scalp, breasts, and buttocks, rare areas for benign acquired nevi. Both lesions are usually associated with similar lesions (10 to 40 on average for benign nevi, often > 100 in the case of dysplastic nevi). Dysplastic nevi are larger (> 6 mm) and have irregular pigmentation and borders. *(Braunwald, p. 556)*

75. **(E)** Prerenal azotemia usually has urine osmolality over 500, urine creatinine over 40, and fractional excretion of sodium less than 1. The urinary sediment in prerenal azotemia reveals hyaline casts. In intrinsic renal azotemia, muddy brown granular casts are seen. *(Braunwald, p. 1546)*

76. **(D)** The behavioral respiratory control system of the brain drives the hyperventilation, which leads to decreased P_{CO_2} and increased pH. If alkalemia is present with the hypocarbia, symptoms can be quite significant. They include dizziness, visual impairment, syncope, and seizures secondary to cerebral vasoconstriction; parasthesias, carpopedal spasm, and tetany (secondary to decreased free serum calcium); muscle weakness (secondary to hypophosphatemia); and cardiac arrhythmias (secondary to alkalemia). *(Braunwald, pp. 1519–1520)*

77. **(D)** Early ischemic changes are tall, peaked T waves that then develop into inverted T waves. Elevated ST segments and Q waves also occur early. *(Braunwald, pp. 1267–1269)*

78. **(B)** Renal elimination of phenobarbital is enhanced by alkalinization of the urine to a pH of 8 with sodium bicarbonate and fluids. Hemodialysis and hemoperfusion are reserved for extreme cases with refracting hypotension. Short-acting barbiturates are metabolized in the liver, so fluid administration and alkalinization are not helpful. Activated charcoal absorbs barbiturates very effectively and is useful in decontamination of the GI tract. *(Braunwald, p. 2604)*

79. **(E)** Exposure to ionizing radiation is more likely to cause cancer if it occurs at an early age. Radiation-induced malignancy tends to occur at the same age as the same malignancy in the general population. This suggests that radiation is not the only factor. *(Braunwald, p. 2590)*

80. **(D)** Men are affected twice as frequently as women. The most apparent sign of the supranuclear ophthalmoplegia is failure of voluntary saccadic gaze in the downward direction. Tremor is unusual, but dementia is common. Medications may help somewhat, but their impact is limited and rarely sustained. *(Braunwald, p. 2403)*

81. **(D)** The loop diuretics inhibit tubular reabsorption of sodium, potassium, and chloride in the loop of Henle and can continue to cause diuresis even during volume contraction. The likely site of action of furosemide is in the thick ascending limb of the loop of Henle. *(Braunwald, pp. 1325–1326)*

82. **(D)** INH acts as a pyridoxine antagonist and causes polyneuropathy in slow acetylators. Both sensory and motor involvement occurs. Treatment with pyridoxine can improve symptoms. *(Braunwald, p. 1019)*

83. **(B)** The first stage of Lyme disease is an acute infection with the spirochete *Borrelia burgdorferi*, usually transmitted by tick bite. It is most common in the summer in rural, wooded areas. About 60% of patients who have not received antibiotic therapy will develop arthritis months later. The typical pattern is intermittent attacks of oligoarthritis lasting weeks to months. The knees are the most common joints involved. *(Braunwald, pp. 1062–1063)*

84. **(A)** AZT is beneficial to patients with HIV infection, but the best time at which to commence therapy is still controversial. Common side effects include fatigue, macrocytic anemia, neutropenia, and myopathy. Treatment regimens now include protease inhibitors as well. Monotherapy with AZT results in development of resistance. *(Braunwald, p. 1901)*

85. **(C)** The mortality from acute myocardial infarction is greater in women, particularly African-American women. It is unclear whether this correlation is independent of age and disease severity. Ischemic heart disease, not breast cancer, is the leading cause of death in U.S. women. The relative benefit of thrombolytic therapy seems similar in men and women. Estrogen therapy's major effect

in decreasing mortality is via its reduction (40 to 50%) in deaths due to ischemic heart disease. This has not yet been verified in prospective trials. Estrogen therapy has not been shown to be beneficial in secondary prevention of heart disease in women. Immune-related disorders (rheumatoid arthritis, lupus, multiple sclerosis, thyroid disease, etc.) are usually more common in women. *(Braunwald, pp. 22–23)*

86. **(D)** Alpha-methyldopa has been used extensively throughout pregnancy, with no evidence of harm to the fetus. ACE inhibitors are associated with increased fetal loss. Preeclampsia and eclampsia are diseases of the end of pregnancy. There is no evidence that pregnancy affects the course of essential hypertension. Gestational hypertension has a high rate of recurrence in subsequent pregnancies. *(Braunwald, p. 26)*

87. **(B)** CMV is the most common congenital viral infection, affecting 1 to 2% of all U.S. newborns. Only a small minority of these infants are abnormal. *N. gonorrhoeae* infection can be transmitted in utero, during delivery, or in the postpartum period. Asymptomatic bacteriuria occurs in up to 7% of all pregnancies. Treatment can prevent about 75% of all acute pyelonephritis in pregnancy; thus, screening is warranted. HIV infection is usually transmitted during the perinatal period. Although postpartum infections are a significant cause of maternal mortality, the most important are thromboembolic disease, hypertension, ectopic pregnancy, and hemorrhage. *(Braunwald, pp. 29–31)*

88. **(E)** This story of daily attacks of periorbital pain with annual recurrence in a man between age 30 to 50 is typical of cluster headaches. The recurrent bouts last days to weeks. The headaches can be provoked by alcohol and relieved by oxygen administration. Prophylactic treatment, however, is preferred. *(Braunwald, pp. 78–79)*

89. **(E)** Wernicke's aphasia involves disease (most commonly infarction) in the distribu-

tion of the lower division of the middle cerebral artery. It is frequently associated with parietal lobe sensory deficits and hemianopsia; motor disturbance is not part of the syndrome. The condition may improve with time. *(Braunwald, pp. 141–142)*

90. **(C)** The ECG reveals diffuse ST elevation with characteristic concave upward shape and PR depression in the precordial leads. This is more typical of pericarditis than of myocardial infarction. The presentation, symptoms, and age of the patient are all typical for viral pericarditis. *(Braunwald, pp. 1365–1369)*

91. **(B)** Community-acquired pneumonia in previously healthy young people is commonly caused by *S. pneumoniae, Mycoplasma,* viruses, or *Chlamydia*. The pattern of dense right upper lobe consolidation in this case strongly suggests a typical bacterial pneumonia, such as *S. pneumoniae*. A follow-up CXR in 6 weeks is appropriate to ensure that no underlying abnormality is the cause of the problem. *(Braunwald, p. 1479)*

92. **(D)** The CXR is typical of COPD, with flattened diaphragms, hyperlucent lungs, and increased retrosternal air space. *(Braunwald, p. 1495)*

93. **(E)** Renal, musculoskeletal, and peripheral nerve involvement are the most common manifestations of PAN. Generally, if no tissue is easily available for biopsy, an arteriogram is a better diagnostic test than a blind biopsy. This arteriogram reveals multiple aneurysmal dilatations, the classic finding in PAN. *(Braunwald, pp. 1958–1959)*

94. **(D)** The x-ray reveals typical evidence of sacroiliitis, with widening of the joints, sclerosis, and evasions. Similar findings can be seen in psoriatic and enteropathic spondyloarthropathy. *(Braunwald, p. 1951)*

95. **(C)** The articular calcification chondrocalcinosis is typical for pseudogout or calcium pyrophosphate disease (CPPD). The most common joint involved is the knee, but the wrist,

shoulder, ankle, elbow, and hand are also frequently involved. Definitive diagnosis depends on finding typical rhomboid-shaped crystals with weak positive birefringence in the synovial fluid, but chondrocalcinosis in the correct setting allows a presumptive diagnosis. Numerous diseases are associated with CPPD, but the most common predisposing factor is advancing age. *(Braunwald, pp. 1995–1996)*

96. **(B)** The x-ray reveals a Zenker's diverticulum. Halitosis, aspiration (perhaps explaining his pneumonia), regurgitation of old meals, and dysphagia are typical symptoms. Surgical treatment involves a cricopharyngeal myotomy. At times, a diverticulectomy is also required. *(Braunwald, p. 1648)*

97. **(C)** The film shows hypochromic, microcytic red cells, suggesting iron deficiency. Although thalassemia can mimic iron deficiency, the normal hemoglobin 1 year earlier makes this unlikely. Anemia of chronic disease is unlikely because there are no signs of such a chronic disease. Thus, blood loss from the GI tract is the most likely cause. *(Braunwald, p. 662)*

98. **(A)** The macrocytic cells and hypersegmented neutrophil are characteristic of megaloblastic anemia. Vitamin B_{12} and folate deficiency are the most common cause. Lack of intrinsic factor because of gastrectomy will eventually result in B_{12} deficiency. *(Braunwald, p. 677)*

99. **(D)** The medical expert need never have seen the claimant and may testify based on a review of the records. *(Fuster, p. 2522)*

100. **(C)** The plaintiff must show that the defendant's conduct breached a duty and that the victim's negligence did not contribute to the injury. *(Fuster, p. 2521)*

101. **(B)** Beta-adrenergic receptors become less sensitive with advancing age. Higher rates of isoproterenol infusion are required in the elderly to achieve an increased resting heart rate. Clinically, higher doses of propranolol have been shown to be required in the elderly to achieve similar degrees of beta blockade as in the young. *(Grimley Evans, pp. 132–133)*

102. **(A)** The response to benzodiazepines is more pronounced in the elderly, even when corrected for pharmacokinetics. Prior impairment is a factor in this response. *(Grimley Evans, pp. 132–133)*

103. **(A)** Despite similar pharmacokinetics, the dose of warfarin to provide effective anticoagulation is lower in the elderly. *(Grimley Evans, p. 132)*

104. **(E)** The elderly have more body fat and less body water. A water-soluble drug such as lithium will have a considerably smaller volume of distribution. Thus, dosages should be decreased in the elderly to prevent toxicity. *(Grimley Evans, p. 130)*

105. **(A)** Failure to correct for the elderly's increased sensitivity to narcotics can result in significant toxicity. *(Grimley Evans, p. 132)*

106. **(A)** Tricyclic antidepressants and SSRIs are both effective treatments for depression, but their side effect profiles are different. Tricyclics can promote weight gain while weight loss is more common with SSRIs. *(Grimley Evans, pp. 993–994)*

107. **(C)** Diuretics promote urinary losses of magnesium, zinc, and potassium. Zinc deficiency is also seen in liver cirrhosis, type 2 diabetes, and lung cancer. *(Grimley Evans, p. 163)*

108. **(D)** INH can result in pyridoxine (vitamin B_6) deficiency, particularly in malnourished individuals. It is recommended that patients who are elderly, or have diabetes mellitus, poor nutrition, alcoholism, seizure diathesis, or uremia, take pyridoxine while on INH. *(Grimley Evans, p. 538)*

109. **(G)** Corticosteroids impair calcium absorption. They are useful in managing hypercalcemia, but bisphosphonates are the usual drug of choice. *(Grimley Evans, p. 183)*

110. **(E)** Both phenytoin and phenobarbital can cause altered vitamin D metabolism and can even result in osteomalacia. Calcium absorption from the gut is also blocked directly. *(Grimley Evans, p. 628)*

111. **(B)** Sleep becomes more shallow with the loss of deep stages of sleep, resulting in more frequent arousals. Specific sleep disturbances such as sleep apnea and periodic leg movements increase with advancing age as well. *(Grimley Evans, p. 758)*

112. **(B, F)** Neurodegenerative disorders can cause a change in normal circadian rhythm by causing a breakdown in the temporal organizing of sleep–wake cycling. This alteration in time of sleeping can be very disruptive to family members. The sleep pattern can be polyphasic, with multiple irregularly distributed periods of sleep, rather than one long sleep period at night. This can result in the patient's awakening during the night, which is also very disruptive. *(Grimley Evans, pp. 756–758)*

113. **(E)** Sleep apnea syndrome is the most common cause of daytime sleepiness in the elderly. The prevalence (at least in sleep disorder centers) increases with advancing age. Narcolepsy (usually having started earlier in life) and periodic limb movement disorder (restless legs) are other common causes of excessive daytime sleepiness. *(Grimley Evans, p. 750)*

114. **(C)** The lack of focal neurological findings suggests that the confusion is secondary to delirium. Bilateral asterixis is frequently seen in metabolic encephalopathy, particularly in cases of hepatic encephalopathy, hypercapnia, or drug ingestion. In this case, the most urgent investigations would be to rule out pneumonia with respiratory failure. *(Braunwald, p. 133)*

115. **(E)** Although impaired attention is the hallmark of delirium (along with impaired consciousness), it can also be impaired in dementia. In very mild cognitive impairment, deficits in attention might differentiate delirium from dementia, but in the usual hospitalized patient, fluctuation in performance (particularly with regard to attention and level of consciousness) is probably more helpful. *(Braunwald, p. 132)*

116. **(B)** The progressive nature of the disorder suggests a degenerative dementia, and the predominance of disinhibited behavior suggests the frontal lobes are involved. Frontal dementias can result from trauma, tumor, or ischemia, but this history suggests a degenerative disorder. Alzheimer's can involve the frontal lobes and mimic a frontal dementia. *(Braunwald, p. 151)*

117. **(D)** In frontal dementia, and others as well, behavioral disturbances are often the reason for institutionalization. *(Braunwald, p. 154)*

118. **(E)** In fronto temporal dementia (FTD), amyloid plaques are not present. The predominant abnormality is the presence of neurofibullary tangles. If Pick's disease is the cause of the FTD, specific neuropathological changes can be found. *(Braunwald, p. 151)*

References

Beutler E, Lichtman MA, et al: *Hematology*, 6th ed. New York, McGraw-Hill, 2001.

Braunwald E, Fauci A, et al: *Harrison's Principles of Internal Medicine*, 15th ed. New York: McGraw-Hill, 2001.

Devita VT, Hellman S, Rosebenberg SH: *CANCER Principles and Practice of Oncology*, 6th ed. Philadelphia: Lippincott Williams & Wilkins, 2001.

Felig P, Frohman LA: *Endocrinology & Metabolism*, 4th ed. New York: McGraw-Hill, 2001.

Fitzpatrick TB, Johnson RA, Wolff K: *ColourAtlas & Synopsis of Clinical Dermatology*, 4th ed. New York: McGraw-Hill, 2001.

Fuster V, Alexander RW, O'Rourke RA, et al: *The Heart*, 10th ed. New York: McGraw-Hill, 2001.

Goldman L, Bennett JC: *Cecil Textbook of Medicine*, 21th ed. Philadelphia, PA: W.B. Saunders Co., 2000.

Grimley Evans J, Williams TF, Beattie BL, et al: *Oxford Textbook of Geriatric Medicine*, 2nd ed. Oxford: Oxford University Press, 2000.

Hardman JG, Limbird LE: *Goodman and Gilman's The Pharmacological Basis of Therapeutics*, 9th ed. New York: McGraw-Hill, 2001.

Victor M, Ropper AH: *Adams and Victor's Principles of Neurology*, 7th ed. New York: McGraw-Hill, 2001.

Index